Florida Regional

SECOND EDITION

Common EMS Protocols

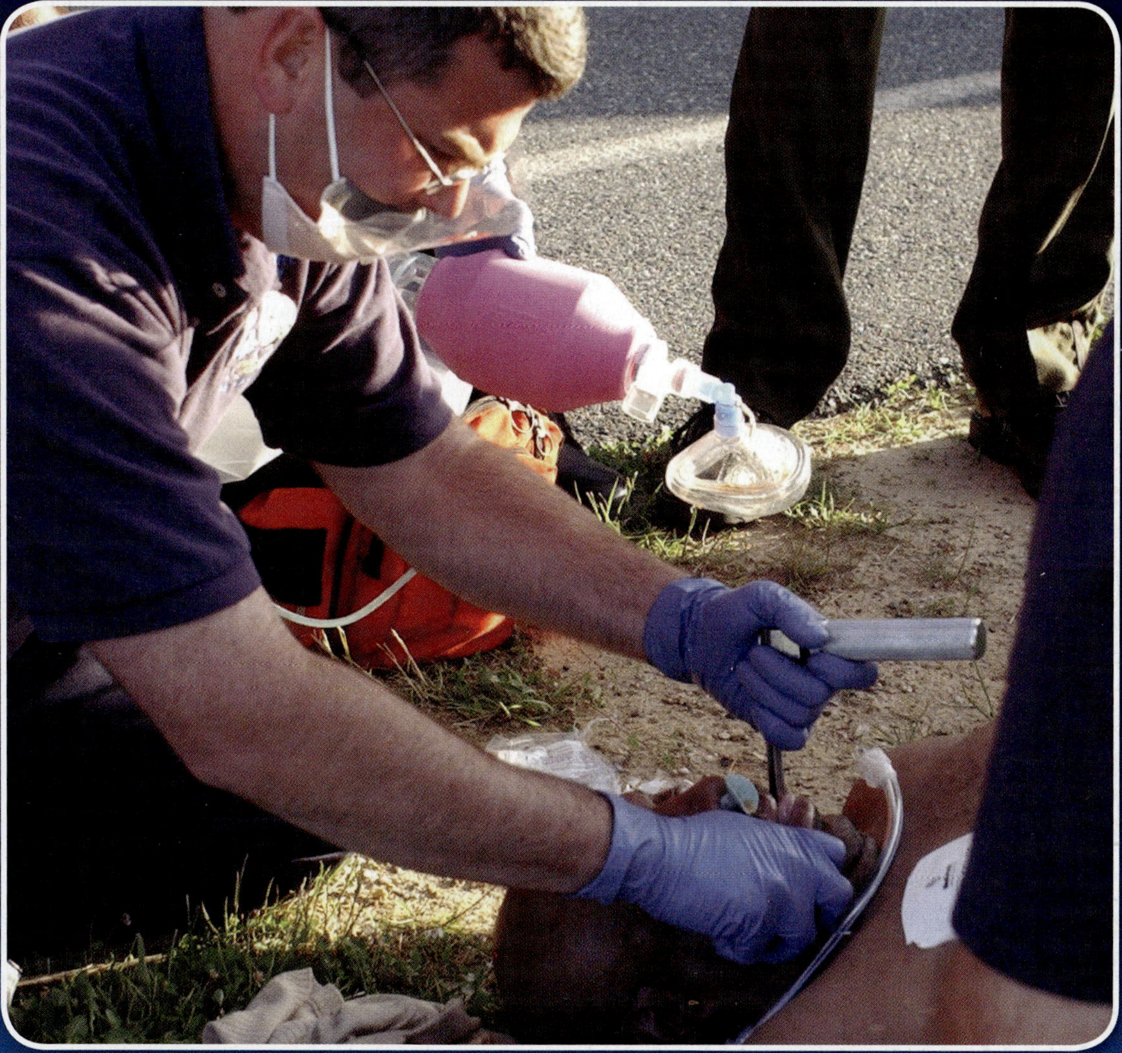

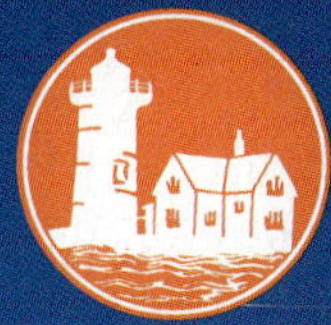

JONES AND BARTLETT PUBLISHERS

Sudbury, Massachusetts

BOSTON TORONTO LONDON SINGAPORE

World Headquarters
Jones and Bartlett Publishers
40 Tall Pine Drive
Sudbury, MA 01776
978-443-5000
info@jbpub.com
www.jbpub.com

Jones and Bartlett Publishers Canada
6339 Ormindale Way
Mississauga, Ontario L5V 1J2
Canada

Jones and Bartlett Publishers
International
Barb House, Barb Mews
London W6 7PA
United Kingdom

Jones and Bartlett's books and products are available through most bookstores and online booksellers. To contact Jones and Bartlett Publishers directly, call 800-832-0034, fax 978-443-8000, or visit our website, www.jbpub.com.

Substantial discounts on bulk quantities of Jones and Bartlett's publications are available to corporations, professional associations, and other qualified organizations. For details and specific discount information, contact the special sales department at Jones and Bartlett via the above contact information or send an email to specialsales@jbpub.com.

The procedures and protocols in this book are based on the most current recommendations of responsible medical sources. The Fire Chiefs Association of Broward County and the publisher, however, make no guarantee as to, and assume no responsibility for, the correctness, sufficiency, or completeness of such information or recommendations. Other or additional safety measures may be required under particular circumstances.

This textbook is intended solely as a guide to the appropriate procedures to be employed when rendering emergency care to the sick and injured. It is not intended as a statement of the standards of care required in any particular situation, because circumstances and the patient's physical condition can vary widely from one emergency to another. Nor is it intended that this textbook shall in any way advise emergency personnel concerning legal authority to perform the activities or procedures discussed. Such local determination should be made only with the aid of legal counsel.

Additional photographic and illustration credits appear on p. 555, which constitutes a continuation of the copyright page.

Production Credits
Chief Executive Officer: Clayton Jones
Chief Operating Officer: Don W. Jones, Jr.
President, Higher Education and Professional Publishing: Robert W. Holland, Jr.
V.P., Design and Production: Anne Spencer
V.P., Manufacturing and Inventory Control: Therese Connell
Publisher: Kimberly Brophy
Associate Editor: Lindsay Murdock
Associate Production Editor: Sarah Bayle
Director of Marketing: Alisha Weisman
Director, Public Safety Group: Matthew Maniscalco
Composition: diacriTech
Text Design: Anne Spencer
Cover Design: Kristin E. Parker
Photo Research and Permissions Manager: Kimberly Potvin
Assistant Photo Researcher: Bridget Kane
Cover Image: © Mark C. Ide
Printing and Binding: Courier Corporation
Cover Printing: Courier Corporation

Library of Congress Cataloging-in-Publication Data
Florida regional common EMS protocols/Fire Chiefs Association of Broward County. -- 2nd ed.
p. ; cm.
ISBN-13: 978-0-7637-7748-7
ISBN-10: 0-7637-7748-X
1. Emergency medical services--Florida--Handbooks, manuals, etc. 2. Medical protocols--Florida--Handbooks, manuals, etc. I. Fire Chiefs Association of Broward County.
[DNLM: 1. Emergency Medical Services--Florida--Practice Guideline. 2. Emergency Treatment--methods--Florida--Practice Guideline. WB 105 F636 2010]
RA645.6.F6F566 2010
362.1809759--dc22

2009006105

6048

Printed in the United States of America
13 12 11 10 09 10 9 8 7 6 5 4 3 2 1

TABLE OF CONTENTS

Participating Agencies

Broward County EMS Agencies

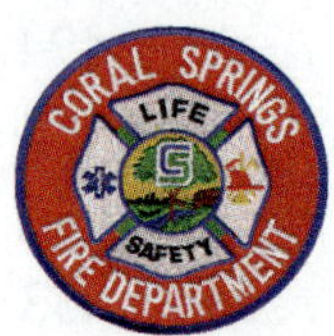

Coral Springs Fire Rescue
Fire Chief – Mark Curran.
Medical Director – Wayne Lee, MD, FACEP

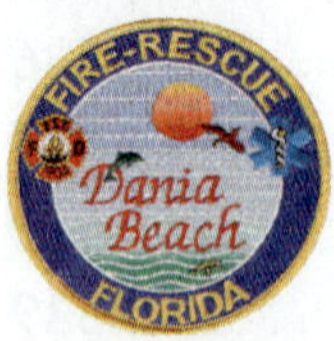

Dania Beach Fire Rescue
Fire Chief – Jack McCartt
Medical Director – L. Scott Ulin, MD

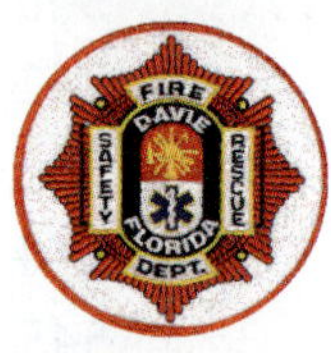

Davie Fire Rescue Department
Fire Chief – Joseph Montopoli
Medical Director – Wayne Lee, MD, FACEP

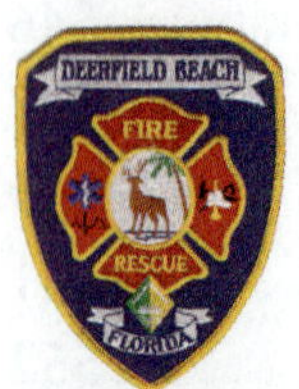

Deerfield Beach Fire Rescue
Fire Chief – Tony Stravino, BS
Medical Director – Richard Paley, MD, FACEP

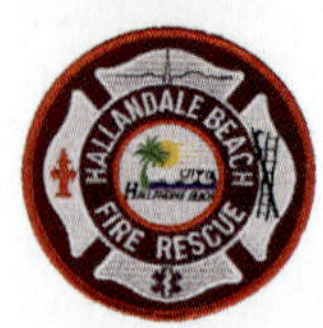

Hallandale Beach Fire Rescue
Fire Chief – Daniel P. Sullivan
Medical Director – Sat P. Punyani, MD, FACEP

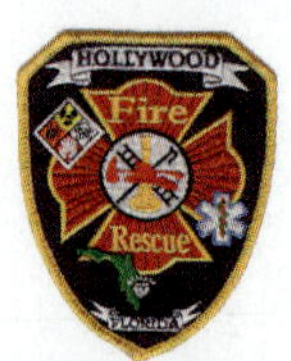

Hollywood Fire Rescue
Fire Chief – Virgil Fernandez
Medical Director – Richard Dellerson, MD

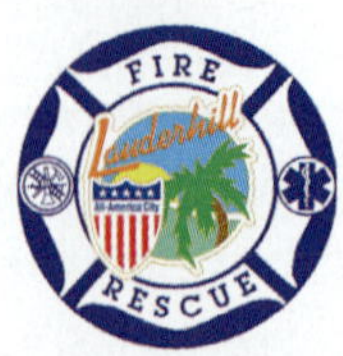

Lauderhill Fire Rescue
Fire Chief – Edward Curran
Medical Director – L. Scott Ulin, MD

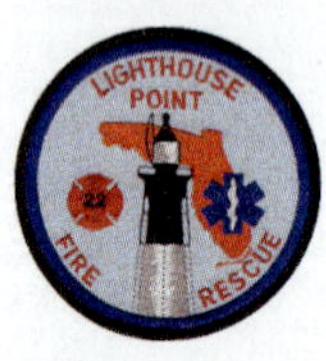

Lighthouse Point Fire Rescue
Fire Chief – David Donzella
Medical Director – Richard Paley, MD

Broward County EMS Agencies (*continued*)

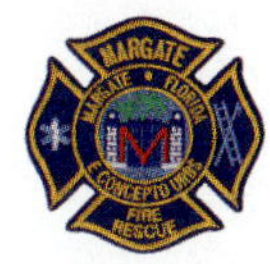

Margate Fire Rescue
Fire Chief – Garrison Westbrook
Medical Director – Wayne Lee, MD, FACEP

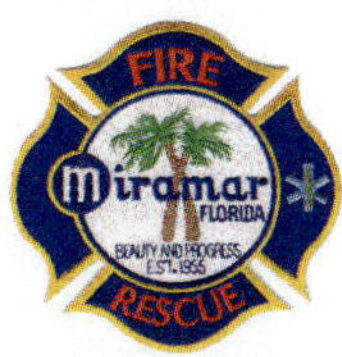

Miramar Fire Rescue
Fire Chief – James Hunt
Medical Director – Barry Feingold, DO, FACEP
Associate Medical Director – Antonio Gandia, MD

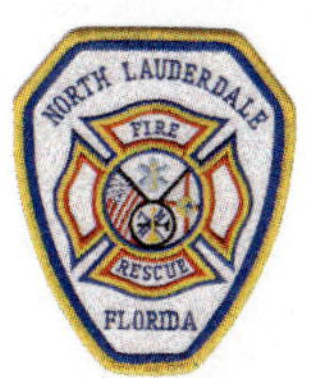

North Lauderdale Fire Rescue
Fire Chief – Kevin Bowman
Medical Director – Wayne Lee, MD, FACEP

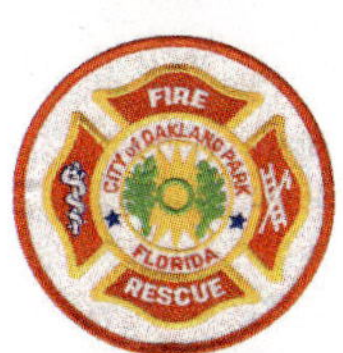

Oakland Park Fire Rescue
Fire Chief – Donald P. Widing
Medical Director – Wayne Lee, MD, FACEP

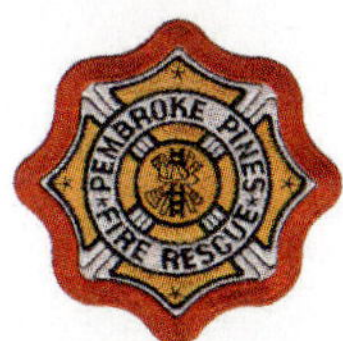

Pembroke Pines Fire Rescue
Fire Chief – John Picarello
Medical Director – Richard Dellerson, MD

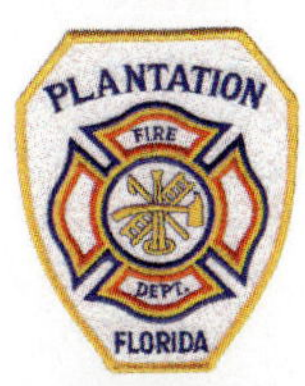

Plantation Fire Department
Fire Chief – Robert Pudney
Medical Director – Wayne Lee, MD, FACEP

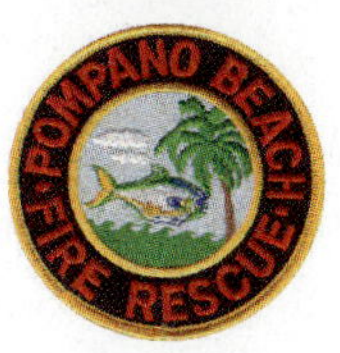

Pompano Beach Fire Rescue
Fire Chief – Harry Small
Medical Director – Michael Farrell, MD, FACEP

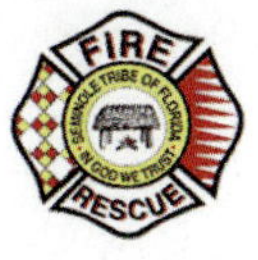

Seminole Tribe of Florida Fire-Rescue
Fire Chief – Donald Dipitrillo
Medical Director – Wayne Lee, MD, FACEP

Broward County EMS Agencies (continued)

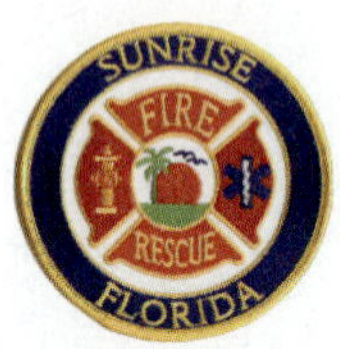

Sunrise Fire Rescue
Fire Chief – Norman Ryning
Medical Director – Wayne Lee, MD, FACEP

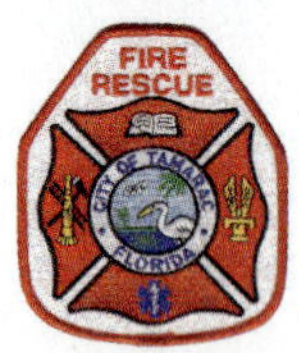

Tamarac Fire Rescue
Fire Chief – Jim Budzinski
Medical Director – L. Scott Ulin, MD

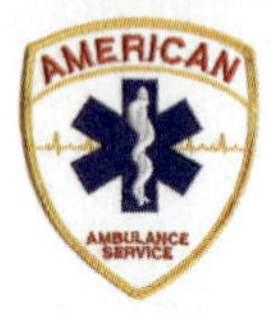

American Ambulance – Broward
Operations Manager – Mary Albin
Medical Director – L. Scott Ulin, MD

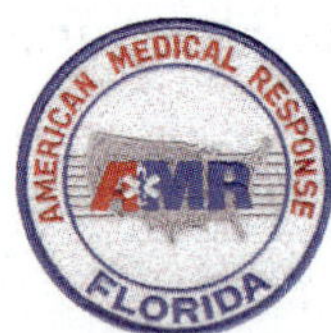

American Medical Response – Broward
Operations Manager – William Hall
Medical Director – Joe A. Nelson, DO, MS, FACOEP, FACEP

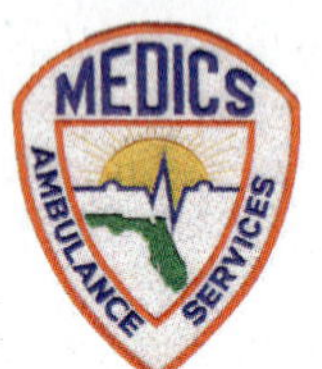

Medics Ambulance Services
Operations Manager – Robert Eberhardt
Medical Director – Currin Nichols, MD

Miami-Dade County EMS Agencies

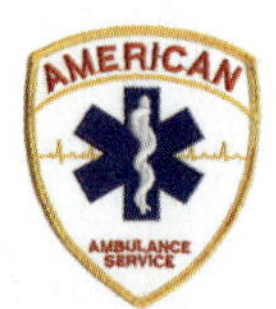

American Ambulance – Miami-Dade
Operations Manager – Mary Albin
Medical Director – L. Scott Ulin, MD

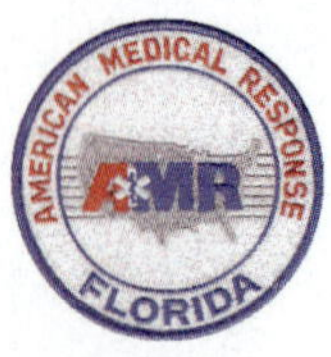

American Medical Response – Miami-Dade
Operations Manager – Tami Tehrani
Medical Director – Joe A. Nelson, DO, MS, FACOEP, FACEP

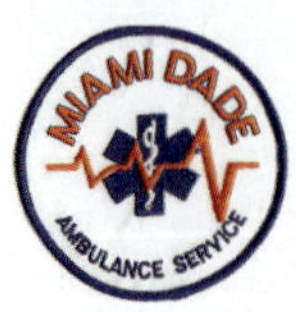

Miami-Dade Ambulance
Operations Manager – Ray Espinosa
Medical Director – Rudolph Moise, DO

Monroe County EMS Agencies

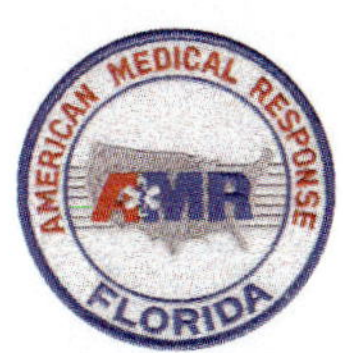

Key West Rescue – AMR
Operations Manager – Tami Tehrani
Medical Director – Joe A. Nelson, DO, MS, FACOEP, FACEP

West Florida EMS Agencies

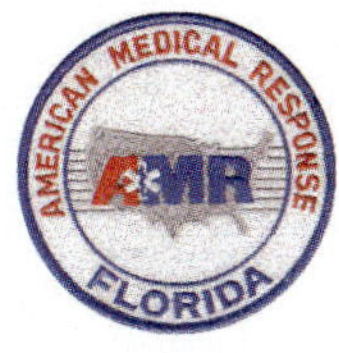

American Medical Response
Operations Manager – Tomas Diaz
Medical Director – Joe A. Nelson, DO, MS, FACOEP, FACEP

Medical Director Authorization

The *Florida Regional Common EMS Protocols 2009* have been approved by the following Medical Directors for use in the EMS agencies listed below.

Richard S. Dellerson, MD
Hollywood Fire Rescue
Pembroke Pines Fire Rescue

Michael Farrell, MD
Pompano Beach Fire Rescue

Barry Feingold, DO, FACEP
Miramar Fire Rescue

Antonio Gandia, MD
Miramar Fire Rescue

Wayne Lee, MD, FACEP
Davie Fire Rescue
Coral Springs Fire Rescue
Margate Fire Rescue
North Lauderdale Fire Rescue
Oakland Park Fire Rescue
Plantation Fire Department
Seminole Tribe Fire Rescue
Sunrise Fire Rescue

Rudolph Moise, DO
Miami-Dade Ambulance

Joe A. Nelson, DO, MS, FACOEP, FACEP
American Medical Response – Florida
Key West Rescue – State of Florida Medical Director

Currin Nichol, MD
Medics Ambulance Services

Richard Paley, MD
Deerfield Beach Fire Rescue
Lighthouse Point Fire Rescue

Sat P. Punyani, MD FACEP
Hallandale Beach Fire Rescue

L. Scott Ulin, MD
Dania Beach Fire Rescue
Lauderhill Fire Rescue
Tamarac Fire Rescue
American Ambulance

Acknowledgements

Editor

Bill Huff, EMT-P, BPA
Principal Author/Chair—Editing Committee
EMS Chief—Miramar Fire Rescue

Contributing Editors

Ernest G. Bertha, MD, MBA, CPE, FAAP
Senior Medical Officer, Pediatrics—Phoenix Physicians, LLC

Dan Blundy, EMT-P
Training Officer—Hollywood Fire Rescue

Richard Boulger, EMT-P
Division Chief—Lauderhill Fire Rescue

Richard Dellerson, MD
Medical Director—Hollywood, Pembroke Pines Fire Rescue

David Donzella, EMT-P
Fire Chief—Lighthouse Point Fire Rescue

Julie Downey, RN, EMT-P
Assistant Chief—Davie Fire Rescue

Mike Farrell, MD
Medical Director—Pompano Beach Fire Rescue

Barry Feingold, DO, FACEP
Medical Director—Miramar Fire Rescue

Antonio Gandia, MD
Associate Medical Director—Miramar Fire Rescue

Michael Hohl, EMT-P, MPA
Division Chief—Pompano Beach Fire Rescue

Denise Johnson, NREMT-P
Battalion Chief—Plantation Fire Department

Frederick Keroff, MD, FACEP
Medical Director—Hialeah, Miami Beach Fire Rescue
District Medical Director of Emergency Services—Memorial

Wayne Lee MD, FACEP
Medical Director—Coral Springs, Margate, Oakland Park, Plantation Fire Department, Seminole Tribe, Sunrise Fire Rescue Healthcare System

Joe A. Nelson, DO, MS, FACOEP, FACEP
Medical Director—American Medical Response, State of Florida Medical Director

Richard Paley, MD
Medical Director—Deerfield Beach, Lighthouse Point Fire Rescue

Andrew Popick, BPA, NREMT-P
Battalion Chief—Davie Fire Rescue

Doug Rider, RN, CEN, EMT-P
EMS Program Instructor—Broward Community College

Tim Roche, EMT-P
Training Captain—Miramar Fire Rescue

Sharon Snyder, EMT-P
Captain—Broward Sheriff's Office Department of Fire Rescue

Scott Ulin, MD
Medical Director—Dania Beach, Lauderhill, Tamarac Fire Rescue, American Ambulance

Michael Vincent, EMT-P
EMS Chief—Pembroke Pines Fire Rescue

Charles Wohlitka, EMT-P, CFO
EMS Chief—Margate Fire Rescue

Ad Hoc Committees

Toxicology/Hazardous Materials Exposure

Michael Hohl, EMT-P, MPA
Committee Chair
Division Chief (EMS)—Pompano Beach Fire Rescue

Richard S. Weisman, Pharm.D., FAACT
Director—Florida Poison Information Center/Miami
Research Associate Professor of Pediatrics
University of Miami, Miller School of Medicine

Jeffery Bernstein, MD, FACEP, FACMT
Medical Director—Florida Poison Information Center/Miami
Attending Physician Emergency Care Center—Jackson Memorial Hospital, University of Miami, Miller School of Medicine

Joe Nelson, DO, MS, FACOEP, FACEP
Medical Director—American Medical Response Florida Operations/Key West Rescue

Kathleen Schrank, MD, FACEP
Medical Director—Key Biscayne, Miami Fire Rescue
Chief—Division of Emergency Medicine, Professor of Clinical Medicine, University of Miami, Miller School of Medicine

Armando Bevelacqua, EMT-P, BS
District Chief (Homeland Security and Special Operations)—Orlando Fire Department
WMD Medical Protocol Committee—Rocky Mountain Poison Control Center/Department of Homeland Security (Former)

Al Cruz, EMT-P
Chief Fire Officer (Special Operations Administrative Chief)—Miami-Dade Fire Rescue

Mark Steele, EMT-P, BS
Battalion Chief (Training)—Hollywood Fire Rescue

Richard Stilp, RN, MA
Director—Central Florida Fire Academy
WMD Medical Protocol Committee—Rocky Mountain Poison Control Center/Department of Homeland Security (Former)

Ad Hoc Committees

MCI/Triage

Julie Downey, RN, EMT-P
Committee Chair
Assistant Chief—Davie Fire Rescue

Lou Romig, MD, FAAP, FACEP
Emergency Physician—Miami Children's Hospital
Medical Advisor—Miami-Dade Fire Rescue
Medical Director—Team Life Support, Inc.
Medical Director—S. Florida Regional Disaster Medical Assistance Team (FL-5 DMAT)
Author—JumpSTART Triage

New Port Beach Fire Department and Hoag Hospital
S.T.A.R.T. Triage

Pediatrics

Ernest G. Bertha, MD, MBA, CPE, FAAP
Committee Chair
Senior Medical Officer, Pediatrics—Phoenix Physicians, LLC

Anna Airy, MSN, ARNP
Nurse Manger—Pediatric Emergency Department, Memorial Hospital Miramar

John Fischer EMT-P
Lieutenant—Palm Beach County Fire Rescue

Marianne Gausche-Hill, MD, FACEP, FAAP
Professor of Medicine
David Geffen School of Medicine at UCLA
Director of EMS and Pediatric Emergency Medicine Fellowships
Harbor—UCLA Medical Center
Department of Emergency Medicine

William P. Horvath, CEN, RN
Assistant Nurse Manager
Coral Springs Medical Center
Pediatric Emergency Department

Deborah Ann Mulligan, MD, FAAP, FACEP
President—Florida Chapter American Academy of Pediatrics
Director—Institute for Child Health Policy
Professor Pediatrics COM Nova Southeastern University

Lou Romig, MD, FAAP, FACEP
Emergency Physician—Miami Children's Hospital
Medical Advisor—Miami-Dade Fire Rescue
Medical Director—Team Life Support, Inc.
Medical Director—S. Florida Regional Disaster Medical Assistance Team (FL-5 DMAT)

Michael Eric Weis, MD
Physician Liaison—Joe DiMaggio Children's Hospital

Ad Hoc Committees

Air Rescue Transport

Kenneth Kronheim, MS, EMT-P
Committee Chair
Chief of special Operations/Training Bureau—Broward Sheriff's Office Air Rescue

Casey Brady
Commander—Miami-Dade Fire Rescue

James Hasselman
Pilot—Broward Sheriff's Office Air Rescue

Randall Ovcen, EMT-P
Lieutenant—Broward Sheriff's Office Air Rescue

Dabra Swensson,
Captain—Miami-Dade Fire Rescue

Airway Management

Tom Sheridan
Committee Chair
Division Chief, Tamarac Fire Rescue

Dan Blundy, EMT-P
Training Officer—Hollywood Fire Rescue

Randy Gonzalez
Division Captain—Miramar Fire Rescue

Steve Grasso
Lauderhill Fire Rescue

William Huff, EMT-P
Battalion Chief—Miramar Fire Rescue

Tim Roche, EMT-P
Training Captain—Miramar Fire Rescue

Scott Ulin, MD
Medical Director—Dania Beach, Lauderdale Lakes, Lauderhill, and Tamarac Fire Rescue

Infectious Disease

Wayne Lee, MD, FACEP
Committee Co-Chair
Medical Director—Coral Springs, Fort Lauderdale, Margate, Oakland Park, Plantation, Sunrise Fire Rescue

Thomas Dibernardo, EMT-P
Deputy Chief—Sunrise Fire Rescue

Nancy Zanotti, RN, BSN, MPH, CIC
Director of Infection Control
Westside Regional Medical Center

Ad Hoc Committees

Infectious Disease (continued)

Bruce Caruso, EMT-P
Battalion Chief—Dania Beach Fire Rescue

Lamar Davis, EMT-P
Division Chief (EMS)—Hollywood Fire Rescue

Joshua Perper, MD, LL.B., M.Sc.
Chief Medical Examiner—Broward County Medical Examiner and Trauma Services

George Danz, MPA
Director of Trauma Services/Chief of Operations—Broward County Medical Examiner and Trauma Services

Cardiac/Stroke Care and Transport

Sharon Snyder, EMT-P
Committee Chair
Captain—Broward Sheriff's Office Department of Fire Rescue & Emergency Services

Howard S. Bush, MD, FACC
Chairman—Department of Cardiology, Cleveland Clinic Hospital Weston

Henry Cusnir, MD

Greg Blue, EMT-P
Community Training Program Coordinator—Broward Sheriff's Office Department of Fire Rescue

Mark Caputo, MD
Director of Emergency Services—Holy Cross Hospital, Ft. Lauderdale

Mike Farrell, MD
Medical Director—Pompano Beach Fire Rescue

Oscar Gonzalez, EMT-P
Firefighter Paramedic—Lauderhill Fire Rescue

Jonathan Harris, MD
Neurologist, Stroke Program Director—North Broward Medical Center

William Huff, EMT-P, BPA
EMS Chief—Miramar Fire Rescue

Lou Isaacson, DO
Medical Director—Florida Medical Center, Emergency Department

Frederick Keroff, MD, FACEP
Medical Director—Hialeah/Miami Beach Fire Rescue/Memorial Healthcare Emergency Services

Alvaro Pedilla, MD
Department of Neurology—Memorial Regional Hospital, Hollywood

Tim Roche, EMT-P
Training Captain—Miramar Fire Rescue

Ad Hoc Committees

Cardiac/Stroke Care and Transport (*continued*)

Debbi Stanfield, RN
Senior Account Consultant—Physio-Control

Scott Ulin, MD
Medical Director—Dania Beach, Lauderdale Lakes, Lauderhill, Tamarac Fire Rescue, American Ambulance

Trauma Care and Transport

Eddie Carrillo, MD
Committee Co-Chair
Trauma Director—Memorial Regional Hospital, Hollywood

Michael Vincent, EMT-P
Committee Co-Chair
EMS Chief—Pembroke Pines Fire Rescue

William Huff, EMT-P, BPA
EMS Chief—Miramar Fire Rescue

George Danz, MPA
Director of Trauma Services/Chief of Operations—Broward County Medical Examiner and Trauma Services

Ivan Puente, MD
Trauma Director—Broward General Medical Center

Joshua Perper, MD, LL.B., M.Sc.
Chief Medical Examiner—Broward County Medical Examiner and Trauma Services

Other Contributors

Baruch Krauss, MD, Ed.M., FAAP
Division of Emergency Medicine—Children's Hospital Boston
Assistant Professor—Department of Pediatrics, Harvard Medical School

Special Thanks
Tim Arnwine—Former EMT-P and father of Shane Arnwine, for his assistance in developing Medical Procedure 4.34—TREATING THE AUTISTIC PATIENT.

Supporting Agencies

Fire Chiefs Association of Broward County, Inc.

Broward Regional EMS Council

Broward County Trauma Agency

Broward Community College

The Florida Department of Health, Bureau of Emergency Medical Services sponsored the printing of this manual for Broward County EMS Agencies.

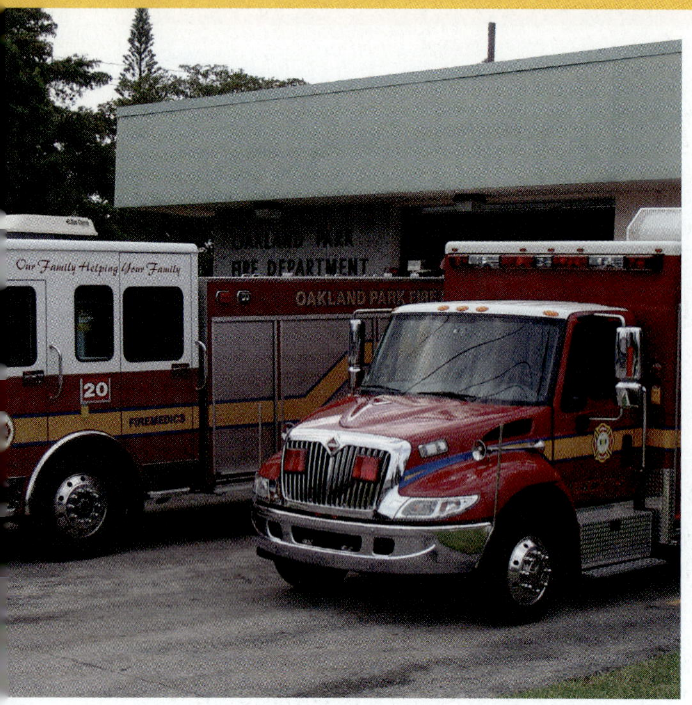

chapter 1

General Protocols

1.1 Intent and Use of Protocols

These medical treatment protocols have been developed as a part of the medical direction program for participating Emergency Medical Services (EMS) agencies. The medical director of an individual EMS provider may choose to modify certain treatment recommendations. In addition, some patients may require therapy not specified in these protocols. The treatment protocols should not be construed as prohibiting such flexibility. The paramedic/EMT must use his/her judgment in administering treatment in the following manner:

- The paramedic may determine that no specific treatment is needed; or
- The paramedic may consult medical direction before initiating any specific treatment; or
- The paramedic may follow the appropriate treatment protocol and then consult medical direction.
- The paramedic/EMT may contact medical direction at any time he/she deems necessary.

When the paramedic/EMT is unable to make contact with other forms of medical direction, he/she may contact the receiving hospital for consultation with the emergency department physician. It is recommended that the paramedic/EMT make contact with the physician for consultation on complicated patients whenever possible. When the paramedic is unable to make contact with a physician for medical direction, the paramedic may administer BLS treatment according to his/her judgment. In this instance, the paramedic may administer ALS treatment only as authorized in the treatment protocols.

The treatment protocols are divided into adult and pediatric sections, each with three parts:

Supportive Care

Actions authorized for the EMT or paramedic that are supportive in nature. EMT (BLS) and paramedic (BLS and ALS) actions are specified within each of these protocols.

ALS Level 1

Actions authorized prior to physician contact.

ALS Level 2

Actions authorized only for the paramedic that require a physician consult.

Authorization of procedures prior to physician contact in Level 1 allows the paramedic to initiate care promptly while getting a better idea of the patient's condition and evaluating his/her response to initial treatment.

The general protocols outline care for a typical case. As the protocol continues, the assumption is usually made that previous steps were ineffective. For example, the protocol for ventricular fibrillation authorizes three countershocks; however, the second countershock and third countershock are given only if the previous countershock was unsuccessful and the patient remains in ventricular fibrillation. If the patient went into PEA following the first countershock, the second countershock would not be given. The paramedic would then use the PEA protocol to guide further treatment. In this or other situations where a switch is made to a different protocol during the course of care, the paramedic's

1.1 Intent and Use of Protocols

judgment must determine where entry into the new protocol sequence is appropriate. It would be impractical to write protocols that specify every possible sequence of events. **The order of treatment listed here may not be appropriate for all situations. In fact, not all treatment options may be indicated in every situation.** The paramedic's judgment must be relied upon to determine which of the authorized treatment procedures are appropriate for a given situation. The treatment guidelines are given in bulleted list form as a general order of the steps necessary to treat the patient; however, it is assumed that interventions such as patient assessment, airway management, establishing medication access, applying AED/heart monitor, and so forth can be performed simultaneously.

Orders listed in ALS Level 2 may be expected from the physician. They may or may not be the orders that are actually given, however. The intention in listing ALS Level 2 orders is to allow for appropriate preparation and to guide the paramedic who wishes to request specific orders. The physician directing care in the field retains discretion in ordering specific treatment, even if that treatment conflicts with these protocols. **ALS Level 2 orders require consultation with a physician.** The name of the physician authorizing ALS Level 2 orders must be documented in the patient care report (PCR). Physicians authorized to approve ALS Level 2 orders include the following individuals:

1. EMS provider's medical director (a).
2. Receiving hospital emergency department physician (a).
3. Physician present in his/her own office (b).
4. Online medical control physician (a).
5. Bystander physician personally known to the paramedic (c).
6. Bystander physician who presents a valid M.D. or D.O. Florida license and a nationally recognized ACLS card (c).
7. Poison information center (d).

NOTE

(a) Contact for ALS Level 2 orders by the EMS provider's medical director, online medical control physician, or emergency department physician should be initiated in the following order:
   1. Medcom.
   2. Telephone.
   3. Relay of information via dispatch.

(b) Only verbal or written orders that are signed by the physician that are given directly to the paramedic by a physician in his/her office are acceptable.

(c) A bystander physician, as described above, must accept full responsibility for patient care and accompany the patient in the ambulance to the hospital to give Level 2 orders.

(d) The Poison Information Center is authorized to direct all medical care (Supportive Care, ALS Level 1, and ALS Level 2) for the toxicology and hazardous material exposure patient. The Poison Information Center must be contacted via telephone at 800-222-1222.

1.1 Intent and Use of Protocols

All patients who receive ALS care should be transported to the hospital, unless the patient refuses transport and signs a release (see General Protocol 1.8). Contact with the receiving hospital emergency department is required for all patients transported, even in situations where ALS care has not been initiated. This policy is intended to provide emergency departments with sufficient notification of incoming patients to allow appropriate preparations to be made. Direct contact with the physician in the emergency department needs be made only when seeking consultation or authorization for ALS Level 2 orders.

NOTE

An EMT or paramedic should evaluate all patients on responses to 911 emergencies, as deemed appropriate by the individual EMS provider's medical director.

The treatment protocols have been designed as clinical guides, not as educational documents. The therapeutic rationale behind the treatment protocols reflects the general principles of field care outlined in the following standard EMS references:

References

General Care

Porter R, et al.: *Essentials of Paramedic Emergency Care,* Brady, Englewood Cliffs, NJ, 2006.

Cardiac Care

American Heart Association: Guidelines for Cardiopulmonary Resuscitation and Emergency Cardiovascular Care 2005: *Supplement to Circulation* 112: 24, December 13, 2005.

American Heart Association: *ACLS Provider Manual,* Dallas, TX, 2006.

American Heart Association/American Academy of Pediatrics: *Textbook of Pediatric Advanced Life Support,* Dallas, TX, 2006.

Walraven, G: *Basic Arrhythmias,* 6th edition, Brady, Englewood Cliffs, NJ, 2005.

Trauma

NAEMT, Frame, Salomone: *Pre-hospital Trauma Life Support,* 6th edition, Mosby, St. Louis, MO, 2006.

Campbell JE: *Basic Trauma Life Support, Advanced Pre-hospital Care,* 5th edition, Brady, Englewood Cliffs, NJ, 2004.

Pain Control

Paris P, Stewart R: *Pain Management in Emergency Medicine,* Appleton & Lange, Norwalk, CN, 1988.

McCaffrey M, Pasero C: *Pain Clinical Manual,* 2nd edition, Mosby, St. Louis, MO, 1999.

1.1 Intent and Use of Protocols

Toxicology and Hazardous Materials Exposure

Shannon M, et al.: *Clinical Management of Poisoning and Drug Overdose,* 4th edition, W.B. Saunders Company, Philadelphia, PA, 2007.

Stilp R, Bevelacqua A: *Emergency Medical Response to Hazardous Materials Incidents,* Delmar Publishers, Albany, NY, 1996.

Walter GG, ed.: *Advanced HAZMAT Life Support Provider Manual,* 3rd edition, University of Arizona, Tucson, AZ, 2003.

USAMRICID: *Medical Management of Biological Casualties Handbook,* 4th edition, U.S. Army, Frederick, MD, 2001.

USAMRICID: *Medical Management of Chemical Casualties Handbook,* 3rd edition, U.S. Army, Aberdeen Proving Ground, MD, 2001.

Additional educational materials, supplementary to these references, are included in this manual as Chapter 4 Medical Procedures. Chapter 5 contains Drug Summaries for each of the drugs authorized in the treatment protocols. These documents are provided to clarify protocol items and issues that might differ from the preceding references, or in which conflicts between references may occur.

1.2 Behavioral Emergencies

Guiding Principles

1. Respect the dignity of the patient.
2. Assure physical safety of the patient and EMS personnel.
3. Diagnose and treat organic causes of behavioral disturbances such as hypoglycemia, hypoxia, or poisoning.
4. Use reasonable physical restraint **only** if attempts at verbal control are unsuccessful. Every attempt should be made to avoid injury to the patient when using physical restraint (see Medical Procedure 4.43).
5. Teamwork between EMS personnel and law enforcement will improve patient care.

General Approach

1. Communicate in a calm and nonthreatening manner.
2. Offer your assistance to the patient.
3. Use reasonable physical force via law enforcement if the patient is a threat to himself/herself or to others.

Use of Restraints

1. Physical.
   a. Use standard restraining techniques and devices (see Medical Procedure 4.43, Physical Restraints).
   b. Use sufficient padding on extremity restraints on elderly patients or others with delicate skin.
2. Chemical.
   a. Use chemical restraints in conjunction with physical restraints if the latter are unsuccessful in controlling violent behavior.
   b. Agents (see Adult Protocol 2.5.2, Violent and/or Impaired Patient).
3. Any type of restraints.
   a. Constantly monitor and observe the patient to prevent injury. If physical and/or chemical restraints are used, place the patient on an ECG monitor and pulse oximeter.
   b. Carefully document the rationale for the use of restraints.

Treatment Protocol

See Adult Protocol 2.5.2, Violent and/or Impaired Patient, for specific treatment protocols.

It may be appropriate for law enforcement to execute an involuntary certificate for psychiatric examination (Baker Act—FS Chapter 394.463). However, such a certificate shall not be an absolute condition for hospital transport.

1.2 Behavioral Emergencies

Transportation

1. All individuals being transported for psychological evaluation under the premises of the Baker Act should be accompanied by a police officer. The paramedic in charge shall determine whether the police officer will ride in the back or follow behind the Rescue Unit.
2. In those situations where a female patient is being transported and a female is not part of the rescue crew, the paramedic should attempt to have a female police officer accompany the patient to the hospital. (This is imperative in situations such as possible rape.) Also document the beginning and ending mileages with dispatch via radio communication.

Baker Act

Florida Statute Chapter 394.463—Mental Health relates to the authorization of police, physicians, and the courts to dictate certain medical care for persons who pose a threat to themselves or to others.

Incapacitated Persons Law

Florida Statute Chapter 40.445 allows for examination and treatment of incapacitated persons in emergency situations. (Patients who are not capable of informed consent as provided in FS Chapter 766.103 cannot refuse medical care.)

Florida Statutes may be viewed online at http://www.flsnate.gov/Statutes/index.cfm?Tab=statutes&submenu=1.

1.3 Critical Incident Stress Management

Purpose

Critical Incident Stress Management (CISM) is a comprehensive, integrated, multicomponent, systematic program of crisis intervention. Its purpose is to provide education, support, assessment, and intervention for emergency service personnel who are often exposed to and/or affected by critical incidents. CISM was born out of emergency services and has become a world standard of care for first responders. Formulated and standardized by the International Critical Incident Stress Foundation (ICISF), CISM has proven to be effective in mitigating many of the common symptoms of critical incident stress. The goal when applying any of the CISM components is to assess, educate, and intervene as necessary and return individuals to their work with the tools and support needed to reduce the effects of a critical incident. The benefits of the intervention include a reduction in symptoms of post-traumatic stress, quicker return to normal productive functioning, increased job satisfaction, reduced worker's compensation claims, reduced absenteeism and presenteeism, reduced errors, enhanced group cohesion, increased personal confidence and extended longevity.

Overview

The Broward County CISM Team (Broward Region X CISM) is made up of trained and credentialed members of law enforcement, fire/rescue, corrections, communications, and others, as well as trained, credentialed, and licensed mental health professionals, all of whom have completed at least three (3) of the core ICISF courses. Broward's CISM Team is independent of any other organization or department in Broward County. The team is designed and organized to respond to any incident that occurs in any emergency services department or agency in Broward County on a 24 × 7 × 365 basis, within a maximum of two (2) hours after a critical incident has occurred and CISM services are requested. The team meets on a periodic basis for additional training and information.

Confidentiality

Florida Statute 401.30(3)(e) protects the discussions held during a CISM intervention as being "confidential and privileged communication under section 90.503." Therefore, all information shared during any part of a CISM intervention is held in the strictest of confidence.

1.3 Critical Incident Stress Management

CISM Services

The following types of services can be provided by the Broward CISM Team.

A. Pre-event planning and preparation.
   1. Educational and informational programs about CISM.
   2. Pre-incident planning and education.

B. Strategic planning and assessment.
   1. Pre- and post-incident assessment of needs.
   2. Development and implementation of a strategic plan for major events.

C. Individual intervention.
   1. One-on-one services with a qualified CISM team member.
   2. Individual support and follow-up.

D. Small group defusing.
   1. Recommended within the first 12 hours after a critical incident occurs.
   2. Best delivered as soon as possible after a critical incident.
   3. Homogeneous groups.
   4. Assessment and education with possible referral and follow-up.

E. Small group debriefing.
   1. 12–72 hours post-critical incident.
   2. Prior to demobilization from extended deployment or upon return home from extended deployment.
   3. Events of significant personal loss (expanded-phase defusing within first 12 hours).

F. Crisis management briefing.
   1. Appropriate for large incidents, incidents with high media involvement, respite/rehab centers, and demobilizations.
   2. Best for large groups or mixed groups.
   3. Primary focus on assessment and information.

G. Family crisis intervention.

H. Organizational consultation.

I. Assessment of organizational needs.

J. Development and recommendation for coordination and delivery of services.

K. Pastoral/spiritual crisis intervention.

L. Referral and follow-up.

1.3 Critical Incident Stress Management

CISM Call-Out Basis

A critical incident is any situation that is either out of the norm or that challenges or would appear to challenge a person's normal coping mechanisms. Examples include the following situations:

- Pediatric injury or death
- Multiple youth fatalities
- Events with severe operational challenges
- Line-of-duty death or line-of-duty injury
- Officer involved in a shooting
- Off-duty death, suicide, homicide, or injury
- Events with multiple or mass casualties
- Prolonged events with loss of life
- Events when the victim(s) is (are) known
- Events with excessive media interest
- Any incident that could perceivably cause emotional impact

Emergency responders work under stressful conditions and situations. Training and continuing education about stress management contribute to the development and maintenance of improved emotional health, stress resistance, and resilience. Statistics demonstrate significantly higher instances of drug and alcohol abuse, marital and family strife, intimate-partner and domestic violence, heart attack, and suicide rates among emergency services personnel compared to the general population. These facts underscore the need for CISM services in any situation similar to those in the preceding list. Because one of the positive benefits of a group intervention is stronger group cohesion, all members of the group are encouraged to be present.

CISM Activation Process Example (Broward County)

A. Requesting agency officer contacts the Communications Captain on duty at Broward Regional Communications Center, requesting CISM Team response.

B. Communications Center number: 954-765-5100.

C. Requesting agency shall supply the following information:
   1. Agency name.
   2. Type of incident.
   3. Number of members involved.
   4. Call-back contact number or pager number.

D. The Communications Captain shall page out the on-call CISM Team Leader.

1.3 Critical Incident Stress Management

CISM Call-Out Procedure

1. When a critical incident event occurs or when an on- or off-scene command determines that an incident may or could have an emotional impact on the responding personnel, department, or agency, any person authorized to do so contacts the Broward Sheriff's Office (BSO) Communications at 954-765-5100 and requests a CISM response, giving a brief description of the event, the caller's name, and his/her contact information.
2. BSO Communications contacts the on-call CISM Team coordinator and, at the same time, pages and/or sends a text message to all members on the CISM Team list.
3. The CISM Team Coordinator contacts the CISM Team Clinical Director or designee and provides the incident contact name and number. The CISM Team Coordinator then begins assembling peer team members for a response. No team member from the affected department, agency, or organization will be part of the responding CISM Team.
4. The CISM Clinical Director contacts the site or incident contact person, receives details about the incident, and advises the contact of the appropriate type and timing of the response.
5. Once the type, timing, and location of the response are determined, the Clinical Director contacts the Team Coordinator with the information necessary to conduct the appropriate intervention. The Clinical Director then contacts mental health members for the intervention as needed.
6. Upon arrival at the determined site, the CISM Team members assemble for a briefing with the Team Leader and then meet with the contact person or designee.
7. Personnel are assembled according to type, in a quiet and secure location. All personnel shall be either off-duty or out of service for the duration of the intervention and related services.
8. In the case of a critical incident stress defusing or debriefing, personnel are assembled according to rank, involvement in the incident, proximity to the incident, as determined by the responding Team Leader.
9. No written, audio, or video recording of the intervention shall be permitted.
10. The CISM Team consults with the contact person to provide general recommendations or for possible follow-up.
11. The CISM Team gathers for a team debriefing.

1.4 Death in the Field

This protocol is divided into separate sections that cover the different situations involving death in the field that the paramedic will encounter. All patients found in cardiac arrest *will* receive cardiopulmonary resuscitation unless an exception is met as outlined in the following sections:

I. Advanced Directives/Do Not Resuscitate Orders (DNRO).

II. Determination of Death.

III. Discontinuance of CPR.

I. Advanced Directives/Do Not Resuscitate Orders (DNRO)

A. Legislative authority.
Under Chapter 401.45, Florida Statutes (F.S.) "Denial of Emergency Treatment Civil Liability," a competent adult, or an incompetent adult, through a healthcare surrogate who was previously chosen, or a proxy or guardian, has the right to be able to control decisions regarding medical care, including the withdrawal or withholding of life-prolonging procedures. This legislation authorizes EMS personnel to honor a prehospital Do Not Resuscitate Order (DNRO). This legislative authority does not include a "living will."

B. Valid Do Not Resuscitate Orders.
   1. An original yellow DNRO (DOH Form 1896) executed as required by State Statute (with original signatures).
   2. A copy on yellow paper (or similar color to the original) of DNRO DOH Form 1896 executed as required by State Statute (with original signatures).
   3. The patient is wearing a bracelet that identifies the patient and indicates the patient has executed a DNRO in accordance with DOH Form 1896.
      a. In this instance, EMS personnel MUST receive the original DNRO DOH Form 1896 or a copy on yellow paper that contains original signatures (attach to the EMS Run Report).
   4. A DNRO document from a licensed healthcare facility or hospice facility, either the original or a copy. For a paramedic to honor a facility's DNRO, it must:
      a. State that it is a DNRO and provide instructions that the patient is not to be resuscitated in the event of cardiac or respiratory arrest.
      b. Have an effective date, which predates the date the assistance is requested.
      c. Include the patient's full legal name, either typed or printed.
      d. Be signed by the patient's attending physician and include the physician's medical license number, telephone number, and date completed.
      e. Be signed and dated by the patient if competent or, if the patient is incompetent, by the patient's healthcare surrogate, legal guardian, or proxy.
      f. Be signed and dated by at least two witnesses.

1.4 Death in the Field

5. *Oral* orders from nonphysician staff members or telephoned requests from an absent physician do not adequately assure paramedics that the proper decision-making process has been followed and are NOT acceptable.

C. Confirmation and documentation.

1. The paramedic must confirm the identity of the patient with a DNRO through a driver's license, other photo identification, or from a witness in the presence of the patient. If a witness is used to identify the patient, this fact shall be documented in the EMS Run Report, which must include the following information:
   a. The full name of the witness.
   b. The address and telephone number of the witness.
   c. The relationship of the witness to the patient.

II. Determination of Death

The EMT or paramedic may determine that the patient is dead/non-salvageable and decide not to resuscitate the patient under the following guidelines.

A. The patient may be determined to be dead/non-salvageable and will not be resuscitated or transported if all four (4) presumptive signs of death *and* at least one (1) conclusive sign of death are identified.

1. The four presumptive signs of death that MUST be present are:
   a. Unresponsiveness.
   b. Apnea.
   c. Pulseless.
   d. Fixed dilated pupils.
2. In addition to the four presumptive signs of deaths, at least one (1) of the following conclusive signs of death MUST be present:
   a. Injuries incompatible with life (e.g., decapitation, massive crush injury, incineration).
   b. Tissue decomposition.
   c. *Rigor mortis* of any degree with warm air temperature.
      1) Hardening of the muscles of the body, making the joints rigid.
   d. Liver mortis (lividity) of any degree.
      1) Venous pooling of blood in dependent body parts causing purple discoloration of the skin, which does blanch with pressure.
3. Patients with suspected hypothermia, barbiturate overdose, or electrocution require full ALS resuscitation unless they have injuries incompatible with life or tissue decomposition.

1.4 Death in the Field

4. EMS personnel may contact medical direction for a "determination of death" whenever support in the field is desired. Clearly state the purpose for the contact as part of the initial hailing.
5. Children are excluded from this protocol unless EMS personnel make contact with medical direction for consultation. Only in cases of obvious, prolonged death should CPR not be started or discontinued on infants, children, or young adults, or in cases in which an unexpected death has occurred.

B. A trauma victim who does not meet the "Determination of Death" criteria listed above may be determined to be dead/non-salvageable based on the following criteria:
   1. Pulselessness and apnea associated with asystole (confirmed in two leads) and
      a. Blunt trauma arrest.
      b. Prolonged extrication time (more than 15 minutes) where no resuscitative measures can be initiated prior to extrication.
         1) An additional rhythm assessment is required, followed by at least one reassessment after 15 minutes.
      c. Arrest from primary brain injury or with no brain stem reflexes; arrest from blunt multiple injuries.
   2. If there is any concern regarding leaving the patient at the scene, begin resuscitation and transport.
   3. Consideration should be given for the possibility of organ harvest; however, this should not be the sole reason for resuscitation.

C. Absence of pulse or spontaneous respiration in a *multiple-casualty* situation where EMS resources are required for stabilization of living patients.

The local law enforcement agency that has jurisdiction will be responsible for the body once death has been determined. The body is to be left at the scene until a disposition has been made by the Medical Examiner's Office or the local jurisdiction.

III. Discontinuance of CPR

A. Resuscitation that is started in the field by EMS personnel cannot be discontinued without an order from medical direction. EMS personnel are not obligated to continue resuscitation efforts that were started inappropriately by others at the scene. *However,* contact with medical direction is necessary to cease resuscitative efforts in ALL situations.

B. When there is a delay in presenting a DNRO to EMS personnel, resuscitation must be started. However, once the DNRO is presented to EMS personnel, the EMT or paramedic with an order from medical direction may terminate resuscitation.

1.4 Death in the Field

C. A paramedic with an order from medical direction may terminate resuscitation provided the following criteria are met:
   1. Appropriate BLS and ALS have been attempted without restoration of circulation and breathing.
   2. Endotracheal intubation has been successfully accomplished.
   3. Intravenous (IV, IO, ETT) medication and countershocks for ventricular fibrillation have been administered according to the appropriate treatment protocol(s) (see Adult Protocols or Pediatric Protocols).
   4. Persistent asystole or agonal ECG patterns are present and no reversible causes are identified.
      a. Patients with suspected hypothermia, barbiturate overdose, or electrocution require full ALS resuscitation, unless they have injuries incompatible with life or tissue decomposition.

D. Provide appropriate grief counseling or support to the patient's immediate family, bystanders, or others at the scene.
   1. Provide family members with appropriate referral information, if available.

E. Patient preparation.
   1. Once it has been determined that the patient has died and resuscitation will not continue, cover the body with a sheet or other suitable item. *Do not* remove any property from the body or the scene for any purpose.
   2. Immediately notify the appropriate law enforcement agency (if not done already), and remain on scene until their arrival.
   3. Complete the EMS Run Report, documenting the previously mentioned criteria, and leave a copy with the patient for the Medical Examiner's Office or fax a copy to the Medical Examiner's Office via the Department's EMS Division.
   4. ECG rhythm documentation must be attached to the EMS Run Report.
   5. Endotracheal (ET) tube placement may be verified by two paramedics for patients who are determined to be dead in the field or for whom resuscitation measures have ceased. The ET tube should be left in place and its confirmation should be recorded on the EMS Run Report. Improperly placed ET tubes should be left in place and reported to the appropriate personnel. (Proper ET tube placement *must* be confirmed prior to terminating resuscitation.)
   6. Consult the patient's family for "organ donor" information, if appropriate.
   7. If the death is a suspected homicide (criminal scene), do not cover the body (see General Protocol 1.13).

1.5 Emergency Worker Rehabilitation

Medical Evaluation of Emergency Workers on Emergency Incidents or Training Evolutions

A. **Purpose:** Emergency operations require significant physical activity, but no rescuer will be required to perform emergency operations beyond safe levels of physical or mental endurance. This protocol is intended to examine and evaluate the physical and mental status of emergency workers working on an emergency incident or a training exercise and determine which treatment, if any, is necessary. Personnel rehabilitation using appropriate protocols in this area will decrease injury risk and enhance recovery for later emergency operations.

B. **Implementation:** A Rehabilitation Area (Rehab Area) will be set up at the discretion of the Incident Commander. It is recommended that a Rehab Area be utilized at all working incidents to provide a staging area for on-scene personnel, as well as an immediate source of personnel for rescue or aid, and an area for recovery and rehabilitation of emergency workers. When a Rehab Area has been deemed necessary by the Incident Commander (IC), the first available EMS unit will be responsible for the management and coordination of the Rehab Area.

C. **Location:** Establish a Rehab Area away from environmental hazards (e.g., in a shady, cool place that is, upwind and away from smoke and traffic) that is readily accessible to rescue personnel for transport and supplies. Air truck and canteen service will be stationed in this area. Multiple Rehab Areas may be needed on large incidents. If a specific location has not been designated by the IC, the Rehab Officer shall select an appropriate location based on the following site characteristics:
   1. The Rehab Area should be in a location that will provide physical rest by allowing the body to recuperate from the demands and hazards of the emergency operation or training evolution.
   2. It should be far enough away from the scene that members may safely remove their turnout gear and self-contained breathing apparatus (SCBA) and be afforded mental rest from the stress and pressure of the emergency operation or training evolution.
   3. It should provide suitable protection from the prevailing environmental conditions. During hot weather, it should be in a cool, shaded area. During cold weather, it should be in a warm, dry area.
   4. It should enable members to be free of exhaust fumes from apparatus, vehicles, or equipment (including those involved in the rehabilitation group operations).
   5. It should be easily accessible by EMS units.
   6. It should allow prompt reentry back into the emergency operation upon complete recuperation.

1.5 Emergency Worker Rehabilitation

D. **Resources:** The Rehab Officer shall secure all necessary resources required to adequately staff and supply the rehabilitation area. The supplies should include the following items:
   1. Fluids—water, activity beverages, oral electrolyte solutions, and ice.
   2. Food (for extended operations where crews are engaged for 3 hours or more)—soup, broth, or stew in hot/cold cups.
   3. Medical equipment—blood pressure cuffs, stethoscopes, oxygen administration devices, cardiac monitors, intravenous solutions, thermometers, and pulse oximeters (which include the ability to monitor SpCO).
   4. Other—awnings, "cool zone" misting fans, cooling chairs, heaters (according to climate), towels, and tarps.

E. **Manning:** Assign a minimum of two rescue personnel to monitor and assist fire fighters in the Rehab Area. An appointed rehab area command will oversee rehab operations. Their responsibility is to oversee provision of food, fluids, oxygen, and appropriate environment for rehab and rehabilitation operations in the area. These personnel will oversee the rehabilitation and availability for work of all emergency responders placed in this area.

F. **Medical evaluations:** When the Incident Commander has established a Rehab Area, fire fighters and other emergency responders shall be evaluated following (a):
   1. The use of two SCBA bottles and/or 30 minutes of strenuous activity (e.g., use of chemical PPE, advancing hose lines, forcible entry, ventilation) (b).
   2. SCBA failure.
   3. Weakness, dizziness, chest pain, muscle cramps, nausea/vomiting, altered mental status, difficulty breathing, and other stress-related symptoms (c).
   4. At the discretion of the Incident Commander, Rehab Officer, Safety Officer, CISM Coordinator, and Company Officer.

NOTE

(a) A medical evaluation form shall be completed on all personnel entering the Rehab Area and before they return to emergency work.

(b) This does not preclude an officer from having a rescue team member evaluated if he/she deems it appropriate. A member may be evaluated any time he/she feels it necessary.

(c) All personnel receiving ALS treatment and transport will have a patient care report completed for them.

1.5 Emergency Worker Rehabilitation

G. **Examination:** EMS personnel should evaluate persons arriving to the Rehab Area as they appear. Arriving emergency workers must be questioned regarding any medical symptoms, be asked about any injury resulting from incident work, and have assessment of appropriate vital signs. Examination shall occur at 10-minute intervals and will involve a minimum of:
   1. Glasgow Coma Scale score.
   2. Pupillary response.
   3. Vital signs (BP, P, R, CR).
   4. ECG (if applicable).
   5. Lung sounds.
   6. Skin condition.
   7. Signs and symptoms.
   8. Oral temperature.
   9. Pulse oximetry.
      a. Arterial oxygen saturation (SpO_2).
      b. Carboxyhemoglobin saturation (SpCO).

   An EMS Run Report and a Casualty Report shall be completed for each fire fighter or other emergency worker who is not routinely returned to emergency operations.

H. **Guidelines for rehab:** The following will occur:
   1. Normal presentations: The emergency responder will rehydrate and rest before reporting to Manpower. Rest shall not be less than 15 minutes.
   2. Abnormal presentations:
      a. Blood pressure values that are higher or lower than the person's usual level.
      b. SpO_2 values $\leq 92\%$.
      c. Values for the pulse rate in an emergency responder will normally be less than 100 beats per minute (BPM) at rest and less than 120 BPM at a working incident. At no time should the pulse exceed 180 BPM.
      d. Values for carbon monoxide oximetry will normally be 5% for a nonsmoker and less than 8% for a smoker. A carbon monoxide oximetry reading of more than 12% indicates moderate carbon monoxide inhalation; a reading of more than 25% indicates severe inhalation of carbon monoxide.
      e. Body temperature greater than 100.6°F.

1.5 Emergency Worker Rehabilitation

3. Management.
   a. The emergency responder will rehydrate and rest. The emergency responder will report to Manpower when presentations are normal. Presentations should return to normal within 15 minutes.
   b. If a team member's heart rate exceeds 110 BPM, an oral temperature should be taken. If the oral temperature exceeds 100.6°F, the member should not be permitted to wear protective equipment and should be treated for heat stress and monitored for worsening of the heat emergency (i.e., heat exhaustion and heat stroke).
   c. The emergency responder will receive ALS treatment and transport if presentations are abnormal for more than 15 minutes. Abnormal presentation includes the following signs and symptoms:
      1) SpO_2 value $\leq$ 92%.
      2) Persistent heart rate greater than 120 BPM (lasting for 15 minutes or longer).
      3) Any emergency worker with a carbon monoxide oximetry reading of more than 8% but less than 15% must be given the opportunity to breathe ambient air for 5 minutes.
      4) If the carbon monoxide oximetry reading is still higher than 8%, the emergency worker should be given oxygen via mask until the value drops below 5%. Any worker with a carbon monoxide oximetry reading of more than 25% must be completely evaluated and removed to a hospital, preferably one that has a hyperbaric chamber. No emergency worker should leave the Rehab Area until his/her CO level is less than 8%.
      5) Blood pressure above or below the emergency worker's normal level.
      6) Symptoms of heat stroke.
      7) Oral temperature > 100.6°F, lasting longer than 15 minutes (after oxygen administration).
   d. Any emergency responder with chest pain, difficulty breathing, and altered mental status will receive immediate ALS treatment and transport.
   e. Any other abnormal presentation not specified herein, where the examining paramedic's judgment determines a need for treatment and transport, will be managed accordingly.

1.5 Emergency Worker Rehabilitation

I. **Treatment:** Treatment will consist of one or more of the following measures. Prior to taking anything orally, the fire fighter or other emergency responder will clean his/her hands and face. On-scene rescue personnel will provide water and a cleaning agent.
   1. Rest.
   2. Oral rehydration and nutrition (air truck, canteen service); minimum of 1 to 2 quarts of fluids over a 15-minute time period (e.g., half-strength Gatorade®). Avoid any substance containing caffeine (e.g., Coke®, Pepsi®, sodas, coffee, tea).
      a. Members should consume at least 1 quart of water per hour.
      b. Members shall rehydrate with at least 8 ounces of fluid while SCBA cylinders are being changed.
   3. Oxygen (humidified, nebulizer).
   4. Cool environment utilizing "cool zone" fans and/or "cooling chairs" if available (e.g., shade, electric fan, air conditioning, removal of bunker gear, showers).
   5. For extended operations lasting 3 or more hours, the Rehab Area should provide food such as soup, broth, or stew; these items are digested much faster than sandwiches and fast-food products. In addition, foods such as apples, oranges, and bananas provide supplemental forms of energy replacement. Fatty and/or salty foods should be avoided.
   6. Follow ALS/BLS protocols for further treatment.

J. **Return to emergency duties:** Members assigned to the rehabilitation group shall enter and exit the Rehab Area as a crew. The crew designation, number of crew members, and the times of entry to and exit from the Rehab Area shall be documented by the Rehab Officer or his/her designee on the company check-in/out sheet. Crews shall not leave the Rehab Area until authorized to do so by the Rehab Officer. Report to Manpower or Incident Commander when the following criteria have been met:
   a) Vital signs within normal limits.
   b) Absence of abnormal signs and symptoms.
   c) Minimum period of 15 minutes for rest and rehydration.
   d) Released by Rehab Officer.

K. **Documentation:** A Rehab Medical Evaluation Form shall be completed for all personnel evaluated in the Rehab Area and forwarded to the appropriate Rescue (EMS) Division following all applicable patient confidentiality guidelines (e.g., HIPAA). A complete patient care report (PCR) shall be completed for any member who receives treatment/transport.

See the Online Forms for the Strenuous Activity—Medical Evaluation form.

1.5 Emergency Worker Rehabilitation

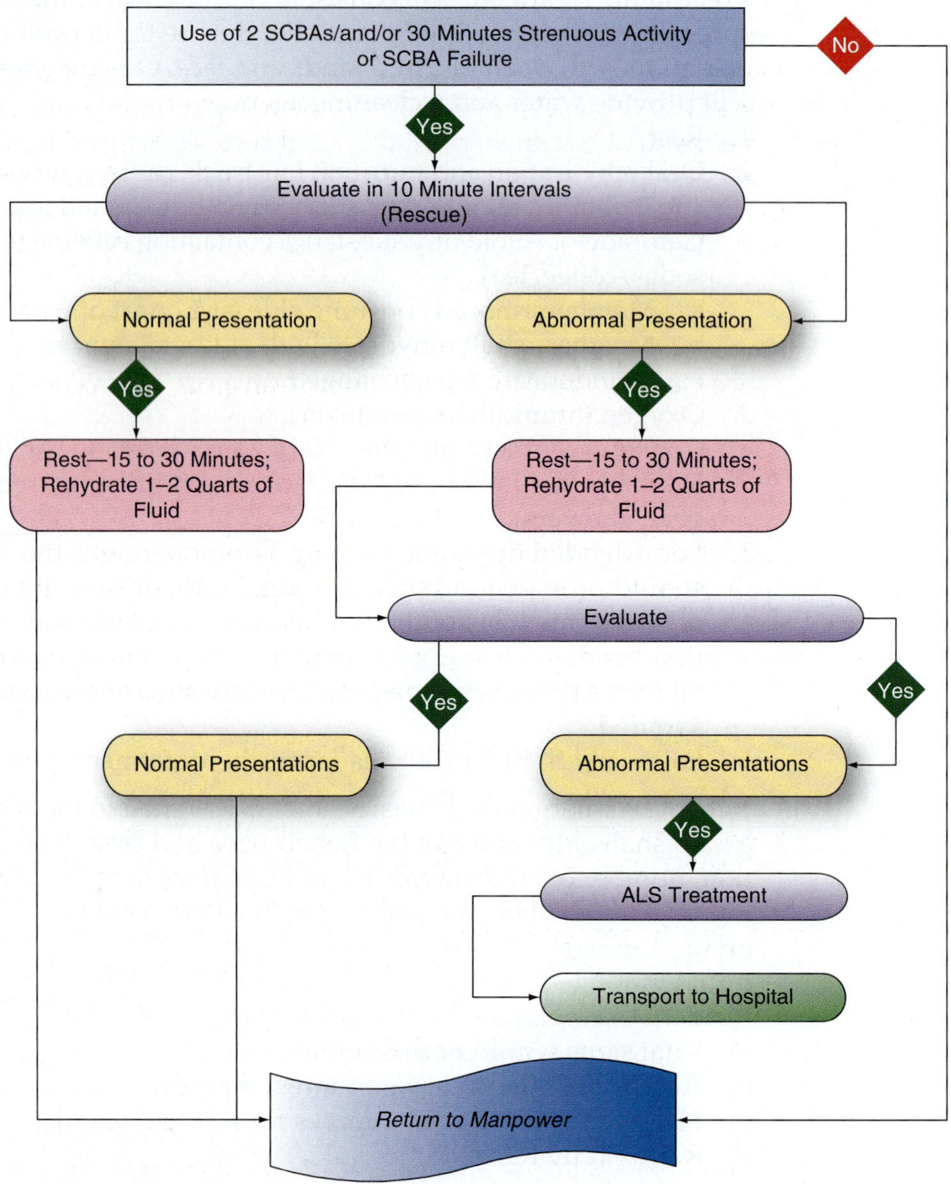

SCBA failure chart.

1.6 Helicopter Safety

Communication Procedures

The standard dispatch for an Air Rescue assignment should be one (1) engine company and one (1) rescue. The need for additional units should be dictated by the incident circumstances. It should be kept in mind that the unit assigned as the heli-spot (HS) group may need all of its personnel to properly secure the HS site. This may create the need for additional units to address patient care needs. Dispatchers *should not* take it upon themselves to modify this assignment, nor should they suggest modification of the assignment. As with any Fire Department assignment, the only personnel who can modify the assignment are Uniformed Fire Department Officers.

See General Protocol 1.10, Trauma Transport, Helicopter Transport Protocol.

Heli-Spot Procedures

Rescue Units, when requesting an Air Rescue assignment, should not concern themselves with an HS unless they know of one at or very near the incident site. The rescue personnel should concern themselves with proper and rapid patient packaging. In the event that the unit assigned as the HS group experiences difficulties in finding an HS, they should wait until Air Rescue arrives. Air Rescue has a better vantage point in choosing an HS, and its personnel will advise the HS group.

In the event that the HS is remotely located and appears to be safe for landing, the Pilot in Command (PIC) may elect to land without the assistance of an HS sector. This *does not* mean that the unit assigned to the HS should be canceled. These team members will be utilized for security, safety, and patient loading once the helicopter is on the ground. The Pilot in Command (PIC) is both legally and operationally responsible for the safety of the aircraft. *Therefore, the final decision of the suitability of the HS site is that of the PIC.*

When setting up an HS, there are several things to keep in mind:

1. The HS should be set up as to facilitate takeoffs and landings into the wind. (*Do not* rely on dispatch for correct wind direction; use visual indicators.)
2. If the HS group Officer in Command (OIC) is not sure of the wind direction or the direction from which the helicopter should approach, then he/she should wait until the helicopter is in the area and confer with the Air Crew on this decision.
3. The approach and departure ends of the HS should be clear of obstacles (any object more than 40 feet tall that is within 100 feet of the HS).
4. Debris such as wood, cans, and plastic should be removed from the HS. Flying debris can do damage to both the helicopter and personnel on the ground.
5. To minimize the hazard of blowing sand and dust, the HS should be hosed down (may be hosed down as necessary).
6. Once the helicopter has landed, the Marshaller should post a minimum of **one tail rotor guard** (two, if available). This person should be someone other than the Marshaller. The Marshaller shall remain at his/her post until the aircraft departs.
7. *No unauthorized* personnel shall be permitted to approach the helicopter. This is the general responsibility of all Fire Department personnel, but it is most definitely the overall combined responsibility of the PIC and the HS group OIC.

1.6 Helicopter Safety

8. The HS group should assure that the Rescue Unit personnel are supplemented with an appropriate number of personnel to assist in the safe and efficient loading of patients into the helicopter.
9. Once the helicopter has landed, the Marshaller should confer with the Air Crew as to the helicopter's departure.
10. It is not necessary to have a hose line pulled and charged. In the event of a catastrophic event involving the helicopter, tactics and strategy will be left up to the Incident Commander.

The Marshaller is one of several tools that are at the disposal of the PIC for the accomplishment of a safe landing and departure. The PIC considers several factors when making an approach or departure into a confined area. As a consequence, he/she may not always follow the exact direction of the Marshaller. Note that most approaches will be to the ground, not to a hover. The PIC, at his/her discretion, may elect to land without the assistance of a Marshaller and may request that the Marshaller remain clear of the HS until after the helicopter has landed. If the PIC does not follow the exact direction of the Marshaller, be assured there are reasons for his/her actions.

Review Your Marshalling Hand Signals

A. Marshalling.
   1. Positioning.
      a. The Marshaller will stand at the outer edge of the HS perimeter on the windward side, with his/her back to the wind.
      b. The Apparatus Lieutenant/Captain will have the primary responsibility for the marshalling duties.
      c. An additional fire fighter who is assigned to the Marshaller will maintain constant radio contact with the helicopter as well as visual and verbal contact with the Marshaller.
      d. Remain in eye contact with the pilot at all times.
      e. *Do not* approach the helicopter; remain vigilant at your post.
   2. Equipment.
      a. Helmet with chin strap tightly secured.
      b. Goggles on or visor down.
      c. Gloves.
      d. Full bunker gear with collar up.
      e. Flash lights with wands for night operations.

1.6 Helicopter Safety

3. Safety precautions and procedures.
   a. **Stay well clear of the tail rotor area.**
   b. Use caution when traversing uneven terrain.
   c. Approach the helicopter in the pilot's field of vision and ONLY after an "All Clear" signal has been given by a helicopter crewmember.
   d. Use low crouch when approaching and departing the helicopter.
   e. *Do not* use road flares. *Do not* shine spotlights or headlights at the helicopter or into the HS. The pilot will utilize the "night sun" to light up the HS as needed. Shining lights or strobes at the HS may cause vertigo, night blindness, or seizures of the pilot.

Rescue Unit Procedures

The Rescue Unit OIC has the primary responsibility of patient care and should not become overly concerned with the availability of an appropriate HS. The following points should be kept in mind when deciding on Air Rescue as the mode of transport for the patient:

1. Make the decision to transport by air early. Have Air Rescue dispatched by the Incident Commander. Even if you are not sure that a patient meets the established criteria for air transport, place Air Rescue on standby status. You can always cancel the standby.
2. It is imperative that the ground Rescue Unit contact the receiving facility prior to Air Rescue's on-scene arrival. This will preclude any delay in transportation in the event the receiving facility cannot accept the patient. This early advisory is also necessary to allow the hospital time to prepare for an Air Rescue arrival. Air Rescue may monitor the medical channel and receive patient information while it is given to the receiving facility from the ground Rescue Unit.
3. Relaying information concerning HS location and any hazards is a priority (this information may be relayed to the Air Rescue team after they are airborne). The only patient information that the Rescue Unit needs to advise the Incident Commander about when requesting Air Rescue is the number of patients and the designated receiving facility. *The ground Rescue Unit should not spend time advising Air Rescue of patient conditions over the incident frequencies.* That time would be better spent communicating with the receiving facility.
4. There is no reason to provide the Air Rescue crew with a completed EMS Run Report. This may create an undue delay in the transportation of the patient. A "hard copy" of whatever information you do have should be provided to the Flight Medic.
5. All bandages and dressings shall be affixed securely.

1.6 Helicopter Safety

6. The patient will be secured to a backboard with a *minimum* of three (3) straps, unless contraindicated by his/her medical condition. If the patient is unruly, place an additional strap above the knees. Having a patient lie on a backboard with the head immobilized and nothing securing the body is *unacceptable*. In the event that straps are not available, another method of securing the patient should be improvised.
7. A *minimum of four (4) personnel,* one of whom will be a member of the Air Rescue crew, will carry the stretcher. Each member of this team should have a helmet with face shield and chin strap in place when loading the patient.
8. If the patient is difficult to carry, a stretcher may be utilized, provided the sheets, pillow, and mattress are removed.
9. The key to saving a trauma patient who requires surgical intervention is *speed. Do not* delay transport for invasive procedures other than those necessary to maintain the patient's airway. Most invasive procedures can be done while en route to the Trauma Center.
10. Be aware of the time you are on the scene with the patient. Attempts at certain procedures may be perceived as progressing at a rapid pace, but in reality they are taking an extended period of time that can better be used in moving the patient.
11. Advise the Air Rescue Unit if you have any need for additional equipment or assistance (e.g., for managing patient airway difficulties).
12. Remain at the incident side (or at least 100 feet from the HS) until the helicopter has landed.
13. *Absolutely no personnel should approach the helicopter unless cleared "in" by an Air Rescue crew member.*
    a. Do not approach the helicopter with a patient unless escorted by an Air Rescue crew member.
    b. It is the responsibility of *all* Fire/Rescue/EMS personnel to ensure that any and all unauthorized persons are prevented from approaching the helicopter. This is usually accomplished with visual and verbal warnings, but in some instances may require physical intervention.
14. In the event that the Air Rescue crew requires assistance with patient care, the ground paramedic in charge of patient care will accompany the patient during air transport. In this event, the ground paramedic, with Air Crew approval, will bring any equipment necessary to affect patient care during air transport. Any additional Fire/Rescue personnel will be determined by the Air Rescue crew and the ground paramedic in charge of patient care.

References

Broward County Aeromedical Transport Program

Miami-Dade Air Rescue Assignment Procedures

U.S. Coast Guard Helicopter Procedures

1.6 Helicopter Safety

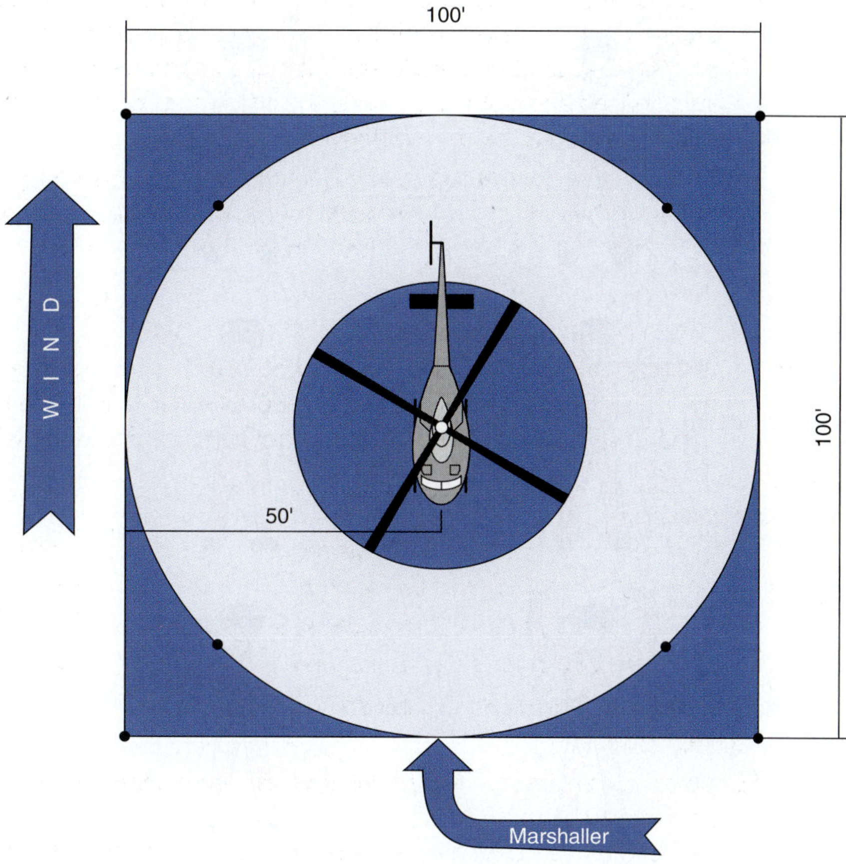

● *Indicates positioning of markers*

The heli-spot shall be a minimum of 100′ × 100′ (HS size may be increased by local protocol).

1.6 Helicopter Safety

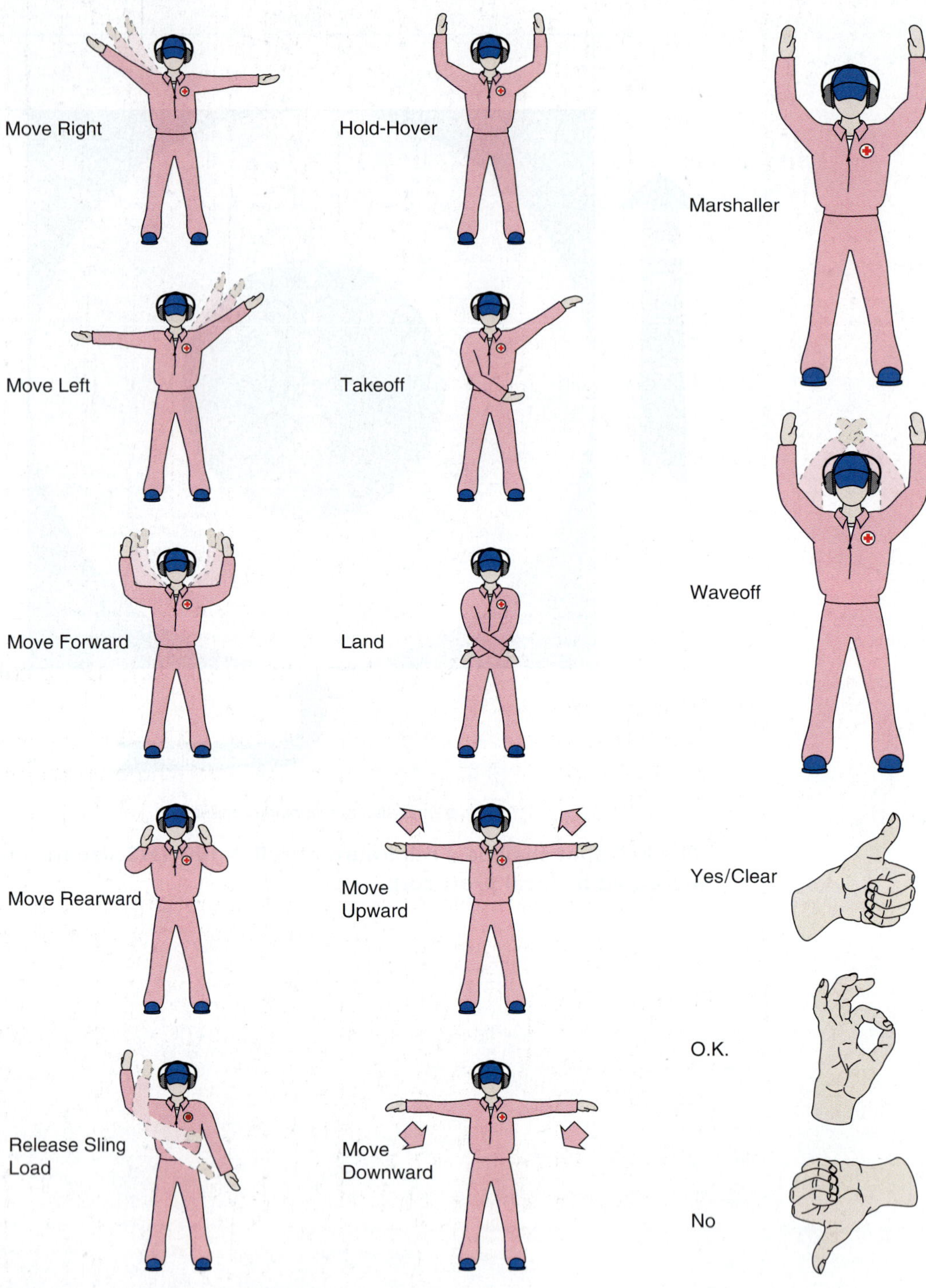

Helicopter safety motions.

1.9 Mass-Casualty Incidents

C. **Triage Officer.**
   1. Radio designation = "Triage." Follow FOG #3.
   2. Organize the Triage Team to begin initial triaging of victims, utilizing the START/JumpSTART triage system. Assemble the walking wounded and uninjured in a safe area. Use bullhorns or a public address (PA) system if necessary.
   3. Advise Command (or the Medical Branch, if established) as soon as possible if there is a need for additional resources.
   4. Coordinate with Treatment to ensure that priority victims are treated first.
   5. Ensure that all areas around the MCI scene have been checked for potential victims, walking wounded, ejected victims, and so forth.
   6. Supervise the Triage Personnel, Litter Bearers, and Medical Examiner's Office personnel.
   7. Maintain security and control of the triage area. Request the assistance of law enforcement.
   8. Report to Command or the Medical Branch upon completion of duties for further assignments.

D. **Treatment Officer.**

   Reports to Command or the Medical Branch. Supervises the Treatment Managers of the Red, Yellow, and Green Areas. Coordinates the retriage and tagging of all victims and the on-site medical care. Directs the movement of victims to the loading area(s).
   1. Radio designation = "Treatment." Follow FOG #4.
   2. Consider assigning a Documentation Aide to assist with paperwork.
   3. Direct personnel to either begin treatment on the victims where they lay *or* establish a centralized treatment area.
   4. Considerations for a treatment area:
      a. Capable of accommodating the number of victims and equipment.
      b. Consider weather, safety, and the possibility of hazardous materials.
      c. Designate entrance and exit areas, which are readily accessible (funnel points).
      d. On large-scale incidents, divide the treatment area into three distinct areas based on priority. Designate a Treatment Manager for each area (Red, Yellow, Green). Use appropriate-color tarps if available.
   5. Complete a Treatment Log as victims enter the area.

1.9 Mass-Casualty Incidents

6. Ensure that all victims are retriaged through a secondary exam and the assessment is documented on a triage tag (Disaster Management System [DMS]—All Risk Triage tag). The rescuer filling out the All Risk Triage tag will keep a corner of the tag for future documentation.
7. All red-tagged victims will be transported immediately as transport units become available. These victims should not be delayed in the treatment area.
8. Ensure that enough equipment is available to effectively treat all victims.
9. Establish communications with Transport to coordinate proper transport of the appropriate victims. Direct movement of victims to the ambulance loading areas.
10. Provide periodic status reports to Command/Medical Branch.

Note

Red, Yellow, and Green Treatment Manager: Report to the Treatment Officer and are responsible for the treatment and continual retriaging of victims. Notify the Treatment Officer of victim readiness and priority for transportation. Assure that appropriate victim information is recorded.

E. **Transport Officer.**

Reports to Command or the Medical Branch. Supervises the Medical Communication Coordinator and Documentation Aide(s). The Transport Officer is responsible for the coordination of victims and maintenance of records relating to victim identification, injuries, mode of transportation, and destination.

1. Radio designation = "Transport." Follow FOG #5.
2. Assign a Documentation Aide with a radio to assist with paperwork and communications.
3. Assign a Medical Communication Coordinator to establish continuous contact with Medical Control (Medcom or MRCC1).
4. Establish a victim loading area. Advise Staging of the location and direction of travel. Consider requesting law enforcement assistance for ensuring the security of the loading area.
5. Arrange for the transport of victims from the treatment area. Maintain a Hospital Transportation Log #5B. Keep a piece of the triage tag for future documentation.
6. Communicate with the Landing Zone (LZ)/Heli-spot Officer and relay the number of victims to be transported by air. Air-transported victims should be assigned to distant hospitals, unless the victims' needs dictate otherwise (e.g., trauma center, burn unit).

1.9 Mass-Casualty Incidents

F. **Medical Communications Coordinator.**

Reports to the Transport Officer and is responsible for maintaining communication with Medical Control to assure proper victim transport information and destination.

1. Radio designation = "Communication." Follow FOG #5A.
2. Establish communication with Medical Control (Medcom or MRCC1). Advise Medical Control of the overall situation (e.g., smoke inhalation, trauma, burns, hazardous materials exposure) and the number and categories of victims. Medical Control will survey area hospitals to determine their capabilities and capacities and then relay this information to the field. Document this information on the Hospital Capability Worksheet #5C and maintain this document for the duration of the incident.
3. When units are prepared to transport, advise Medical Control and supply of the following information:
   a. The unit transporting.
   b. The number of victims to be transported.
   c. Their priority: Red, Yellow, or Green.
   d. Any victims with special needs (e.g., cardiac, burn, trauma).
4. The Medical Communication Coordinator, in conjunction with Medical Control, will determine the most appropriate facility. Ground-transported victims should be assigned to hospitals on a rotating basis.
5. Once Medical Control receives the information from the Medical Communication Coordinator, Medical Control will notify the appropriate hospital.
6. Transporting units will not contact the individual hospital on their own, unless there is a need for medical direction/care outside of protocols.

NOTE

Medical Resource Coordination Center (MRCC): The MRCC's prime function is to maintain status information—that is, the number of victims and the hospital readiness status to accept victims, to coordinate transportation, and to direct patients to the appropriate hospital during a disaster or other situation characterized by a high demand for medical resources.

G. **Medical Supply Coordinator.**

Reports to the Medical Branch and is responsible for acquiring and maintaining control of all medical equipment and supplies.

1. Radio designation = "Supply." Follow FOG #6.
2. Assure necessary equipment is available on the transporting vehicle.
3. Provide an inventory of medical supplies at the staging area for use on scene.
4. Assure support vehicles are requested. (Broward County has four MCI supply trailers and Region 7 has three large MCI supply trailers available for use during a large-scale MCI.)

1.9 Mass-Casualty Incidents

H. **Staging Officer.**

Reports to Command and is responsible for managing all activities within the staging area.

1. Radio designation = "Staging." Follow FOG #7.
2. Establish the location of a staging area and notify the Communication Center to direct any incoming units.
3. Maintain a Unit Staging Log #7A.
4. Ensure that all personnel stay with their vehicles unless otherwise directed by Command. If personnel are directed to assist in another function, ensure that the keys stay with each vehicle.
5. Coordinate with the Transport Officer the designation of a location for victim loading and the best route to the area.
6. Maintain a reserve of at least two transport vehicles. When the reserve is depleted, request additional units through Command.

Documentation

A. The Incident Commander will, at the completion of the incident, coordinate the gathering of all pertinent documentation.

B. A Post-Incident Analysis (PIA) will be completed.

MCI Kits

Each unit will carry an MCI bag. Included in the bag will be the following items:

A. **Two (2) triage packs with:**

1. Four (4) combine dressings.
2. Four (4) 4 × 4's.
3. Six (6) pairs of gloves.
4. One (1) pediatric face mask, assorted oropharyngeal airways (OPAs) and nasopharyngeal airways (NPAs).
5. Two (2) clip rings containing triage ribbons paired in red and yellow, green and black. There are 15 ribbons of each color per ring.

B. One (1) additional set of triage ribbons.

C. Fifty (50) triage tags—Disaster Management Systems (DMS) All Risk Triage tags.

D. Three (3) mechanical pencils and three (3) grease pencils.

1.9 Mass-Casualty Incidents

E. The following MCI FOGs, logs, and associated paperwork for each officer:
   1. Command FOG #1—White.
   2. Medical FOG #2—Blue.
   3. Triage FOG #3—Yellow.
   4. Treatment FOG #4—Red.
   5. Treatment Area Log #4A—Red.
   6. Transport FOG #5—Green.
   7. Medical Communication FOG #5A—Green.
   8. Hospital Transport Log #5B—Green.
   9. Hospital Capability Worksheet #5C—Green.
   10. Medical Supply FOG #6—Blue.
   11. Staging FOG #7—Orange.
   12. Unit Staging Log #7A—Orange.
   13. MCI-WMD/Terrorist Event FOG #8—Beige.

MCI Supervisor Kit

A. Complete vest set with the following identification vests:
   1. White for Command.
   2. Blue for Medical Officer.
   3. Yellow for Triage Officer.
   4. Red for Treatment Officer.
   5. Green for Transport Officer.
   6. Green Striped for Medical Communication Coordinator.
   7. Blue Striped for Medical Supply Officer.
   8. Orange for Staging Officer.

B. Portfolio for each officer that contains a clipboard, paperwork for each officer, pens, pencils, grease pencils, and a pad of paper.

C. EMS tactical EMS Command Board.

D. Tarp set: red, yellow, green, black tarps.

E. Bullhorn.

1.9 Mass-Casualty Incidents

START System of Triage

This procedure is based on the Simple Triage and Rapid Treatment (START) process for adult victims and the JumpSTART adaptation for pediatric victims. These methods of triage are designed to assess a large number of victims objectively, efficiently, and rapidly and can be used by personnel with limited medical training.

Procedure

A. Initial triage: Using the START or JumpSTART method (described in the following two sections):
   1. Locate and direct all of the walking wounded to one location away from the incident if possible. Assign someone to keep them together (Fire Department personnel, law enforcement officer, or capable bystander).
   2. Begin assessing all non-ambulatory victims where they are found.
   3. Utilize the triage ribbons (color-coded plastic strips). One should be tied to an upper extremity in a *visible* location.
      a. Red: Immediate care.
      b. Yellow: Delayed care.
      c. Green: Ambulatory (minor).
      d. Black: Deceased (non-salvageable).
   4. Independent decisions should be made for each victim. Do not base triage decisions on the perception of too many reds, not enough greens, and so forth.
   5. If borderline decisions are encountered, always triage to the most urgent priority (e.g., for a Green/Yellow patient, tag as Yellow).

B. Secondary triage.
   1. Performed on all victims during the Treatment phase. If a victim is identified in the initial Triage phase as a Red and transport is available, do not delay transport to perform a secondary assessment.
   2. Utilize a triage tag (Disaster Management System [DMS] All Risk Triage tag) and attempt to assess for and complete all information required on the tag (time permitting). Affix the tag to the victim and remove the ribbon.
   3. The Triage priority determined in the Treatment phase should be the priority used for transport. If trauma-related, the trauma transport criteria will be applied to trauma victims during the secondary triage in the Treatment phase.

1.9 Mass-Casualty Incidents

START (Refer to Flowchart on Page 47)

Remember the mnemonic **RPM** (**R**espiration, **P**erfusion, **M**ental status). The first assessment that produces a Red stops further assessment. Only correction of life-threatening problems, such as airway obstruction or severe hemorrhage, should be managed during triage.

A. **Assess Respirations.**
   1. If respiratory rate is 30/min or less, go to the Perfusion assessment.
   2. If respiratory rate is more than 30/min, prioritize as Red.
   3. If the victim is not breathing, open the airway, remove obstructions, if seen, and assess for (1) or (2).
   4. If the victim is still not breathing, prioritize as Black.

B. **Assess Perfusion.**
   1. Performed by assessing a radial pulse.
   2. If radial pulse is present, go to the Mental Status assessment.
   3. If no radial pulse, prioritize as Red.

Note

Any major external bleeding should also be controlled at this time.

C. **Assess Mental Status.**
   1. Assess the victim's ability to follow simple commands and his/her orientation to time, place, and person (CAO 3).
   2. If the victim does not follow commands, is unconscious, or is disoriented, prioritize as Red.
   3. If the victim follows commands and is oriented × 3, prioritize as Green.

Note

Depending on the victim's injuries (burns, fractures, bleeding), it may be necessary to prioritize him/her as Yellow.

JumpSTART Triage (Refer to JumpSTART Flowchart on Page 48)

Physiological differences in children necessitate adaptation of the standard START triage method in children 8 years of age or younger, or in those victims with the anatomical or physiological features of a child in the age group. The same parameters (RPM) are utilized, with the adaptations indicated here.

1.9 Mass-Casualty Incidents

A. **Assess Respirations.**
   1. If the respiratory rate is between 15 and 45/min, go to the Perfusion assessment.
   2. If the respiratory rate is more than 45/min or less than 15/min, prioritize as Red.
   3. If the victim is not breathing, open the airway, remove obstructions, if seen, and assess for (1) or (2).
   4. If the victim is not breathing and no obstructions are present, check a peripheral (radial or pedal) pulse. If a peripheral pulse is present, provide five (5) ventilations (approximately 15 seconds) via any type of barrier device. If spontaneous respirations resume, prioritize as Red.
   5. If the victim is still not breathing, prioritize as Black.

B. **Assess Perfusion.**
   1. Performed by assessing a peripheral pulse.
   2. If a peripheral pulse is present, go to the Mental Status assessment.
   3. If no peripheral pulse is present, prioritize as Red.

NOTE

Any major external bleeding should also be controlled at this time.

C. **Assess Mental Status.**
   1. Assess the child using the AVPU scale. Assess whether the victim is alert, responds to verbal stimuli, responds to painful stimuli, or is unconscious.
   2. If the victim is unconscious or only responds to painful stimuli, prioritize as Red.
   3. If the victim is alert or responds to verbal stimuli, assess for further injuries and prioritize as Yellow or Green.

NOTE

Infants who are developmentally unable to walk should be triaged using the JumpSTART algorithm either during initial triage or in the Green area if carried out by a nonrescuer. During triage, if the infant does not fulfill the criteria of a Red victim and has no other outward signs of significant injury, he/she may be triaged as a Green victim.

NOTE

The START Triage system was developed by Newport Beach Fire Rescue and Hoag Hospital. The JumpSTART Triage system was developed by Dr. Lou Romig.

I.9 Mass-Casualty Incidents

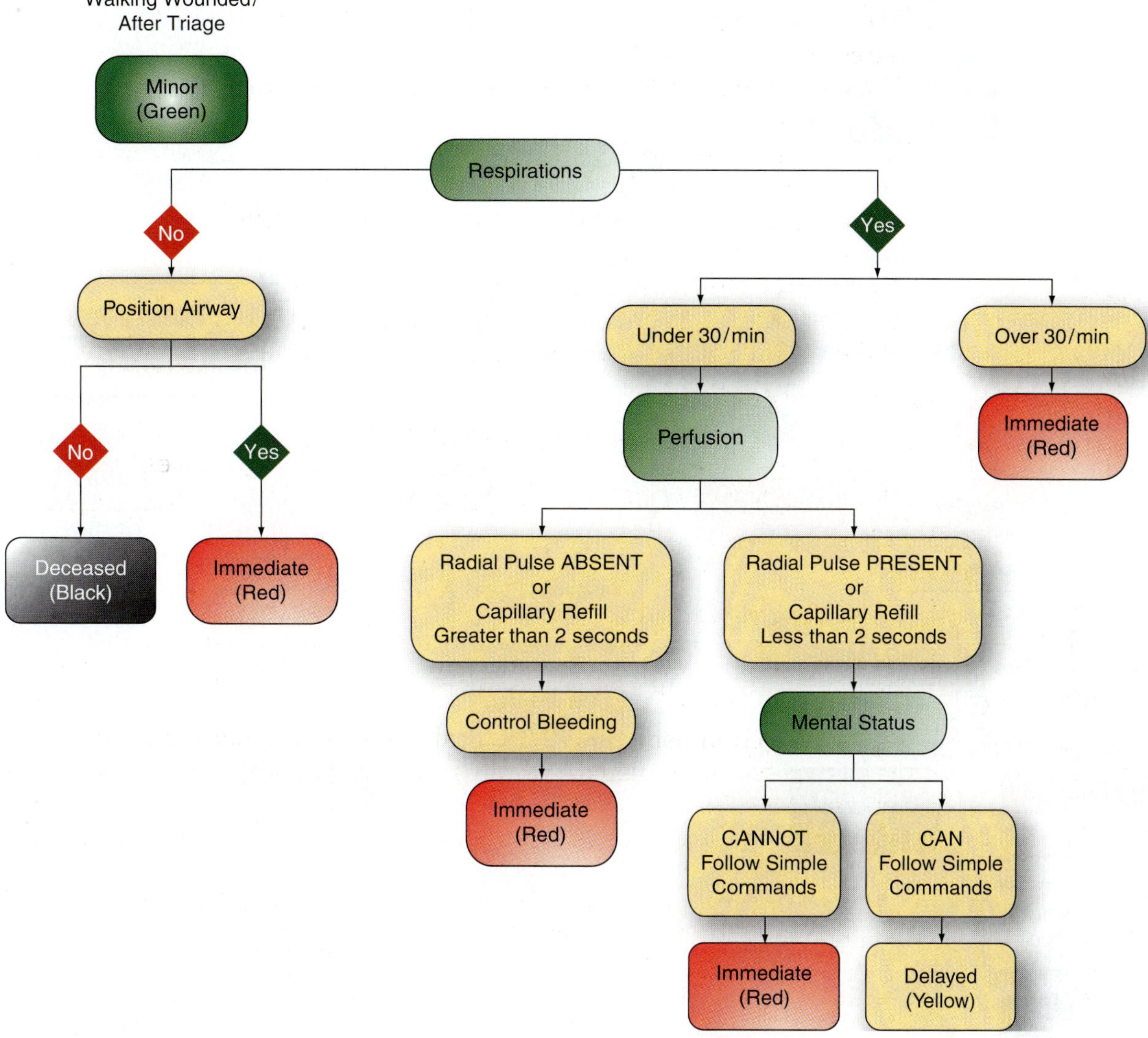

START triage.

1.9 Mass-Casualty Incidents

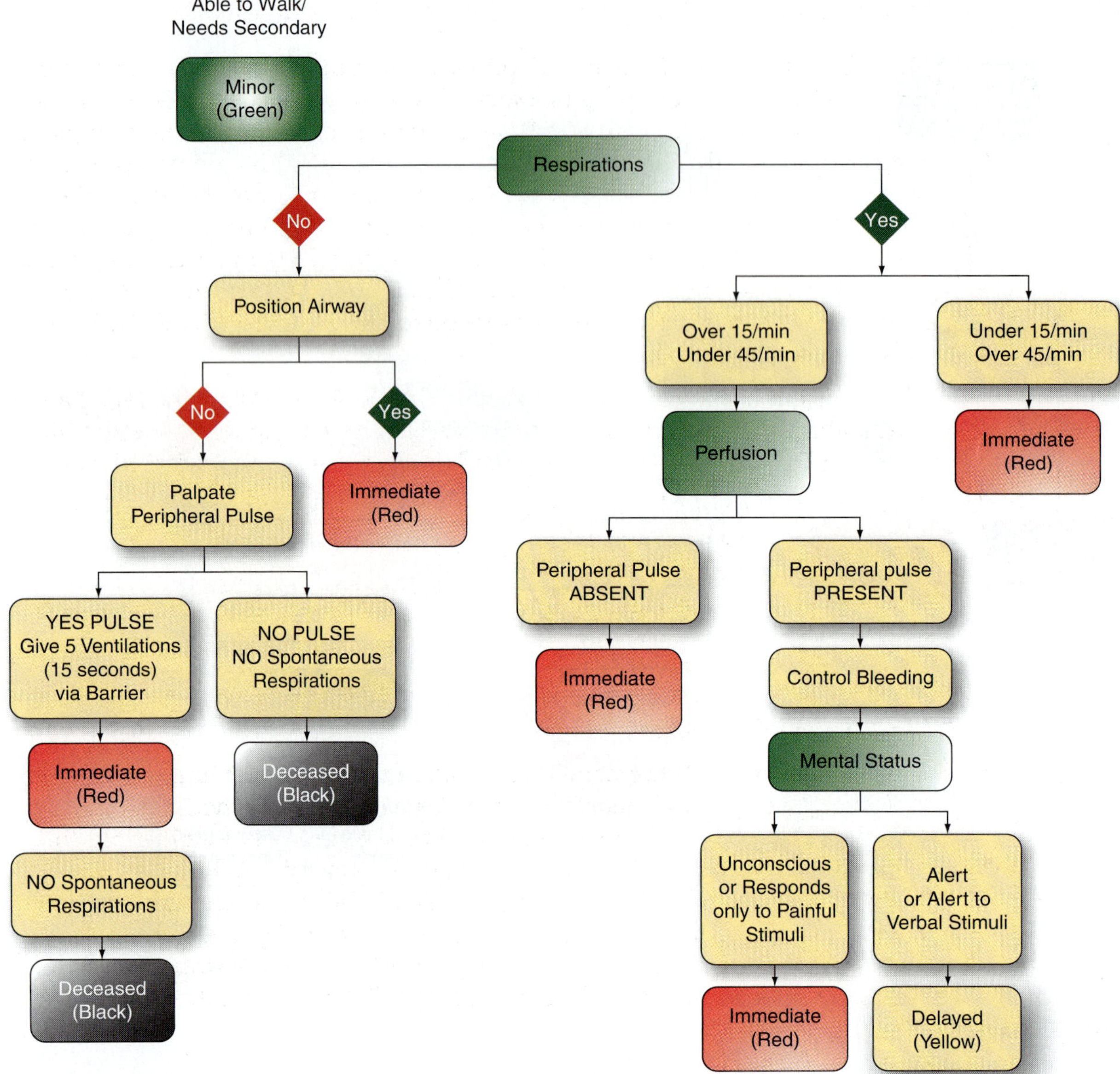

JumpSTART triage.

1.10 Trauma Transport Protocol

Communication (Dispatch) Center Procedure

A. All EMS systems utilize the 911 phone system in conjunction with either manual or computer-aided dispatch (CAD) programs or, if 911 service is not available, the regular telephone communication procedures previously agreed to with the State. All emergency information, including address and call-back data, is confirmed by the call taker prior to the end of the telephone conversation. Emergency information is immediately transmitted to the Fire/Rescue or EMS dispatcher who selects the nearest available unit(s) for response. Units are dispatched at this time by the Fire/Rescue or EMS dispatcher, who provides responding units with all available information concerning the incident.

B. The system has a sufficient number of Fire/Rescue/EMS providers. Patient treatment and transportation to the hospital are provided by the Fire/Rescue/EMS provider's emergency medical technicians and paramedics.

C. Call-taker personnel shall make every attempt to obtain the following information from the 911 caller:
   1. Nature of the emergency.
   2. Location of the incident.
   3. Call-back number.
   4. Number of patients.
   5. Severity of the illness/injury.
   6. Name of the caller.

D. As soon as on-scene personnel recognize a need for other emergency agencies (e.g., law enforcement, fire, EMS, Coast Guard, or other services), they shall notify dispatch immediately. On-scene personnel must identify the agencies needed and the specific amount of personnel, equipment, and other resources required. Fire dispatch shall then make telephone contact with the appropriate services. Mutual aid contracts exist between all adjacent services. Additionally, a master phone list of all available emergency services is maintained at the Central Dispatch Communications Center.

On-Scene Procedure

A. Upon arrival at the scene, paramedic and emergency medical technician (EMT) personnel shall conduct a size-up of the scene, to include the Trauma Alert Criteria as outlined in pages 50–54, including identification of any and all methodologies required by the State, safe entry, severity and number of patients, the need for extrication, and the need for additional help. Multiple patients shall be immediately triaged. Dispatch and the primary receiving hospital will be notified, as soon as possible, of "Trauma Alert" patients. Dispatchers shall immediately transfer this information, using the words "Trauma Alert," to the supervisor on duty.

B. Paramedic personnel shall submit the data on the appropriate State form for each trauma patient.

C. Paramedic personnel shall transport patients to the nearest appropriate trauma center as shown in the catchment area maps in the appropriate trauma plan.

1.10 Trauma Transport Protocol

Helicopter Transport Procedure

Two sets of criteria must be considered. The first is directed toward the safety of the helicopter pilot and crew, the ground personnel, the patient, and bystanders. The second is intended to establish operational guidelines for when the helicopter is to be requested for **Trauma Alert** patients.

A. Safety criteria (helicopter will *not* be used).
   1. Severe weather.
   2. Power lines too close to landing area.
   3. Trees, signs, poles, or other obstacles in immediate landing area.
   4. Large gatherings of civilians in the area.
   5. An expectation that the area may not remain safe.

B. Operational criteria (helicopter *will* be used).
   1. If the trauma center that the patient would be taken to by ground transport is farther away than 20 minutes' driving time (30 minutes for high-index patients).
   2. If ground transportation is not available and is not expected to be available within a reasonable time.
   3. If the helicopter is needed to gain access to the patient or needed to transport the patient out of an inaccessible area.
   4. Extrication time greater than 20 minutes.

Trauma Alert Criteria

The following guidelines are to be used to establish the criteria for a Trauma Alert patient and to determine which patient(s) will be transported to a trauma center. Any patient that meets any *one* of the **Red** criteria will be classified as a Trauma Alert, while any patient that meets any *two* of the **Blue** criteria will be classified as a Trauma Alert.

A. Adult trauma scorecard methodology.
   1. Each EMS provider shall ensure the following actions upon arrival at the location of an incident:
      a. An EMT or paramedic shall assess the condition of each adult trauma patient using the adult trauma scorecard methodology, as provided in this section, to determine whether the patient should be a Trauma Alert.
      b. In assessing the condition of each adult trauma patient, the EMT or paramedic shall evaluate the patient's status for each of the following components: airway, circulation, best motor response (a component of the Glasgow Coma Scale), cutaneous, long-bone fracture, patient's age, and mechanism of injury. The patient's age and mechanism of injury shall be assessment factors only when used in conjunction with assessment criteria included in part (3) of this section.

1.10 Trauma Transport Protocol

2. The EMT or paramedic shall assess all adult trauma patients using the following Red criteria in the order presented. If **any one** of the following conditions is identified, the patient shall be considered a Trauma Alert patient:
   a. Airway: The patient receives active airway assistance beyond the administration of oxygen.
   b. Circulation: The patient lacks a radial pulse with a sustained heart rate greater than 120 beats per minute or has a blood pressure of less than 90 mm Hg.
   c. Best Motor Response (BMR): The patient exhibits a score of 4 or less on the motor assessment component of the Glasgow Coma Scale, or exhibits the presence of paralysis, or there is the suspicion of a spinal cord injury or the loss of sensation.
   d. Cutaneous: The patient has second- or third-degree burns to 15% or more of the total body surface area, or amputation proximal to the wrist or ankle, or any penetrating injury to the head, neck, or torso (excluding superficial wounds where the depth of the wound can be determined).
   e. Long-Bone Fracture: The patient reveals signs or symptoms of two or more long-bone fracture sites (humerus, radius, ulna, femur, tibia, or fibula).
3. Should the patient not be identified as a Trauma Alert using the Red criteria listed in part (2) of this section, the trauma patient shall be further assessed using the **Blue** criteria and shall be considered a Trauma Alert patient when a condition is identified from **any two** of the seven components included in this section.
   a. Airway: The patient has a respiratory rate of 30 or greater.
   b. Circulation: The patient has a sustained heart rate of 120 beats per minute or greater.
   c. BMR: The patient has a BMR of 5 on the motor component of the Glasgow Coma Scale.
   d. Cutaneous: The patient has a soft-tissue loss from a major degloving injury, or a major flap avulsion greater than 5 inches, or has sustained a gunshot wound to the extremities of the body.
   e. Long-Bone Fracture: The patient reveals signs or symptoms of a single long-bone fracture resulting from a motor vehicle collision or a fall from an elevation of 10 feet or greater.
   f. Age: The patient is 55 years of age or older.
   g. Mechanism of Injury: The patient has been ejected from a motor vehicle (excluding any motorcycle, moped, all-terrain vehicle, bicycle, or the open body of a pick-up truck), or the driver of the motor vehicle has made impact with the steering wheel, causing steering wheel deformity.

NOTE

Also see Online Forms for the "Trauma Telemetry Report."

1.10 Trauma Transport Protocol

4. If the patient is not identified as a Trauma Alert case after evaluation of the patient using the criteria in parts (2) and (3) of this section, the trauma patient will be evaluated using all elements of the Glasgow Coma Scale. If the patient's score is 12 or less, the patient shall be considered a Trauma Alert patient (excluding patients whose normal GCS score is 12 or less, as established by the patient's medical history or pre-existing medical condition when known).
5. Where additional local trauma alert criteria have been approved by the Medical Director of the EMS service and presented as part of the State TTP approval process, the use of local trauma alert criteria as the basis for calling a Trauma Alert shall be documented as required. Local trauma assessment criteria can be applied only after the patient has been assessed as provided in parts (2), (3), and (4) of this section.
6. In the event that none of the conditions is identified using the criteria in parts (2), (3), (4), and (5) of this section in the assessment of the adult trauma patient, the EMT or paramedic can call a Trauma Alert if, in his or her judgment, the patient's condition warrants such action. Where EMT or paramedic judgment is used as the basis for calling a Trauma Alert, it shall be documented.
7. The results of the patient assessment shall be recorded and reported in accordance with the requirements of all applicable trauma regulations.

NOTE

Patients who are found to meet the Trauma Alert criteria on arrival at or subsequent to arrival at a nontrauma center will be expeditiously transferred to the appropriate trauma center. See page 54.

B. Pediatric trauma scorecard methodology. Pediatric patients are those individuals age 15 years or younger. Pediatric "Trauma Alert" patients will be transported to the nearest appropriate Pediatric Trauma Center.
   1. The EMT or paramedic shall assess all pediatric trauma patients using the following Red criteria. If **any one** of the following conditions is identified, the patient shall be considered a pediatric Trauma Alert patient:
      a. Airway: To maintain optimal ventilation, the patient is intubated or the patient's breathing is assisted through such measures as manual jaw thrust, continuous suctioning, or use of other adjuncts to assist ventilatory efforts.
      b. Consciousness: The patient exhibits an altered mental status that includes drowsiness, lethargy, the inability to follow commands, unresponsiveness to voice, or total unresponsiveness; or is in a coma; or there is the presence of paralysis; or there is suspicion of a spinal cord injury; or there is a loss of sensation.
      c. Circulation: The patient has a faint or nonpalpable carotid or femoral pulse or the patient has a systolic blood pressure of less than 50 mm Hg.

1.10 Trauma Transport Protocol

   d. Fracture: There is evidence of an open long-bone (humerus, radius, ulna, femur, tibia, or fibula) fracture or there are multiple fracture sites or multiple dislocations (except for isolated wrist or ankle fractures or dislocations).
   e. Cutaneous: The patient has a major soft-tissue disruption, including major degloving injury, or major flap avulsions, or second- or third-degree burns to 10% or more of the total body surface area, or amputation proximal to the wrist or ankle, or any penetrating injury to the head, neck, or torso (excluding superficial wounds where the depth of the wound can be determined).
2. In addition to the red criteria listed in part (1) of this section, a Trauma Alert shall be called when **Blue** criteria are used and **any two** of the components are identified.
   a. Consciousness: The patient exhibits symptoms of amnesia, or there is loss of consciousness.
   b. Circulation: The carotid or femoral pulse is palpable, but the radial or pedal pulses are not palpable or the systolic blood pressure is less than 90 mm Hg.
   c. Fracture: The patient reveals signs or symptoms of a single closed long-bone fracture. Long-bone fractures do not include isolated wrist or ankle fractures.
   d. Size: Pediatric trauma patients weigh 11 kilograms or less, or have a body length equivalent to this weight on a pediatric length and weight emergency tape (the equivalent of 33 inches in measurement or less).

NOTE

Also see the Online Forms for the "Trauma Telemetry Report."

3. In the event that none of these criteria are identified in the assessment of the pediatric patient, the EMT or paramedic can call a Trauma Alert if, in his or her judgment, the trauma patient's condition warrants such action. Where EMT or paramedic judgment is used as the basis for calling a Trauma Alert, it shall be documented as required.

C. High index of suspicion trauma patients (adult and pediatric) (if applicable to local trauma rules). Nontrauma Alert patients who present a high index of suspicion (any of the criteria from the following list), along with significant injury, shall require triage/transport to the nearest appropriate trauma center.
   1. Falls from an elevation greater than 12 feet (adults); falls from an elevation of greater than 6 feet (pediatric patients).
   2. Extrication time of more than 15 minutes.
   3. Rollover motor-vehicle crash.
   4. Death of occupant in the same passenger compartment.

1.10 Trauma Transport Protocol

5. Major intrusion into the passenger compartment.
6. Ejection from a bicycle.
7. Pedestrian struck by vehicles not meeting the preceding automatic criteria (i.e., adults struck by a vehicle going less than 15 mph and pediatric patients struck by a vehicle going less than 5 mph).
8. Age 55 years or older.
9. Paramedic judgment.

Emergency Trauma Interhospital Transfer Procedures

A. Any hospital in the trauma service area may transfer a patient meeting Trauma Alert criteria by simply calling 911 and reporting a Trauma Alert in its ER. A second call from the sending ER physician to the receiving trauma surgeon completes the initiation of the transfer.

B. When 911 or the appropriate emergency number is called, the Fire/Rescue/EMS provider that is responsible for the area where the sending hospital is located responds with an ALS unit to the ER and transports the patient to the nearest appropriate trauma center.

Designated Facilities

Trauma Alert patients will be transported to the nearest appropriate trauma center. If that trauma center is temporarily unable to provide adequate trauma care, the patient will be transported to the next closest trauma center.

Transport Deviation

Any deviation from these Trauma Transport Protocols must be documented and justified on the Run Report.

Run Reports

The Fire/Rescue/EMS crew shall ensure delivery of a copy of the Run Report to the receiving hospital, with the patient.

1.11 Protocol Revision Procedure

Any person may submit input for changes to the Common Protocols. The following procedure will be used to receive and process this input.

Procedure

1. Input may be submitted to the Broward EMS website (www.browardems.com) using the Protocol Update form found in the library.
2. All input will be emailed to the current Chair of the Common Protocol Editing Committee.
3. The Chair of the Common Protocol Editing Committee will convene the committee on an as-needed basis (at least semi-annually, unless deemed urgent) to discuss input for changes to the Common Protocols.
4. The Chair of the Common Protocol Editing Committee will submit recommended changes to the Common Protocols users (EMS Medical Directors, EMS Chiefs, and Hospital ED Directors) via e-mail.
5. When the Protocol Editing Committee submits recommendations for changes to the Common Protocols, a discussion and vote will be held via e-mail to finalize the decision for implementation. If necessary, a meeting will be held for face-to-face discussion and voting. In this instance, the Common Protocols Users Group will be notified of the date, time, and place of the meeting.
6. Once the changes to the Common Protocols have been implemented, they will be posted on the Broward EMS website and all hospitals will be notified. In addition, the Chair of the Protocol Editing Committee will e-mail these changes to all EMS Providers.
7. When approved changes to the Common Protocols are received via e-mail, EMS providers will cause their implementation within their service as soon as possible, subject to their Medical Director's approval.
8. The Medical Director of an individual EMS provider reserves the right to accept or reject changes to the protocols of his/her EMS service.
9. It is the intent of this procedure that every EMS provider implement all approved changes to the Common Protocols.
10. The Medical Director of an individual EMS provider may implement any protocol change he/she deems necessary within his/her individual EMS service with or without the use of this procedure.

1.12 Personal Exposure to Infectious Diseases

Post-Exposure Management

See the Online Forms for exposure forms.

A. Provide first aid.
   1. Secure the area to prevent further contamination.
   2. Remove any contaminated clothing.
   3. Wash the injured area thoroughly with soap and water, or waterless hand cleanser, and apply an antiseptic.
   4. If the eyes, nose, or mouth are involved, flush them thoroughly with large amounts of water.

B. Notification and relief of duty. The worker's supervisor should be immediately notified if a worker experiences an exposure involving potentially infectious source material. The supervisor should determine if the worker needs to be relieved of duty.

C. Assess the level of exposure. An occupational exposure is the "exposure" to another person's body fluids or airborne fluids. There are two types of occupational exposures: nonsignificant and significant.
   1. **Nonsignificant exposure.** Nonsignificant exposures are occupational exposures that have little to no risk of transmission of diseases known at this time. All nonsignificant exposures need to be documented on the Infectious Disease Exposure Report form. If the occupational exposure is later reported by the CDC as having an increased risk, the exposure will have been documented.
   2. **Significant exposure.** Significant exposures have increased risk of transmission and acquiring of disease(s). All significant exposures need documentation and medical follow-up.

D. Assess exposures to blood or body fluids. A significant bloodborne or body fluid exposure is considered a combination of one or more of the types of body fluids and one or more of the injuries listed here.
   1. Body fluids.
      a. Blood, serum, and all fluids visibly contaminated with blood.
      b. Pleural, amniotic, pericardial, peritoneal, synovial, and cerebrospinal fluids.
      c. Uterine/vaginal secretions, semen, feces, and urine.
      d. Saliva.
   2. Action or injury.
      a. Percutaneous (through-the-skin injuries such as a needlestick, laceration, abrasion, or bites).
      b. Mucous membrane (e.g., eyes, nose, mouth).
      c. Non-intact skin (e.g., cut, chapped, or abraded skin). The larger the area and the longer the material is in contact, the more difficult it is to verify that all relevant skin area is intact. Also, an increased risk exists if the exposure occurs within 2 hours of shaving skin, if scabs are less than 24 hours old, or if the skin is still open.

1.12 Personal Exposure to Infectious Diseases

E. Assess the exposure to airborne droplets. A significant airborne exposure is considered a combination of a source exhibiting signs and symptoms of a suspected airborne illness and an incident that would place the worker at risk of droplet or airborne exposure.
   1. **Source:** Any aerosolized exhalations containing droplets, sputum, lung secretions, or saliva, either by the source coughing, spitting, or breathing or by an action of the worker such as suctioning or intubating *and* the worker was not wearing appropriate respiratory protection (HEPA mask, eye protection).
   2. **Action:** Actions by the worker that have increased risk of airborne disease spread include suctioning of nasopharynx or oropharynx, active gag/cough reflex upon suctioning, and insertion of a tracheal tube or supraglotic airway device.

Medical Attention, Counseling, Consent, and Testing

A. **Report the exposure.** The worker or immediate supervisor should promptly complete an Exposure Report and submit it to the Designated Infection Control Officer.

B. **Transport.** A significantly exposed worker should be transported to a designated facility for medical evaluation, counseling, and testing within 2 hours after the exposure. The worker and source patient should be transported to the same medical facility, preferably one that offers rapid HIV testing if the source material consisted of blood or body fluids.

C. **Triage.** The worker should be triaged as quickly as possible. The worker should present to the medical facility an Infectious Disease Exposure Report form and an Employer's Exposure Information form that contains information about the employer, its worker's compensation policy, the Designated Infection Control Officer's contact information, and contact information for the designated medical provider that will provide follow-up care.

D. **Consent and counseling.** Counseling shall be provided to and consent obtained from both the source of the exposure and the exposed worker (29 CFR 1910.1030[f][3]). The worker's compensation carrier will incur the cost of testing for both the source and the worker.
   1. **Informed consent:** Source and exposed worker consent to the physician authorizing testing. The source will not incur any cost of said testing.
   2. **No consent (e.g., the source is unconscious or denies consent):** If consent cannot be obtained from the source of the exposure and a blood sample is available, the facility may conduct testing without consent, and the attending physician documents the need in the medical record of the worker.
      a. Florida's Omnibus AIDS act provides for a court order for the source to comply and have testing completed. In this case, because prophylactic treatment may not be completed in a timely manner, the medical protocol provides for an "unknown source" category.

1.12 Personal Exposure to Infectious Diseases

E. **Post-exposure testing for blood and body fluid exposures.** With airborne droplet exposure, the focus is on alerting the medical facility that a significant exposure has occurred. Testing is administered by the facility, targeting the myriad of airborne diseases. If TB exposure is suspected, a tuberculin skin test (PPD) test should be performed on both the source and the exposed worker. Do not administer a tuberculin skin test (PPD) test if the worker has been tested within the previous 12 weeks or has a history of positive skin test reaction.

F. **Hospital notification.** If no exposure was reported to the medical facility and the medical facility determined through testing that an increased risk of disease transmission may have occurred, the medical facility shall notify the agency of such an event within 48 hours after its determination (Ryan White Act).

G. **Discharge.** The Infectious Disease Exposure Report form should be complete, including a discharge summary that describes all diagnostic tests performed on the worker. A copy of the form is routed to the Designated Infection Control Officer and a copy is provided to the worker.

H. **Post-exposure medical follow-up.** The employer is responsible to provide or make available post-exposure monitoring as directed by the medical provider. Follow-up testing for blood and body fluid exposures will be performed after the initial exposure at 6 weeks, 12 weeks, and 26 weeks. Testing after 1 year may be indicated for high-risk significant exposures.

1.13 Crime Scene Management

This protocol will be used when law enforcement personnel advise EMS that they have responded to a crime scene or EMS determines that a crime scene may exist.

A. **Purpose: To ensure the protection of patient welfare as well as to ensure the ability to conduct an effective and thorough investigation.**

B. **Response/on-scene situations.**
   1. Only those units assigned will respond to the call. Over-response tends to cause confusion at the crime scene and destruction of evidence.
   2. When approaching a potential crime scene that is being protected by law enforcement personnel, the paramedic/EMT may request entry into the area to determine the life status of the individual.
   3. If law enforcement personnel refuse access to the crime scene, do not become confrontational. Notify the EMS Agency Supervisor and complete an incident report as required.
   4. When personnel are allowed access into the scene, the minimum number of required EMS personnel should enter to minimize disturbance of the crime scene.
   5. *Do not* attempt resuscitation if the patient has no pulse, has no spontaneous respiration, *and* meets criteria outlined in General Protocol 1.4, Death in the Field.
   6. If treatment and/or resuscitation are warranted, follow the appropriate protocol.
   7. When on scene:
      a. Keep your medical equipment close to the victim.
      b. Stay close to the body.
      c. Keep your hands out of any blood that has pooled.
      d. Do not wander around the scene.
      e. Minimize destruction of the patient's clothing. If the patient's clothing has a puncture, do not use the hole in the clothing to start cutting. Begin cutting at another part of the garment. Removed clothing should be left with the patient or turned over to law enforcement personnel.
      f. *Do not* go through the victim's personal effects, clean the body, or cover the body with a sheet or other material (if expired).
      g. *Do not* move, take, or handle any object at the scene or litter the crime scene with medical equipment, dressings, bandages, or other supplies.
      h. If resuscitation efforts are deemed necessary, transfer the victim from the scene to the vehicle expeditiously and stabilize the victim in the vehicle, when possible.
      i. If the patient relates any information relating to the crime while in transit to the medical facility, inform law enforcement personnel at once.

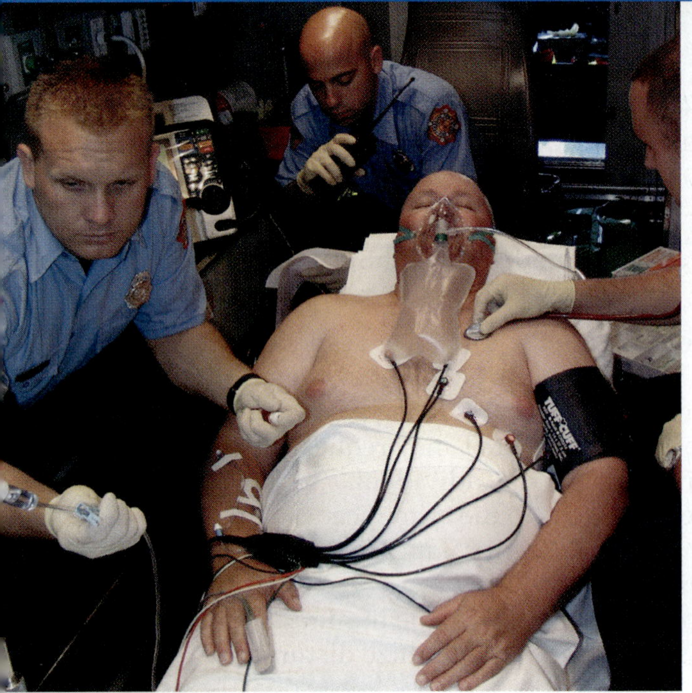

chapter 2

Adult Protocols

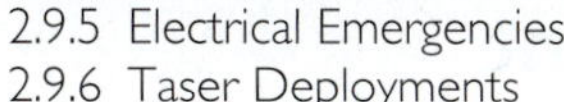

2.1 Adult Initial Assessment and Management

Protocols in Section 2.1 are designed to guide the EMT or paramedic in his or her initial approach to assessment and management of adult patients. Supportive care is specified as being either *EMT and Paramedic* (BLS) or *Paramedic Only* (ALS).

Protocol 2.1.1 should be used on all adult patients for initial assessment. During this assessment, if the EMT or paramedic determines that there is a need for airway management, Protocol 2.1.2 should be used for the management of the adult airway. These protocols are frequently referred to by other protocols, which may or may not override them in recommending more specific therapy.

Protocol 2.1.3 presents the basic components of preparation for transport of medical patients. Due to the significant differences in priorities and packaging in the prehospital care of trauma and hypovolemia cases, a separate Trauma Supportive Care protocol has been developed. After following Protocol 2.1.1, this Medical Supportive Care protocol may be the only protocol used in medical emergency situations where a specific diagnostic impression and choice of additional protocols cannot be made. Judgment must be used in determining whether patients require ALS- or BLS-level care. This protocol is frequently referred to by other protocols, which may or may not override it in recommending more specific therapy.

Protocol 2.1.4 presents the basic components of preparation for transport of trauma patients. Due to the significant differences in priorities and packaging in the prehospital care of medical cases, a separate Medical Supportive Care protocol has been developed. After following Protocol 2.1.1, this Trauma Supportive Care protocol may be the only protocol used in trauma or hypovolemia situations where a specific diagnostic impression and choice of additional protocols cannot be made. Judgment must be used in determining whether patients require ALS- or BLS-level care. This protocol is frequently referred to by other protocols, which may or may not override it in recommending more specific therapy.

Protocol 2.1.5 should be used by paramedics only for pain management.

2.1.1 Initial Assessment

EMT and Paramedic

I. **Scene Size-up.**
   A. Review the dispatch information.
   B. Assess the need for body substance isolation.
   C. Assess for scene safety.
   D. Determine mechanism of injury.
   E. Determine the nature of the illness.
   F. Determine the number and location of patients.
   G. Determine the need for additional resources.
   H. Consider c-spine immobilization.

II. **Initial Assessment.**
   A. General impression of the patient.
   B. Assess mental status (AVPU); maintain spinal immobilization *as needed.*
   C. Assess **airway**.
   D. Assess **breathing**.
   E. Assess **circulation** (rapid evaluation of pulse, major bleeding, skin color, and temperature).
   F. Assess **disability**: movement of extremities. Assess need for **defibrillation**: VF/VT without pulse.
   G. **Expose** and examine the patient's head, neck, chest, abdomen, and pelvis (check the back when the patient is rolled on his/her side).
   H. Identify priority patients.
      1. Poor general impression.
      2. Unresponsive patients.
      3. Responsive but does not or cannot follow commands.
      4. Difficulty breathing.
      5. Hypoperfusion or shock.
      6. Complicated child birth.
      7. Chest pain with a systolic BP < 100 mm Hg.
      8. Uncontrolled bleeding.
      9. Severe pain anywhere.
      10. Multiple injuries.

2.1.1 Initial Assessment

Focused History and Physical Exam			
Trauma Patients		Medical Patients	
Reconsider Mechanism of Injury		Evaluate Responsiveness	
Significant Mechanism of Injury	No Significant Mechanism of Injury	Responsive	Unresponsive
◆ Rapid trauma assessment ◆ Baseline vital signs ◆ SAMPLE history ◆ Reevaluate transport decision (Trauma Alert?)	◆ Focused trauma assessment based on chief complaint ◆ Baseline vital signs ◆ SAMPLE history ◆ Reevaluate transport decision (Trauma Alert?)	◆ History of illness ◆ SAMPLE history ◆ Focused medical assessment based on chief complaint ◆ Baseline vital signs ◆ Reevaluate transport decision (Cardiac Alert/Stroke Alert?)	◆ Rapid medical assessment ◆ Baseline vital signs ◆ SAMPLE history ◆ Reevaluate transport decision

III. **Initial Management.** (See Adult Protocol 2.1.3, Medical Supportive Care, or Adult Protocol 2.1.4, Trauma Supportive Care).

IV. **Secondary Assessment.**
   A. Conduct a head-to-toe survey.
   B. Conduct a neurological assessment.
      1. Pupillary response.
      2. Glasgow Coma Scale score.
   C. Assess vital signs.
      1. Respirations.
      2. Pulse.
      3. Blood pressure.
      4. Capillary refill.
      5. Skin condition.
         a. Color.
         b. Temperature.
         c. Moisture.
      6. Lung sounds.

2.1.1 Initial Assessment

D. Obtain a medical history.
   1. **S**—Symptoms: Assessment of chief complaint.
      a. **O**—Onset and location.
      b. **P**—Provocation.
      c. **Q**—Quality.
      d. **R**—Radiation.
      e. **R**—Referred.
      f. **R**—Relief.
      g. **S**—Severity.
      h. **T**—Time.
   2. **A**—Allergies.
   3. **M**—Medications.
   4. **P**—Past medical history.
   5. **L**—Last oral intake.
   6. **E**—Events leading to illness or injury.

V. **Other Assessment Techniques.**
   A. Cardiac monitoring.
   B. Pulse oximetry (see Medical Procedure 4.29).
   C. Glucose determination (see Medical Procedure 4.39).
   D. Monitor core temperature.
   E. Capnography.

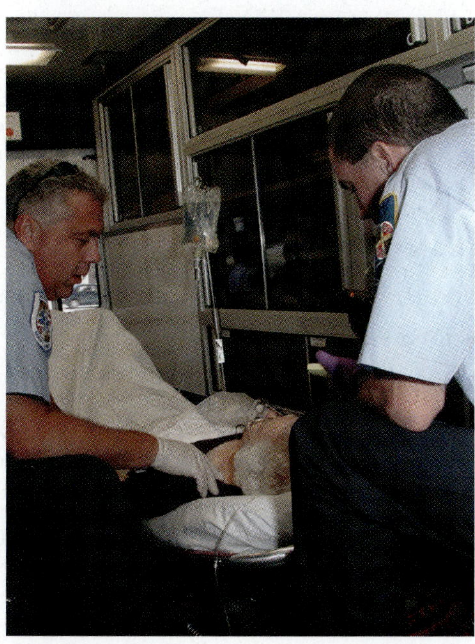

Assessment procedures typically employ direct observations and questions.

2.1.2 Airway Management

Supportive Care

EMT and Paramedic

- Initial Assessment Protocol 2.1.1.

If spontaneous breathing is present without compromise:

- Monitor breathing during transport.
- Administer oxygen via nasal cannula (2–6 L/min) as needed (see Appendix 7.13).

If spontaneous breathing is present with compromise:

- Maintain airway patency (see Medical Procedure 4.5).
- Administer oxygen via non-rebreather mask (10–15 L/min).
- If unconscious, insert oropharyngeal, nasopharyngeal, or supraglottic airway as needed (see Medical Procedures 4.7, 4.8, and 4.13).
- Assist ventilations with a bag-valve device attached to supplemental oxygen at 15–25 L/min as needed (see Medical Procedure 4.4).
- Suction as needed (see Medical Procedure 4.9, Flexible Suctioning, and Medical Procedure 4.10, Rigid Suctioning).
- Apply pulse oximeter and capnography, as soon as possible (see Medical Procedures 4.29 and 4.22).

Paramedic Only

- If patient accepts oropharyngeal airway, consider the need for endotracheal intubation (see ALS Level 1, Advanced Airway Management).

EMT and Paramedic

If spontaneous breathing is absent or markedly compromised:

- Maintain airway patency (see Medical Procedure 4.5).
- Administer oxygen via non-rebreather mask (10–15 L/min).
- If unconscious, insert oropharyngeal, nasopharyngeal, or supraglottic airway as needed (see Medical Procedures 4.7, 4.8, and 4.13).
- Assist ventilations with a bag-valve device attached to supplemental oxygen at 15–25 L/min as needed (see Medical Procedure 4.4).
- Suction as needed (see Medical Procedure 4.9, Flexible Suctioning, and Medical Procedure 4.10, Rigid Suctioning).
- Apply pulse oximeter and capnography, as soon as possible (see Medical Procedures 4.29 and 4.22).

2.1.2 Airway Management

ALS Level 1: Advanced Airway Management

Paramedic Only

- Perform endotracheal intubation and document the following (see Medical Procedure 4.18) (a).
  1. Confirm ETT placement with an end-tidal CO_2 monitoring device.
  2. Additional confirmation methods may include the following options:
     a. Visualization of the tube passing through the vocal cords.
     b. Esophageal detection device (EDD).
     c. Negative epigastric sounds.
     d. Positive bilateral breath sounds.
  3. Secure the ETT with a commercially available device.
     a. Full spinal immobilization is recommended.
  4. Monitor SpO_2 with pulse oximeter.
- *If unable to intubate and patient cannot be adequately ventilated by other means,* perform cricothyroidotomy (see Medical Procedure 4.16) and transport rapidly to the nearest appropriate facility (a).

ALS Level 2

None.

Note

(a) Follow the Universal Airway algorithm on all intubations.

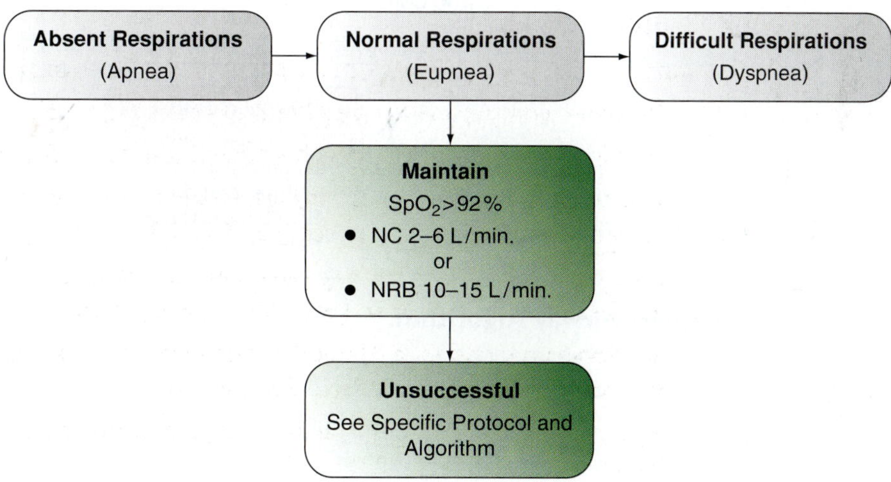

Universal Airway Algorithm.

2.1.2 Airway Management

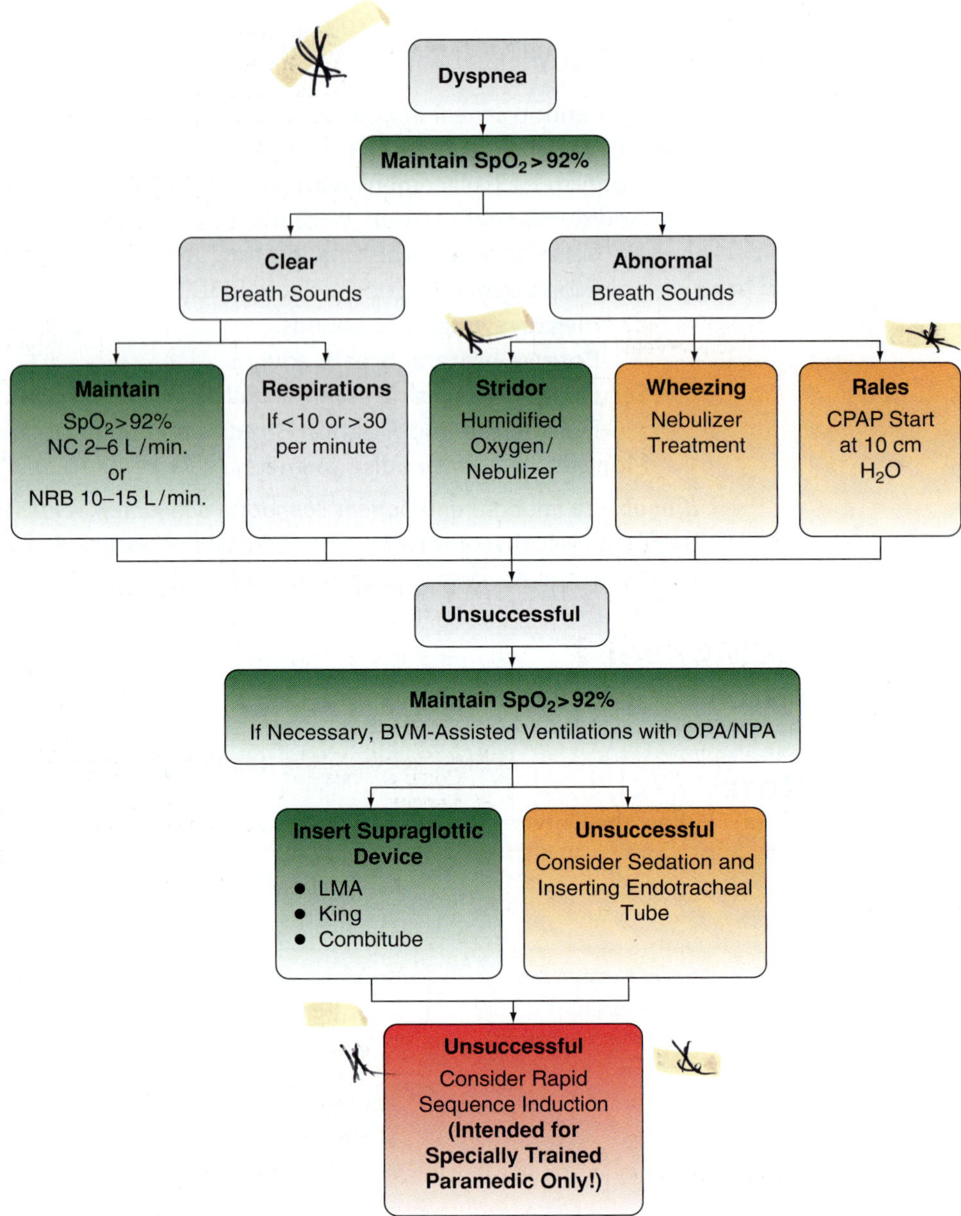

Dyspnea Airway Algorithm.

2.1.2 Airway Management

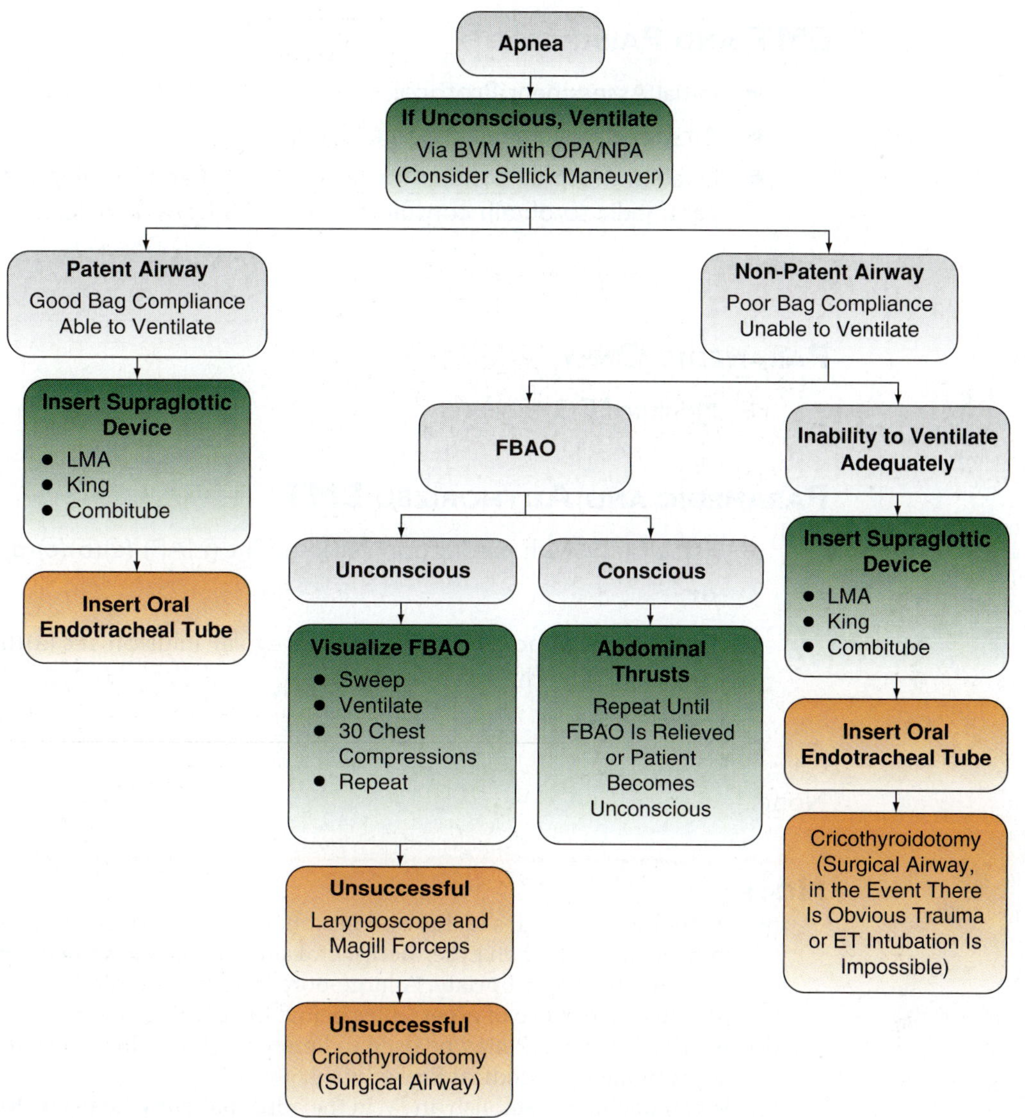

Apnea Airway Algorithm.

2.1.3 Medical Supportive Care

Supportive Care

EMT and Paramedic

- Initial Assessment Protocol 2.1.1.
- Airway Management Protocol 2.1.2.
- Establish hospital contact for notification of an incoming patient and for the paramedic to obtain consultation for ALS Level 2 orders.

ALS Level 1

Paramedic Only

- Monitor ECG *as needed.*

Paramedic and Authorized EMT

- Establish IV with medication access point (MAP) (a)(b)(c)(d).

  or
- Establish IV of normal saline with a regular infusion set (a)(b)(c)(d), unless overridden by the specific protocol.

ALS Level 2

None.

Note

(a) Authorized IV routes include all peripheral venous sites. External jugular veins may be utilized when other peripheral site attempts have been unsuccessful or would be inappropriate. A large-bore intracath should be used for unstable patients. Avoid use of access sites below the diaphragm.

(b) An IV lock or MAP may be used in lieu of an IV bag in some patients, when appropriate (see Medical Procedure 4.60).

(c) When unable to establish an IV in the adult patient who needs to be resuscitated, an intraosseous line may be used by the **paramedic only** (see Medical Procedures 4.58 and 4.59).

(d) An EMT who has been authorized by his/her individual Medical Director may establish an IV.

2.1.4 Trauma Supportive Care

Supportive Care

EMT and Paramedic

- Initial Assessment Protocol 2.1.1. Initiate Trauma Alert, if applicable (see General Protocol 1.10, Trauma Transport).
- Airway Management Protocol 2.1.2. (Manually stabilize c-spine *as needed.*)
- Correct any open wound/sucking chest wound (with an occlusive dressing).
- Immobilize fractures.
- Control bleeding.
- Determine if the patient is taking a "blood thinner" such as Coumadin.

Paramedic Only

- Correct any massive flail segment that causes respiratory compromise (intubate).
- Correct any tension pneumothorax (see Medical Procedure 4.14, Chest Decompression).

EMT and Paramedic

- Control hemorrhage.
- Immobilize c-spine and secure the patient to a backboard *as needed* (see Medical Procedure 4.52, Spinal Immobilization).
- Expedite transport.

The following steps should not delay transport.

- Complete bandaging, splinting, and packaging *as needed.*
- Establish hospital contact for notification of an incoming patient, and obtain consultation for Level 2 orders.

2.1.4 Trauma Supportive Care

ALS Level 1

Paramedic and Authorized EMT

- Establish IV of normal saline with a regular infusion set (a)(b)(c), unless overridden by another specific protocol.

Paramedic

- Monitor ECG *as needed.*

ALS Level 2

None.

Note

(a) Authorized IV routes include all peripheral venous sites. External jugular veins may be utilized when other peripheral site attempts have been unsuccessful or would be inappropriate. Two IVs using large-bore intracaths should be initiated in unstable patients. Avoid use of access sites below the diaphragm. Consider using trauma tubing or blood infusion tubing *as needed.*

(b) When unable to establish an IV in the adult patient who needs to be resuscitated, an intraosseous line may be used by the **paramedic only** (see Medical Procedures 4.58 and 4.59).

(c) An EMT who has been authorized by his/her individual Medical Director may establish an IV.

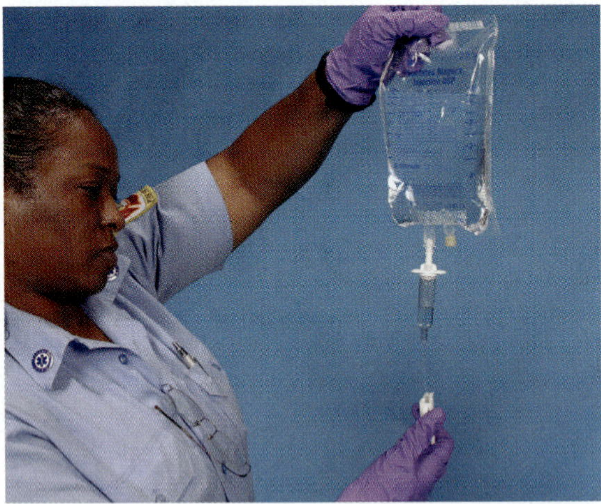

Establish IV of normal saline.

2.1.5 Pain Management

Paramedic Only

This entire protocol is ALS/Paramedic Only.

Isolated Extremity Fracture

The purpose of this procedure is to manage pain associated with isolated extremity fractures but not associated with multisystem trauma or hemodynamic instability.

ALS Level 1

- Patients should be asked to quantify their pain on an analog pain scale (from 0 = least severe to 10 = most severe). This number should be documented and used to measure the effectiveness of analgesia.
- Distal circulation, sensation, and movement in the injured extremity should be noted and recorded.
- The extremity should be immobilized as described in Adult Protocol 2.10.6, Extremity Injuries. **Self-administered** analgesia with nitrous oxide should be given special consideration for pain management during this procedure (see Medical Procedure 4.28, Nitrous Oxide–Nitronox), if available.
- Extremity fractures should be elevated, if possible, and cold applied.
- If pain persists and systolic BP ≥ 90 mm Hg, morphine sulfate may be given via slow IV in 2-mg increments every 3–5 minutes, titrated to pain and BP ≥ 90 mm Hg, up to a maximum of 10 mg (a)(b).

ALS Level 2

None.

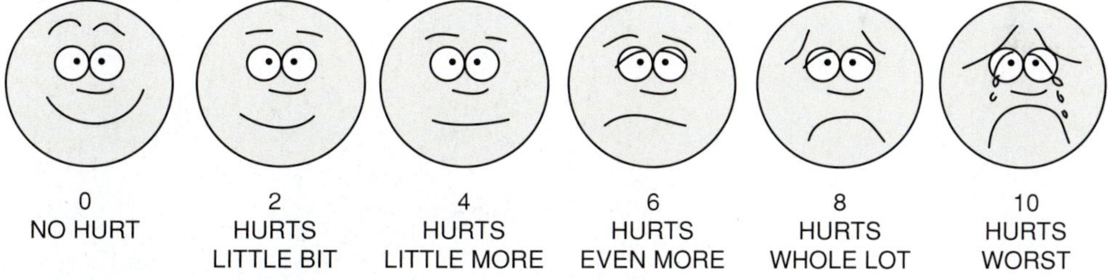

Wong-Baker Faces Scale.

From Hockenberry MJ, Wilson D: *Wong's essentials of pediatric nursing, ed. 8*, St. Louis, 2009, Mosby. Used with permission. Copyright Mosby.

2.1.5 Pain Management

Acute Back Strain

This procedure should be used in the isolated back strain where *an acute abdominal process is not suspected* (see Appendix 7.1, Abdominal Pain Differential).

ALS Level 1

- Patients should be asked to quantify their pain on an analog pain scale (from 0 = least severe to 10 = most severe). This number should be documented and used to measure the effectiveness of analgesia.
- **Self-administered** nitrous oxide may be used (see Medical Procedure 4.28, Nitrous Oxide–Nitronox), if available.
- Secure the patient to a backboard *as needed.*
- If pain persists and systolic BP ≥ 90 mm Hg:
    - Morphine sulfate may be given via slow IV in 2-mg increments every 3–5 minutes, titrated to pain and BP ≥ 90 mm Hg, up to a maximum of 10 mg (a)(b).
- If pain persists and systolic BP ≥ 90 mm Hg, ketorolac tromethamine (Toradol®) may be given as 30 mg IV or 60 mg IM (if patient is > 65 y/o, limit dosage to 15 mg IV or 30 mg IM), if available (c).

ALS Level 2

None.

2.1.5 Pain Management

Renal Colic

This procedure is used for flank pain associated with kidney stones, where an acute abdominal process can be ruled out (see Appendix 7.1, Abdominal Pain Differential).

ALS Level 1

- Patients should be asked to quantify their pain on an analog pain scale (from 0 = least severe to 10 = most severe). This number should be documented and used to measure the effectiveness of analgesia.
- **Self-administered** nitrous oxide may be used (see Medical Procedure 4.28, Nitrous Oxide–Nitronox), if available.
- If pain persists and systolic BP ≥ 90 mm Hg, morphine sulfate may be given via slow IV in 2-mg increments every 3–5 minutes, titrated to pain and BP ≥ 90 mm Hg, up to a maximum of 10 mg (a)(b).
- If pain persists and systolic BP ≥ 90 mm Hg, ketorolac tromethamine (Toradol®) may be given as 30 mg IV or 60 mg IM (if patient is > 65 y/o, limit dosage to 15 mg IV or 30 mg IM), if available (c).

ALS Level 2

None.

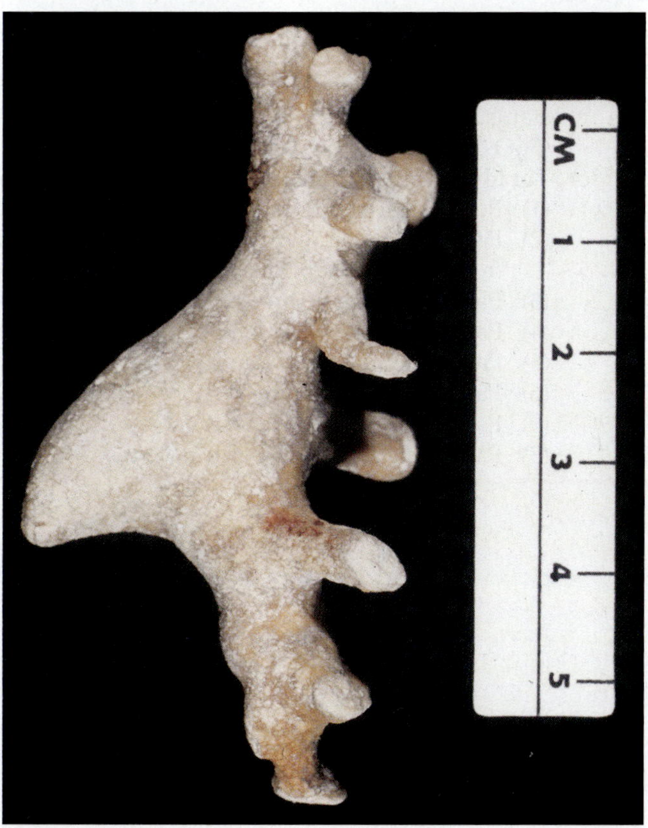

Large staghorn-shaped kidney stone.

2.1.5 Pain Management

Soft-Tissue Injuries, Burns, Bites, and Stings

This procedure is used for pain associated with soft-tissue injuries, burns, bites, and stings **not associated with multisystem trauma or hemodynamic instability.**

ALS Level 1

- Patients should be asked to quantify their pain on an analog pain scale (from 0 = least severe to 10 = most severe). This number should be documented and used to measure the effectiveness of analgesia.
- **Self-administered** nitrous oxide may be used (see Medical Procedure 4.28, Nitrous Oxide–Nitronox), if available.
- If pain persists and systolic BP ≥ 90 mm Hg, morphine sulfate may be given via slow IV in 2-mg increments every 3–5 minutes, titrated to pain and BP ≥ 90 mm Hg, up to a maximum of 10 mg (a)(b).
- If pain persists and systolic BP ≥ 90 mm Hg, ketorolac tromethamine (Toradol®) may be given as 30 mg IV or 60 mg IM (if patient is > 65 y/o, limit dosage to 15 mg IV or 30 mg IM), if available (c).

ALS Level 2

None.

Note

(a) Extreme caution should be used with administering narcotic analgesics to a patient with an $SpO_2 < 92\%$.

(b) When administering morphine sulfate, closely monitor the patient's respiratory status. In the event that the patient's respirations/oxygenation is suppressed ($SpO_2 < 92\%$), administer Narcan 2 mg IV, IM, or intranasal.

(c) **Toradol is contraindicated in the following patients:**
   (1) Potential surgical candidates (e.g., trauma patient).
   (2) Patients with known allergies to nonsteroidal anti-inflammatory drugs (e.g., aspirin, ibuprofen).
   (3) Patients with a history of nasal polyps.
   (4) Patients with angioedema.
   (5) Patients with bronchospastic reactivity (e.g., asthma).
   (6) Patients with bleeding disorders (e.g., ulcers).
   (7) Patients with kidney dysfunction.
   (8) Patients older than 65 years of age.

2.2 Adult Respiratory Emergencies

Assessment of the adult patient in respiratory distress requires specific attention to the function of the respiratory system. The EMT's and paramedic's assessment should be more concentrated in this area, to include the following considerations:

1. Assessment of chest wall movement, including the rate and depth of ventilation as well as the presence of symmetrical rise and fall.
2. Assessment of accessory muscle use.
3. Auscultation of bilateral lung sounds.
4. Use of pulse oximetry.

The paramedic must be able to determine the adequacy of ventilation and understand its relationship to respiration. If signs of hypoxia and respiratory distress are present, immediate airway and ventilatory management should be initiated. These signs include altered mental status, tachypnea, use of accessory muscles, nasal flaring, pursed lips, abnormal lung sounds, tachycardia, and cyanosis. In addition, the general signs of shock may be seen. Other signs of respiratory insufficiency that should alert the paramedic to the need for immediate airway and ventilatory management, including intubation, are respiratory rate < 10/min or > 36/min, and/or $SpO_2 < 92\%$.

In patients with chronic respiratory disease, the paramedic must be able to differentiate between what is chronic and what is acute, as it pertains to the respiratory assessment. Specific questions about the chief complaint and accompanying symptoms may prove to be invaluable in this setting. Assessment of lung sounds should be combined with patient history. For example, a patient with a history of CHF who has wheezing on auscultation of lung sounds should **not** be automatically classified as an "asthma patient." The paramedic must remember that patients with CHF may also present with wheezing. If this patient does not have a history of asthma or allergic reaction, the more prudent assessment would be that of CHF.

Specific treatments for the different causes of respiratory distress are outlined in the following protocols. When the paramedic is unsure as to which protocol to follow, he/she should follow the protocols in Section 2.1 and contact medical control for further direction.

2.2.1 Airway Obstruction

Causes of upper airway obstruction include the tongue, foreign bodies, swelling of the upper airway due to angio-neurotic edema (see Adult Protocol 2.8.1, Allergic Reactions/Anaphylaxis), and trauma to the airway. Differentiation of the cause of upper airway obstruction is essential to determining the proper treatment.

Supportive Care

- Assess mental status (AVPU).
- Assess airway.
- Assess breathing.
- If air exchange is inadequate and there is a reasonable suspicion of foreign body airway obstruction (FBAO), apply abdominal thrusts (see Medical Procedure 4.3) (a).
- Assess circulation—pulse, major bleeding, skin color and temperature.
- Assess disability—movement of extremities.
- Assess exposure and examine the patient's head, neck, chest, abdomen, and pelvis (check the back when the patient is rolled on his/her side).
- Identify the priority for the patient.
- Conduct a secondary assessment (see Adult Protocol 2.1.1).
  - Neurological assessment.
  - Vital signs.
  - OPQRRRST.
  - SAMPLE.
- Perform additional assessments as needed:
  - Cardiac monitoring.
  - Pulse oximetry SpO_2/SpCO.
  - Glucose.
  - Temperature.
  - Capnography.

2.2.1 Airway Obstruction

ALS Level 1

- If unable to relieve FBAO, visualize it with a laryngoscope and extract the foreign body with Magill forceps.
- If the obstruction is due to trauma and/or edema, or if uncontrollable bleeding into the airway causes life-threatening ventilatory impairment, perform endotracheal intubation (see Medical Procedure 4.18, Intubation).
- If unable to intubate and the patient cannot be adequately ventilated by other means, perform a cricothyroidotomy (see Medical Procedure 4.16).
- Establish an IV; give normal saline KVO.

ALS Level 2

None.

NOTE

(a) If air exchange is adequate with a partial airway obstruction, do not interfere; instead, encourage the patient to cough up the obstruction. Continue to monitor the patient for adequacy of air exchange. If air exchange becomes inadequate, continue with the protocol.

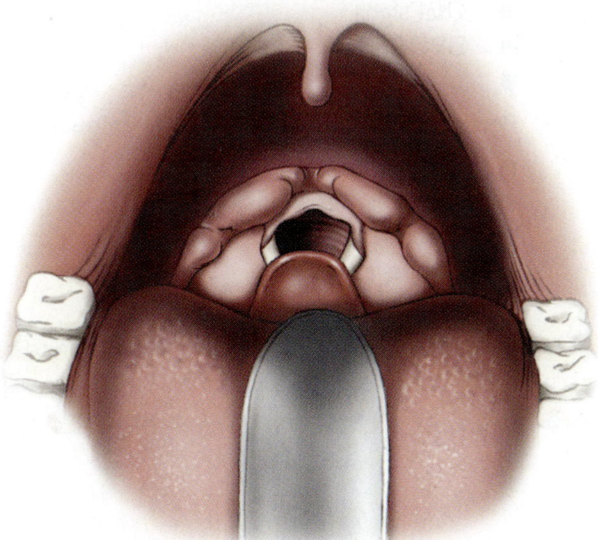

Laryngoscopic view of the vocal cords.

2.2.2 Asthma/Bronchospasm

This protocol is used for patients who are complaining of dyspnea and having wheezing. **A patient with a history of CHF who has wheezing on auscultation of lung sounds should not be automatically classified as an "asthma patient." If the CHF patient does not have a history of asthma or allergic reaction, the more prudent assessment would be that of CHF (cardiac asthma)** (see Adult Protocol 2.2.4, Pulmonary Edema–CHF).

Supportive Care

- Assess mental status (AVPU).
- Assess airway.
- Assess breathing.
- If air exchange is inadequate and there is a reasonable suspicion of foreign body airway obstruction (FBAO), apply abdominal thrusts (see Medical Procedure 4.3).
- Assess circulation—pulse, major bleeding, skin color and temperature.
- Assess disability—movement of extremities.
- Assess exposure and examine the patient's head, neck, chest, abdomen, and pelvis (check the back when the patient is rolled on his/her side).
- Identify the priority for the patient.
- Conduct a secondary assessment (see Adult Protocol 2.1.1).
  - Neurological assessment.
  - Vital signs.
  - OPQRRRST.
  - SAMPLE.
- Perform additional assessments as needed:
  - Cardiac monitoring.
  - Pulse oximetry SpO_2/SpCO.
  - Glucose.
  - Temperature.
  - Capnography.
- Place the patient in Fowler's position and assist ventilations *as needed* (see Medical Procedure 4.4).
- Administer CPAP with 5 cm H_2O PEEP (see Medical Procedure 4.24).

satst tnd

2.2.2 Asthma/Bronchospasm

ALS Level 1

- Establish an IV; give normal saline.
- Give albuterol (Ventolin): one nebulizer treatment containing 2.5 mg of albuterol premixed with 2.5 mL normal saline (see Medical Procedure 4.27). This treatment may be repeated twice *as needed* (a).
- If bronchodilators are administered, may add ipratoprium bromide (Atrovent®) 0.5 mg (0.5 mL) to albuterol nebulizer treatment **on first nebulizer treatment only** (a).
- Consider the need for advanced airway management (see Medical Procedure 4.18).
- If the patient has severe respiratory distress, choose one of the following steroids:
  - Methylprednisolone sodium succinate (Solu-Medrol®) 125 mg IV, if available.

  or

  - Dexamethasone (Decadron®) 10 mg IV, if available.
- If the patient continues to have severe respiratory distress, give epinephrine (1:1000) 0.3 mg SQ (b)(c).
- For severe respiratory distress, give magnesium sulfate 2 g IV (mixed in 50 mL of D_5W given over 5–10 minutes).
- Repeat epinephrine (1:1000) 0.3 mg SQ if the patient has not responded to the previous treatments (b)(c).

ALS Level 2

- Repeat epinephrine (1:1000) 0.3 mg SQ (b)(c).
- If the patient's heart rate ≥ 140, contact medical control for bronchodilator orders.

NOTE

(a) Do not give albuterol or ipratropium bromide if the patient's heart rate ≥ 140.
(b) Caution should be used when the patient is older than 40 years of age or has a history of hypertension or heart disease. Do not administer epinephrine if the patient's heart rate ≥ 140.
(c) If the patient is hypotensive with a delay in capillary refill, consider epinephrine (1:10,000) 0.5 mg via **slow** IV (over 3–4 minutes) or epinephrine (1:10,000) 1 mg ET.

2.2.3 Chronic Obstructive Pulmonary Disease (COPD)

This protocol is used for patients with a history of emphysema and/or chronic bronchitis who complain of dyspnea. If at any point the patient's respiratory status deteriorates, consider intubation and administration of albuterol via the ET tube as a mist, and transport the patient immediately.

Supportive Care

- Assess mental status (AVPU).
- Assess airway.
- Assess breathing.
- If air exchange is inadequate and there is a reasonable suspicion of foreign body airway obstruction (FBAO), apply abdominal thrusts (see Medical Procedure 4.3).
- Assess circulation—pulse, major bleeding, skin color and temperature.
- Assess disability—movement of extremities.
- Assess exposure and examine the patient's head, neck, chest, abdomen, and pelvis (check the back when the patient is rolled on his/her side).
- Identify the priority for the patient.
- Conduct a secondary assessment (see Adult Protocol 2.1.1).
  - Neurological assessment.
  - Vital signs.
  - OPQRRRST.
  - SAMPLE.
- Perform additional assessments as needed:
  - Cardiac monitoring.
  - Pulse oximetry SpO_2/SpCO.
  - Glucose.
  - Temperature.
  - Capnography.
- Place the patient in Fowler's position and assist ventilations *as needed* (see Medical Procedure 4.4).
- Administer CPAP with 5 cm H_2O PEEP (see Medical Procedure 4.24).

2.2.3 Chronic Obstructive Pulmonary Disease (COPD)

ALS Level 1

- Establish an IV; give normal saline KVO.
- Give albuterol (Ventolin): one nebulizer treatment containing 2.5 mg of albuterol premixed with 2.5 mL normal saline (see Medical Procedure 4.27). This treatment may be repeated twice *as needed* (a).
- If bronchodilators are administered, may add ipratoprium bromide (Atrovent®) 0.5 mg (0.5 mL) to albuterol treatment **on first nebulizer treatment only** (a).
- Consider the need for advanced airway management (see Medical Procedure 4.18).
- If the patient has severe respiratory distress, choose one of the following steroids:
  - Methylprednisolone sodium succinate (Solu-Medrol®) 125 mg IV, if available.

  or

  - Dexamethasone (Decadron®) 10 mg IV, if available.

ALS Level 2

None.

Note

(a) Do not give albuterol or ipratropium bromide if the patient's heart rate ≥ 140.

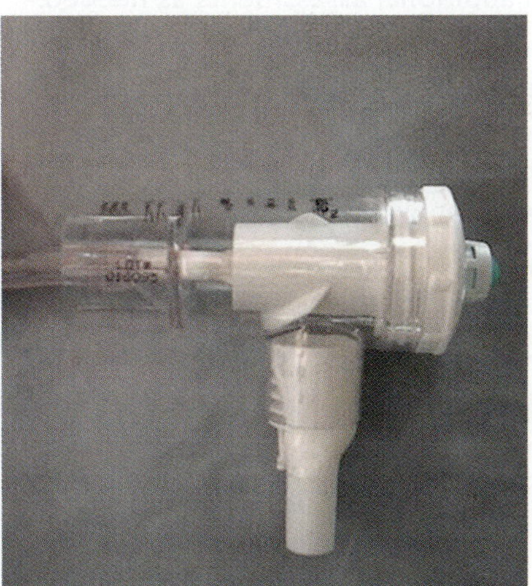

Small-volume nebulizer.

2.2.4 Pulmonary Edema–CHF

This protocol is used for patients who are exhibiting signs of pulmonary edema–CHF, including dyspnea with rales and/or wheezing (cardiac asthma). The patient may also have diminished air exchange. Other treatments for the causes of pulmonary edema–CHF should be considered (e.g., supraventricular tachycardia, myocardial infarction, and cardiogenic shock). **A patient with a history of CHF who has wheezing on auscultation of lung sounds should not be automatically classified as an "asthma patient." The paramedic must remember that patients with CHF may also present with wheezing. If the CHF patient does not have a history of asthma or allergic reaction, the more prudent assessment would be that of CHF (cardiac asthma).**

Supportive Care

- Assess mental status (AVPU).
- Assess airway.
- Assess breathing.
- If air exchange is inadequate and there is a reasonable suspicion of foreign body airway obstruction (FBAO), apply abdominal thrusts (see Medical Procedure 4.3).
- Assess circulation—pulse, major bleeding, skin color and temperature.
- Assess disability—movement of extremities.
- Assess exposure and examine the patient's head, neck, chest, abdomen, and pelvis (check the back when the patient is rolled on his/her side).
- Identify the priority for the patient.
- Conduct a secondary assessment (see Adult Protocol 2.1.1).
  - Neurological assessment.
  - Vital signs.
  - OPQRRRST.
  - SAMPLE.
- Perform additional assessments as needed:
  - Cardiac monitoring.
  - Pulse oximetry SpO_2/SpCO.
  - Glucose.
  - Temperature.
  - Capnography.
- Place the patient in Fowler's position and assist ventilations *as needed* (see Medical Procedure 4.4).
- Administer CPAP with 10 cm H_2O PEEP (see Medical Procedure 4.24) (a).
- If the patient is hypotensive (systolic BP < 90 mm Hg), see Adult Protocol 2.4.1, Cardiogenic Shock (b).

2.2.4 Pulmonary Edema–CHF

ALS Level 1

- If there is no improvement in the patient's pulse oximetry, capnography, and mental status, consider use of an advanced airway (see Medical Procedure 4.18).
- Establish an IV; give normal saline KVO.
- **Do not administer nitroglycerin if:**
  - The patient's systolic BP < 90 mm Hg.
  - The patient has taken erectile dysfunction medications within the last 24 hours (Viagra) or within the last 48 hours (Levitra or Cialis).
- If the patient's systolic BP ≥ 90 mm Hg, give nitroglycerin (Nitrostat® or Nitrolingual® spray) 0.4 mg SL, prior to applying CPAP (b)(c).
- If the patient's systolic BP ≥ 90 mm Hg, apply nitropaste (Nitro-Bid® ointment) 1–2 inches on chest wall (spread nitropaste on the chest to an area the size of the patient's palm) (b).
- If the patient's systolic BP ≥ 90 mm Hg, give furosemide (Lasix®) 1 mg/kg (or 80 mg) IV (b).
- Reevaluate the need for advanced airway management. If there is no improvement in the patient's pulse oximetry, capnography, and mental status, consider use of advanced airway management (see Medical Procedure 4.18, Intubation, and Medical Procedure 4.22, Capnography).
- If the patient is stable, see Adult Protocol 2.4.2.
- If the patient's systolic BP ≥ 90 mm Hg, morphine sulfate may be given via slow IV in 2-mg increments and may be repeated every 3–5 minutes, titrated to BP ≥ 90 mm Hg, up to a maximum of 10 mg *as needed* (b).

ALS Level 2

- Give albuterol (Ventolin): 1 nebulizer treatment containing 2.5 mg of albuterol premixed with 2.5 mL normal saline (see Medical Procedure 4.27) (d).
- If bronchodilators are administered, may add ipratoprium bromide (Atrovent®) 0.5 mg (0.5 mL) to albuterol treatment **on first nebulizer treatment only** (d).
- Repeat furosomide (Lasix®) 1 mg/kg (or 80 mg) IV (b).
- Give nitroglycerin (Tridil®) infusion at 5–20 mcg/min, if available.

Note

(a) The CPAP mask must be tight fitting. Some patients may not tolerate CPAP at 10 cm H_2O PEEP initially. In this instance, 7.5 cm H_2O PEEP should be used. CPAP should not be used if the patient's systolic BP < 90 mm Hg.

(b) Consider withholding if the clinical presentation of the patient indicates signs of hypovolemia (e.g., poor skin turgor, decreased capillary refill, and elevated temperature).

(c) It is preferred to have an IV in place prior to NTG administration. However, if you are unable to establish IV access, NTG may be administered with caution.

(d) Do not give albuterol or ipratropium bromide if the patient's heart rate ≥ 140.

2.2.5 Suspected Pneumonia

Patients complaining of dyspnea should be suspected of having pneumonia when they present with fever, productive cough, possible pleuritic chest pain, history of being bedridden, known immunocompromise, diabetes, elderly age, and lung sounds indicative of consolidation (rales and/or rhonchi with egophony over area of consolidation).

Supportive Care

- Assess mental status (AVPU).
- Assess airway.
- Assess breathing.
- If air exchange is inadequate and there is a reasonable suspicion of foreign body airway obstruction (FBAO), apply abdominal thrusts (see Medical Procedure 4.3).
- Assess circulation—pulse, major bleeding, skin color and temperature.
- Assess disability—movement of extremities.
- Assess exposure and examine the patient's head, neck, chest, abdomen, and pelvis (check the back when the patient is rolled on his/her side).
- Identify the priority for the patient.
- Conduct a secondary assessment (see Adult Protocol 2.1.1).
    - Neurological assessment.
    - Vital signs.
    - OPQRRRST.
    - SAMPLE.
- Perform additional assessments as needed:
    - Cardiac monitoring.
    - Pulse oximetry SpO_2/SpCO.
    - Glucose.
    - Temperature.
    - Capnography.

2.2.5 Suspected Pneumonia

ALS Level 1

- Establish an IV; give normal saline KVO.
- Give albuterol (Ventolin): one nebulizer treatment containing 2.5 mg of albuterol premixed with 2.5 mL normal saline (see Medical Procedure 4.27). This treatment may be repeated twice *as needed* (a).
- If bronchodilators are administered, may add ipratopium bromide (Atrovent®) 0.5 mg (0.5 mL) to albuterol nebulizer treatment **on first nebulizer treatment only** (a).
- Avoid the use of diuretics.

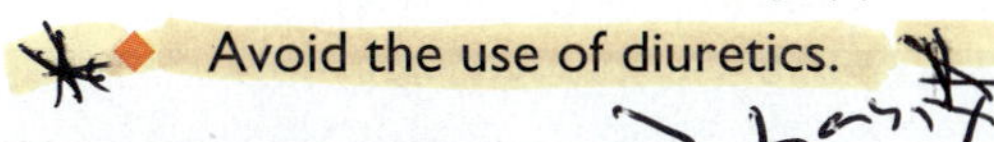

ALS Level 2

- If the patient's heart rate ≥ 140, contact medical control for bronchodilator orders.

NOTE

(a) Do not give albuterol or ipratropium bromide if the patient's heart rate ≥ 140.

2.3 Adult Cardiac Dysrhythmias

Protocols in Section 2.3 follow the ACLS guidelines. The paramedic should use these protocols to guide him/her through the treatment of cardiac patients with specific dysrhythmias and accompanying signs and symptoms. After stabilization of the patient, the paramedic may need to refer to additional protocols for continued treatment (e.g., other cardiac protocols).

In cardiac arrest, a major component of the primary and secondary survey is to consider the secondary, *differential diagnosis* and to think carefully about what could be causing the arrest. The "H's and T's" chart will assist in the recognition of a possible underlying cause.

H's

Cause	Treatment	Protocol
Hypovolemia	Fluid challenge NS 500 mL IV/IO	Shock Protocol
Hypoxia	Airway management	Protocol 2.1.2
Hydrogen ion–acidosis	Airway management, ventilate, consider sodium bicarbonate	Protocol 2.1.2 Drug Summary 5.45
Hyperkalemia	Consider calcium chloride 1 g Consider sodium bicarbonate 1 mEq/kg	Drug Summary 5.9 and 5.45
Hypothermia	Cold-related emergencies	Protocol 2.9.2
Hypoglycemia	If < 60, consider D_{50} or Glucagon	Protocol 2.8.2 Drug Summary 5.13 and 5.22
Hypocalcemia	Consider calcium chloride 1 g	Drug Summary 5.9

T's

Cause	Treatment	Protocol
Tablets	Consult poison control for specific therapy	Protocol 2.6
Tamponade, cardiac	Consider fluid challenge, dopamine drip	Protocol 2.4.1
Tension pneumothorax	Consider chest decompression	Procedure 4.14
Thrombosis, coronary	Consider AMI, cardiogenic shock	Protocol 2.4.2
Thrombosis, pulmonary		Protocol 2.4.1
Trauma		Protocol 2.10

2.3.1 Asystole

Supportive Care

- Consider criteria for death/no resuscitation (see General Protocol 1.4).
- Assess mental status (AVPU).
- Assess airway.
- Assess breathing.
- If air exchange is inadequate and there is a reasonable suspicion of foreign body airway obstruction (FBAO), apply abdominal thrusts (see Medical Procedure 4.3) (a).
- Oxygenate with 15–25 L/min via bag-valve mask with an appropriate airway adjunct device at 8–10 BPM (see Airway Management Protocol 2.1.2) (a).
- Assess circulation—pulse, major bleeding, skin color and temperature.
- If no pulse, begin immediate chest compressions at a rate of 100 per minute for 2 minutes while monitor is being attached.
- Assess disability—movement of extremities.
- Assess exposure and examine the patient's head, neck, chest, abdomen, and pelvis (check the back when the patient is rolled on his/her side).
- Identify the priority for the patient.
- Perform additional assessments as needed:
  - Cardiac monitoring.
  - Pulse oximetry SpO_2/SpCO.
  - Glucose.
  - Temperature.
  - Capnography.
- Do not interrupt CPR to check for a heart rhythm. Continuous uninterrupted compressions are paramount to patient survival.
- Check the heart rhythm; confirm asystole in two leads.
- Resume 2 minutes of continuous compressions at 100 per minute; check the heart rhythm.
- If available, attach an impedance threshold device (ITD).
- Consider the H's and T's.

2.3.1 Asystole

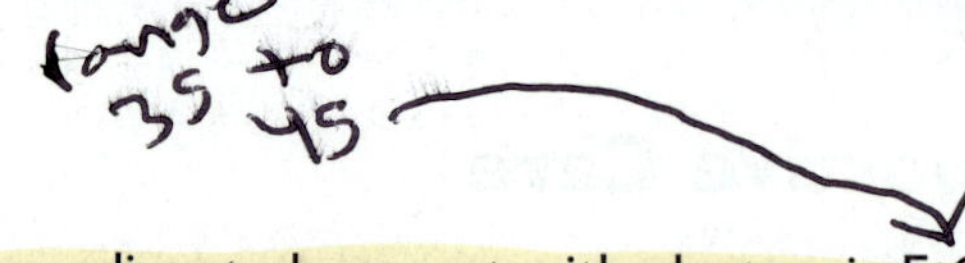

ALS Level 1

- Confirm airway adjunct placement with electronic $EtCO_2$ and waveform on scene, during transport, and during transfer at the hospital.
- Establish IV or IO access; give normal saline KVO.
- When IV or IO line is established, administer a vasopressor:
  - Epinephrine (1:10,000) 1 mg IV/IO; repeat every 3–5 minutes (b).
  - One dose of vasopressin 40 U IV/IO can replace the first or second dose of epinephrine (c).
- Give 2 minutes of chest compressions; check the heart rhythm.
- Give atropine 1 mg IV/IO; repeat every 3–5 minutes, up to 3 doses (d).
- Give 2 minutes of chest compressions; check the heart rhythm.
- Search for and treat possible contributing factors; see the H's and T's charts.
- If the patient is taking a calcium-channel blocker or has known renal failure, give calcium chloride 10% 1 g IV or IO.
- Remove the ITD as soon as the patient regains spontaneous circulation (see Post Resuscitation Protocol 2.3.8).

ALS Level 2

None.

NOTE

(a) Give 1 breath every 6 seconds or 1 breath every 10 compressions.
(b) If IV/IO access is not available, epinephrine 1:1000, 2 mg in 8 mL of normal saline, can be administered via ETT as a last resort. The drug should be injected directly into the ETT.
(c) If IV/IO access is not available, vasopressin can be administered via ETT as a last resort at twice the IV dose. The drug should be diluted in 5–10 mL of normal saline or sterile water and injected directly into the ETT.
(d) If IV/IO access is not available, atropine can be administered via ETT as a last resort at twice the IV dose. The drug should be diluted in 5–10 mL of normal saline or sterile water and injected directly into the ETT.

2.3.2 Bradycardia

Supportive Care

- Patients who present with a heart rate < 60 and are symptomatic (a). Consider the potential causes:

Acute myocardial infarction	Calcium-channel blockers
Well-conditioned athletes	Clonidine
Head injury	Digitalis
Atrio-ventricular block	Toxins
Hypoxia	Sick sinus syndrome
Hypoglycemia	Spinal cord lesion
Medications (beta blockers)	

- Access the ABCs and vital signs.
- Apply an SpO_2 monitor, and administer oxygen to maintain $SpO_2 \geq 92\%$, or assist with bag-valve mask ventilations if indicated.
- Obtain a SAMPLE history and OPQRST.
- Perform a focused exam.
- Consider the H's and T's.

ALS Level 1

- Establish IV access; give normal saline KVO.
- Perform 12-lead ECG. If inferior wall MI is identified, perform additional 12-lead ECG with V4R to confirm/rule out concurrent right ventricular MI (b).
- **If the patient has an acute inferior wall MI with hypotension and clear lungs,** give normal saline 500 cc fluid challenge; may repeat once (see Adult Protocol 2.4.2, Chest Pain—Suspected AMI).
- Begin external pacing if the patient remains hypotensive (SBP < 90 mm Hg), with AMI, altered mental status, chest pain, dyspnea, second-degree AV block type II, or third-degree AV block.
- **If the patient is symptomatic,** consider atropine 0.5 mg IV/IO; repeat every 3–5 minutes, up to a maximum total dose of 3 mg (a)(c)(d)(e).

2.3.2 Bradycardia

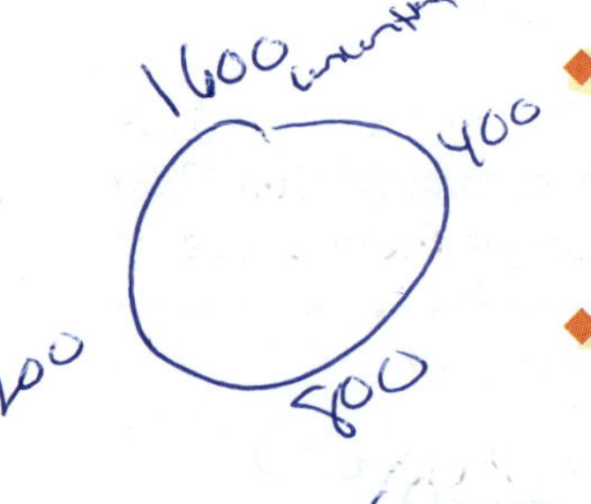

- **If the patient has persistent hypotension/cardiogenic shock,** give dopamine 5–20 mcg/kg/min (1600 mcg/mL infusion concentration = 15–60 gtts/min). Titrate to maintain a minimum systolic BP of 90 mm Hg and maximum BP of 120 mm Hg (maximum dose 20 mcg/kg/min).
- If the patient is conscious and aware of the situation during pacing, administer one of the following benzodiazepines (f):
  - **Diazepam (Valium)** 5 mg IV, IO or intranasal; may repeat once, to a maximum dose of 10 mg (g).

  or

  - **Midazolam (Versed)** 2 mg increments IV, IO, or intranasal, to a maximum dose of 10 mg (g).

  or

  - **Lorazepam (Ativan)** 2 mg IV, IO, or intranasal; may repeat once, to a maximum dose of 4 mg (g).

ALS Level 2

- If the patient displays severe symptoms refractory to ALS Level 1 care, give an epinephrine infusion at 2–10 mcg/min (see Appendix 7.9).

Note

(a) Symptomatic criteria include hypotension (systolic BP < 90 mm Hg) or other signs of shock and congestive heart failure, acute altered mental status, ongoing chest pain, dyspnea, or ischemia/infarction on 12-lead ECG (use with caution in the presence of dyspnea or myocardial ischemia).

(b) **Bradycardia with hypotension may be due to an inferior wall MI associated with right ventricular MI (confirmed on 12-lead ECG as a V4R ST elevation). When an inferior wall MI is associated with right ventricular MI, avoid the use of nitrates (nitroglycerin). If bradycardia and hypotension exist, pacing and IV fluids may improve the patient's hemodynamic status.** Consider pacing and IV fluids prior to the use of atropine. Also refer to Adult Protocol 2.4.2, Chest Pain–Suspected AMI.

(c) **Consider pacing before giving the maximum dose of atropine.**

(d) **For second-degree AV block type II and third-degree AV block, omit atropine and use an external pacer.**

(e) **Use atropine with caution in the presence of myocardial ischemia.**

(f) **Administer benzodiazepines slowly, titrate to effect, and be aware of associated hypotension.**

(g) Intranasal administration of benzodiazepines requires the use of a mucosal atomization device.

2.3.3 Narrow Complex Tachycardia (Supraventricular Tachycardia)

Patients suffering from tachycardia may or may not exhibit symptoms. It is important to note that narrow complex tachycardia has many origins. The atrial rate may be helpful in the differential interpretation of these types of tachycardia. The following rates should be considered:

Sinus tachycardia ranges from 100 to 160 beats per minute.

Junctional tachycardia ranges from 100 to 180 beats per minute.

Atrial tachycardia ranges from 150 to 250 beats per minute (atrial rate).

Atrial flutter ranges from 250 to 350 beats per minute (atrial rate).

Atrial fibrillation starts at 350 beats per minute (atrial rate).

In addition, wide complex tachycardia (QRS ≥ 0.12 seconds) should initially be considered as ventricular in origin, unless proven otherwise (e.g., documented QRS morphology consistent with preexisting BBB; refer to Adult Medical Protocol 2.3.6, Wide Complex Tachycardia with a Pulse).

Those patients who present with SVT may have evidence of cardiovascular dysfunction. Those patients who present with "borderline" symptomatic signs and symptoms may be treated with medications. Those patients who present with "unstable" signs and symptoms should be cardioverted immediately.

The following table shows the range from borderline signs and symptoms to unstable signs and symptoms:

Borderline Symptomatic (Stable)	Critical (Unstable)
Alert and oriented	Decreased level of consciousness
SBP ≥ 90 mm Hg	SBP < 90 mm Hg (shock)
Mild chest discomfort	Chest pain
Shortness of breath	Shortness of breath
	Diaphoresis
	Pulmonary edema

2.3.3 Narrow Complex Tachycardia (Supraventricular Tachycardia)

All Borderline Symptomatic Narrow Complex Tachycardias

Supportive Care

- Assess the ABCs and vital signs.
- Determine hemodynamic stability and symptoms.
- Apply and SpO_2 monitor.
- Administer oxygen to maintain $SpO_2 \geq 92\%$.
- Obtain a SAMPLE history and OPQRST.
- Perform a focused exam.
- Consider the H's and T's.

Borderline Symptomatic SVT, Heart Rate ≥ 150 BPM

ALS Level 1

- Apply the ECG monitor, record a rhythm strip, and obtain a 12-lead ECG.
- Establish IV access; give normal saline KVO.
- If the patient is asymptomatic, provide medical supportive care (Protocol 2.1.3) and transport immediately.
- If necessary, perform vagal maneuvers (see Medical Procedure 4.35).
- If not resolved, administer adenosine triphosphate (Adenocard®) 6 mg rapid IVP, followed by rapid 20 mL NS flush (a).
- If not resolved in 2 minutes, repeat adenosine triphosphate (Adenocard) 12 mg rapid IVP, followed by rapid 20 mL NS flush. This treatment may be repeated a third time at 12 mg (a).

ALS Level 2

- Administer diltiazem (Cardizem®) 0.25 mg/kg IV or IO (over 2 minutes) (20 mg for the average patient) for narrow complex supraventricular tachycardias (b).

2.3.3 Narrow Complex Tachycardia (Supraventricular Tachycardia)

Borderline Symptomatic Atrial Fibrillation or Atrial Flutter and Heart Rate ≥ 150 BPM

ALS Level I

- Apply the ECG monitor, record a rhythm strip, and obtain a 12-lead ECG.
- Establish IV access; give normal saline KVO.
- If the patient is asymptomatic, provide medical supportive care (Protocol 2.1.3) and transport immediately.
- If the patient has borderline symptoms with a SBP of 90–100 mm Hg, consider other causes of hypotension (e.g., hypovolemia or sepsis) prior to the administration of Cardizem.
- Administer diltiazem (Cardizem) 0.25 mg/kg IV over 2 minutes (20 mg for the average patient) (b).
- If the tachyarrhythmia is not resolved in 15 minutes, may repeat diltiazem (Cardizem) 0.35 mg/kg IV or IO (over 2 minutes) (25 mg for the average patient).

All Critical/Unstable Symptomatic Narrow Complex Tachycardias

This patient group includes individuals who are hypotensive with a systolic BP < 90 mm Hg and a heart rate ≥ 150 beats/min and who are symptomatic (clinical evidence of impending cardiac arrest) as evidenced by any of the following:

Diaphoresis	Shortness of breath
Chest pain	Decreased level of consciousness
Pulmonary edema	

Supportive Care

- Assess the ABCs and vital signs.
- Determine the patient's hemodynamic stability and symptoms.
- Apply an SpO_2 monitor and administer oxygen to maintain $SpO_2 \geq 92\%$.
- Obtain a SAMPLE history and OPQRST.
- Perform a focused exam.
- Consider the H's and T's.

2.3.3 Narrow Complex Tachycardia (Supraventricular Tachycardia)

ALS Level 1

- Provide advanced airway management, if necessary (c).
- Establish IV access; give normal saline KVO.
- Evaluate lung sounds. If they are clear, administer a fluid challenge of normal saline 500 cc IV or IO.
- If the patient is conscious and aware of the situation, consider sedation with one of the following benzodiazepines (d):
  - **Diazepam (Valium)** 5 mg IV, IO, or intranasal; may repeat once, up to a maximum dose of 10 mg (e).

  or
  - **Midazolam (Versed)** 2 mg increments IV, IO, or intranasal, up to a maximum dose of 10 mg (e).

  or
  - **Lorazepam (Ativan)** 2 mg IV, IO, or intranasal; may repeat once, up to a maximum dose of 4 mg (e).
- Perform synchronized cardioversion at 50 joules for SVT and atrial flutter, and at 100 joules for atrial fibrillation. Escalate the second and subsequent shock doses as needed to 100, 200, 300, and 360 joules.

ALS Level 2

None.

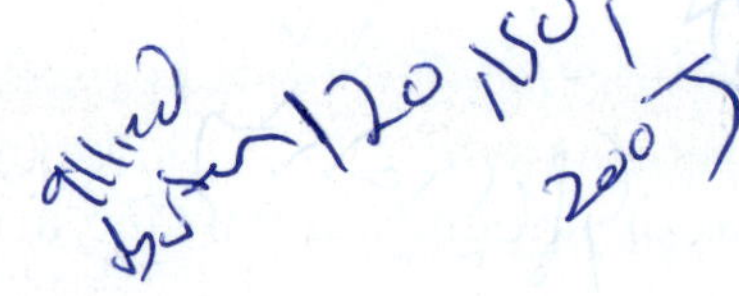

Note

(a) Adenosine triphosphate should not be given to patients with known atrial flutter or atrial fibrillation.

(b) Do not give diltiazem (Cardizem®) to patients with a known history of Wolfe-Parkinson-White (WPW) syndrome.

(c) Confirm airway adjunct placement with electronic $EtCO_2$ and waveform on scene, during transport, and during transfer at hospital.

(d) Administer benzodiazepines slowly, titrate to effect, and be aware of associated hypotension.

(e) Intranasal administration of benzodiazepines requires the use of a mucosal atomization device.

2.3.4 Premature Ventricular Ectopy (PVC)

Treatment of ventricular arrhythmias after MI has been a controversial topic for two decades. Similarly, management of ventricular arrhythmias during the acute phase of MI continues to evolve as treatment strategies are reviewed in the context of new information and changing epidemiological data during the era of adjunctive medical and reperfusion therapy. **At present, the treatment of asymptomatic premature ventricular ectopy (PVC) is not recommended.** Current ACLS protocols recommend amiodorone for the treatment of hemodynamically stable VT and prevention of recurrent VF.

Supportive Care

- Medical Supportive Care Protocol 2.1.3: 100% oxygen via nonrebreather mask at 10–15 L/min.

ALS Level 1

None.

ALS Level 2

If the patient is symptomatic, contact the physician for further orders.

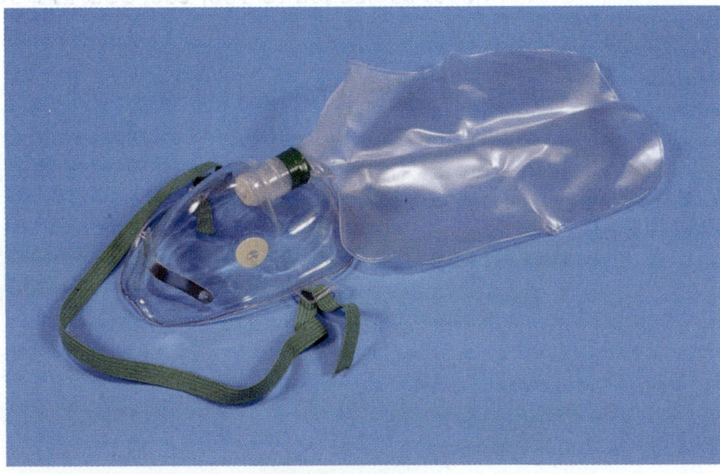

Nonrebreathing mask.

2.3.5 Pulseless Electrical Activity (PEA)

This protocol is used for electromechanical dissociation (EMD), pseudo-EMD, idioventricular rhythms, bradyasystolic rhythms, and post-defibrillation idioventricular rhythms.

Supportive Care

- Determine the patient's (un)responsiveness and check the ABCs.
- Oxygenate with 15–25 L/min via bag-valve mask with an appropriate airway adjunct device at 8–10 BPM (see Airway Protocol 2.1.2) (a).
- Begin immediate chest compressions at a rate of 100 per minute for 2 minutes while the monitor is being attached.
- Do not interrupt CPR to check for a heart rhythm. Continuous uninterrupted compressions are paramount to patient survival.
- Check the heart rhythm. Confirm PEA (absent apical heart sounds).
- Resume 2 minutes of continuous compressions at 100 per minute; check the heart rhythm.
- If available, attach an impedance threshold device (ITD).
- Obtain a SAMPLE history.
- Perform a focused exam.
- Consider the H's and T's.

ALS Level 1

- Establish IV or IO access; give normal saline KVO.
- Confirm airway adjunct placement with electronic $EtCO_2$ and waveform on scene, during transport, and during transfer at hospital.
- When an IV or IO line is established, administer a vasopressor.
  - Give epinephrine (1:10,000) 1 mg IV/IO; repeat every 3–5 minutes (b).
  - One dose of vasopressin 40 U IV/IO can replace the first or second dose of epinephrine (c).
- Give 2 minutes of chest compressions; check the heart rhythm.
- Give atropine 1 mg IV/IO if the PEA rate is bradycardic; repeat every 3–5 minutes, up to 3 doses (d).
- Give 2 minutes of chest compressions; check the heart rhythm.
- **Search for and treat possible contributing factors; see the H's and T's charts.**
- If the patient is taking a calcium-channel blocker or has known renal failure, give calcium chloride 10% 1 g IV or IO.
- Remove the ITD as soon as the patient has a return of spontaneous circulation (ROSC) (see Post-Resuscitation Protocol 2.3.8).

2.3.5 Pulseless Electrical Activity (PEA)

ALS Level 2

None.

NOTE

(a) Give 1 breath every 6 seconds or 1 breath every 10 compressions.
(b) If IV/IO access is not available, epinephrine can be administered via ETT as a last resort at twice the IV dose. The drug should be diluted in 5–10 mL of normal saline or sterile water and injected directly into the ETT.
(c) If IV/IO access is not available, vasopressin can be administered via ETT as a last resort at twice the IV dose. The drug should be diluted in 5–10 mL of normal saline or sterile water and injected directly into the ETT.
(d) If IV/IO access is not available, atropine can be administered via ETT as a last resort at twice the IV dose. The drug should be diluted in 5–10 mL of normal saline or sterile water and injected directly into the ETT.

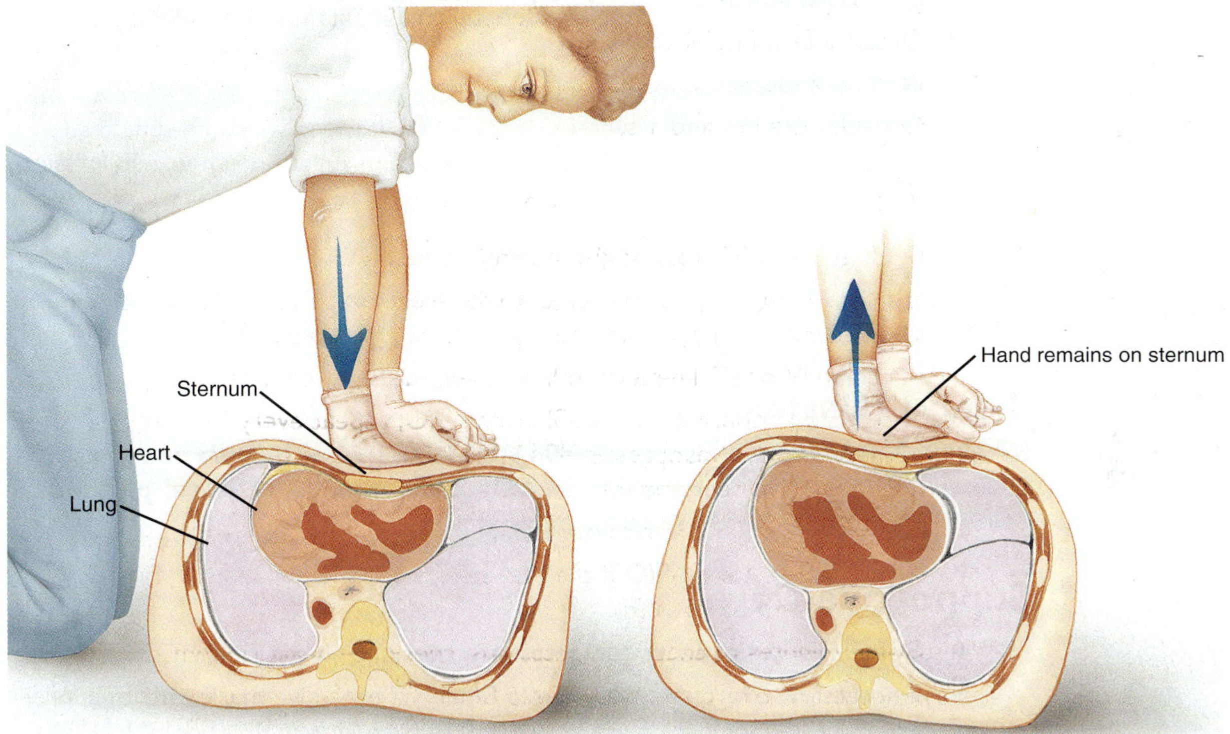

Compression and relaxation should be rhythmic and of equal duration. Pressure on the sternum must be released so that the sternum can return to its normal resting position between compressions. However, do not remove the heel of the hand from the sternum.

2.3.6 Wide Complex Tachycardia with a Pulse (Ventricular Tachycardia)

Borderline Symptomatic (Stable)

Supportive Care

- Determine the patient's (un)responsiveness and check the ABCs.
- Give oxygen via nasal cannula (2–6 L/min).
- Obtain a SAMPLE history.
- Perform a focused exam.
- Consider the H's and T's.

ALS Level 1

- Monitor the ECG.
- Establish IV access; give normal saline KVO.
- Give amiodarone 150 mg in 50 mL of D_5W over 10 minutes IV, if available. Repeat every 10 minutes as needed, up to a maximum dose of 2.2 g in 24 hours.
- If the patient has torsades de pointes, administer magnesium sulfate 2 g in 50 mL of D_5W infused over 1–2 minutes IV. If the magnesium sulfate successfully converts the rhythm, start magnesium sulfate maintenance infusion (1 g in 250 mL of D_5W) at 30–60 gtts/min.

ALS Level 2

None.

Critical (Unstable)

Heart rate > 150 beats/min and systolic blood pressure < 90 mm Hg with one of the following signs and symptoms: chest pain, dyspnea, pulmonary edema, diaphoresis, and altered mental status.

Supportive Care

- Determine the patient's (un)responsiveness and check the ABCs.
- If necessary, oxygenate with 15–25 L/min via bag-valve mask with an appropriate airway adjunct device at 8–10 BPM (see Airway Protocol 2.1.2) (a).
- Confirm airway adjunct placement.
- Obtain a SAMPLE history.
- Perform a focused exam.
- Consider the H's and T's.

2.3.6 Wide Complex Tachycardia with a Pulse (Ventricular Tachycardia)

ALS Level 1

- Monitor the ECG.
- Establish IV or IO access; give normal saline KVO.
- If the patient is conscious and aware of the situation, consider sedation with one of the following benzodiazepines (b):
  - **Diazepam (Valium)** 5 mg IV, IO, or intranasal; may repeat once, up to a maximum dose of 10 mg (c).

  or

  - **Midazolam (Versed)** 2 mg increments IV, IO, or intranasal, up to a maximum dose of 10 mg (c).

  or

  - **Lorazepam (Ativan)** 2 mg IV, IO, or intranasal; may repeat once, up to a maximum dose of 4 mg (c).
- Perform synchronized cardioversion at 100, 200, 300, or 360 joules (d).

ALS Level 2

None.

Note

(a) Give 1 breath every 6 seconds or 1 breath every 10 compressions.
(b) Administer benzodiazepines slowly, titrate to effect, and be aware of associated hypotension.
(c) Intranasal administration of benzodiazepines requires the use of a mucosal atomization device.
(d) If an antiarrhythmic medication was not administered prior to cardioversion, administer amiodarone 150 mg in 50 mL of D_5W over 10 minutes IV, if available. Repeat every 10 minutes as needed, up to a maximum dose of 2.2 g in 24 hours.

2.3.7 Wide Complex Tachycardia Without a Pulse and Ventricular Fibrillation

Supportive Care

- Determine the patient's (un)responsiveness and check the ABCs.
- Oxygenate with 15–25 L/min via a bag-valve mask with an appropriate airway adjunct device at 8–10 BPM (see Airway Protocol 2.1.2) (a).
- Begin immediate chest compressions at a rate of 100 per minute for 2 minutes while the monitor is being attached. If the event was witnessed arrest, defibrillate immediately.
- Do not interrupt CPR to check for a heart rhythm. Continuous uninterrupted compressions are paramount to patient survival.
- Check the heart rhythm. Confirm the rhythm and shock accordingly (b).
- If available, attach an impedance threshold device (ITD).
- Obtain a SAMPLE history.
- Perform a focused rapid assessment.
- Consider the H's and T's.

ALS Level I

- Confirm placement of the airway adjunct with electronic $EtCO_2$ and waveform while on scene, during transport, and during transfer at hospital.
- Establish IV or IO access; give normal saline KVO.
- Defibrillate at **200 joules** for a biphasic device and **360 joules** for a monophasic device. Continue CPR while the defibrillator is charging.
- Immediately resume continuous chest compressions at a rate of 100 per minute for 2 minutes.
- Check the heart rhythm. If it is a shockable rhythm, defibrillate at **300 joules** for a biphasic device and **360 joules** for a monophasic device. Continue CPR while the defibrillator is charging.
- When an IV or IO line is established, administer a vasopressor:
  - Give epinephrine (1:10,000) 1 mg IV/IO; repeat every 3–5 minutes for the duration of the arrest (c).
  - One dose of vasopressin 40 U IV/IO can replace the first or second dose of epinephrine (d).
- Immediately resume continuous chest compressions at a rate of 100 per minute for 2 minutes.
- Check the heart rhythm. If it is a shockable rhythm, defibrillate at **360 joules** for a biphasic or monophasic device. Continue CPR while the defibrillator is charging.
- Immediately resume continuous chest compressions at a rate of 100 per minute for 2 minutes.
- Administer amiodarone 300 mg IV/IO once. If V-Fib/pulseless V-Tach continues, consider additional 150 mg IV/ IO once. Administer during CPR.

2.3.7 Wide Complex Tachycardia Without a Pulse and Ventricular Fibrillation

- Check the heart rhythm. If it is a shockable rhythm, defibrillate at **360 joules** for a biphasic or monophasic device. Continue CPR while the defibrillator is charging.
- Immediately resume continuous chest compressions at a rate of 100 per minute for 2 minutes.
- Check the heart rhythm.
- If the patient has torsades de pointes, administer magnesium sulfate 2 g in 50 mL of D_5W infused over 1–2 minutes IV/IO (e).
- Continue treatment until there is a return of spontaneous circulation (ROSC), a rhythm change, or termination of efforts.
- If the patient has ROSC, see Post-Resuscitation Protocol 2.3.8

ALS Level 2

None.

NOTE

(a) Give 1 breath every 6 seconds or 1 breath every 10 compressions.
(a) The EMT should apply the AED. The paramedic should proceed to ALS Level 1 defibrillation.
(c) If IV/IO access is not available, epinephrine can be administered via ETT as a last resort at twice the IV dose. The drug should be diluted in 5–10 mL of normal saline or sterile water and injected directly into the ETT.
(d) If IV/IO access is not available, vasopressin can be administered via ETT as a last resort at twice the IV dose. The drug should be diluted in 5–10 mL of normal saline or sterile water and injected directly into the ETT.
(e) If magnesium sulfate successfully converts the heart rhythm, start magnesium sulfate maintenance infusion (2 g in 500 mL NS) at 30–60 gtts/min.

2.3.8 Post-Resuscitation Protocol

Post-resuscitation is an extremely unstable period for the patient, so the patient should be monitored closely and reassessed frequently. The immediate goals of post-resuscitation care are as follows:

- Provide cardio-respiratory support to optimize tissue perfusion, especially to the brain.
- Institute antiarrhythmic therapy to prevent recurrence of the arrest.
- Attempt to identify the precipitating cause of the arrest.
- Rapidly transport the patient to the closest appropriate facility.

When responding to a facility that provides therapeutic hypothermia, implement the hypothermia protocol if the patient has a return of spontaneous circulation (ROSC) and remains unconscious.

Supportive Care

- Reassess the ABCs and vital signs.
- Remove the ITD as soon as the patient has a ROSC.
- Obtain a SAMPLE history.

ALS Level I

- Maintain an open airway with an appropriate airway adjunct device, administer 100% O_2 to maintain $SpO_2 \geq 92\%$, and monitor with electronic $EtCO_2$ capnography/waveform. Ventilate at 8–10 BPM; **avoid hyperventilation.**
- Determine the patient's hemodynamic stability. If systolic blood pressure < 90 mm Hg:
  - If the patient's lungs are clear, administer IV NS 500 mL; may repeat once to maintain systolic blood pressure ≥ 90 mm Hg (a).

  If systolic BP remains < 90 mm Hg:
  - Give a dopamine infusion at 10 mcg/kg/min; titrate to maintain blood pressure ≥ 90 mm Hg.
- Manage dysrhythmias according to the specific protocol.

2.3.8 Post-Resuscitation Protocol

- If the cardiac arrest was the result of VF or VT, manage the patient as follows:
  - If an antiarrhythmic medication was *not* used to convert the heart rhythm, administer amiodarone 150 mg in 50 mL of D_5W over 10 minutes IV/IO (a).
  - If amiodarone was administered during resuscitation, do *not* administer additional amiodarone.
  - If the patient is having frequent PVC or runs of VT, or if the transport time will exceed 30 minutes, start an amiodarone drip (150 mg in 50 mL of D_5W = 3:1 concentration). Using a 60 gtt/mL set, initiate the flow at 1 gtt every 3 seconds.
  - Proceed to Therapeutic Hypothermia Protocol 2.3.9.
- Transport the patient to the closest interventional cardiac facility (c).

ALS Level 2

None.

Note

(a) If rales or crackles are auscultated in the lungs or the patient's systolic blood pressure remains less than 90 mm Hg despite fluid therapy, proceed directly to dopamine administration.

(b) Do not use amiodarone if the patient has a heart rate < 60, second-degree type II AV block, or third-degree AV block.

(c) If the patient's airway is compromised or crews are unable to manage the patient, transport the patient to the nearest facility.

2.3.9 Therapeutic Hypothermia

Cardiac arrest outside of the hospital is a common occurrence and typically results in a poor outcome for the patient. Those patients who do have a return of spontaneous circulation (ROSC) will often have a poor neurological outcome as a result of cerebral reperfusion injury. The American Heart Association (AHA) has recognized this fact and offers the following recommendation: "Unconscious adult patients with ROSC after out-of-hospital cardiac arrest should be cooled to 32°C to 34°C (89.6°F to 93.2°F) for 12 to 24 hours when the initial rhythm was ventricular fibrillation/pulseless ventricular tachycardia (Class IIa)."

Inclusion Criteria	Exclusion Criteria
ROSC after a nontraumatic **witnessed** cardiac arrest, when the rhythm was V-Fib/pulseless V-Tach	Pregnant
Adults ≥ 18 years old	Age < 18 years old
No purposeful pain response following neurological assessment	Down time > 15 minutes prior to EMS arrival
Endotracheal Intubation, $EtCO_2$ > 20 mm Hg and patient remains comatose	Known history of drugs and/or alcohol addiction
Initial temperature > 98°F (34°C)	Terminal illness

Supportive Care

- Reassess the ABCs and vital signs.
- Remove the ITD as soon as the patient has a ROSC.
- Confirm therapeutic hypothermia inclusion/exclusion criteria.
- Obtain a SAMPLE history.
- Transport the patient to the nearest hospital providing therapeutic hypothermia resuscitation.

ALS Level I

- The patient must be intubated and have an $EtCO_2$ > 20 mm Hg prior to proceeding with therapeutic hypothermia treatment.
- Maintain SpO_2 ≥ 92% and attempt to maintain an $EtCO_2$ of 35–45 mm Hg. Avoid hyperventilation.
- Conduct a neurological assessment. Document and reassess:
  - Pupils (size, reactivity, equality).
  - Motor response to pain.
- Remove the patient's clothing.
- Attempt to place an IV line of NS, if not already in place.

2.3.9 Therapeutic Hypothermia

The following steps are intended for those agencies establishing therapeutic hypothermia in the field:

- Apply cold packs to the patient's head, axilla, and groin.
- Sedate the patient with one of the following benzodiazepines (a):
  - **Diazepam (Valium)** 5 mg IV, IO, or intranasal; may repeat once, up to a maximum dose of 10 mg.

  or

  - **Midazolam (Versed)** 2-mg increments IV, IO, or intranasal, up to a maximum dose of 10 mg.

  or

  - **Lorazepam (Ativan)** 2 mg IV, IO, or intranasal; may repeat once, up to a maximum dose of 4 mg.
- If available, give vecuronium 0.1 mg/kg IV or IO, up to a maximum dose of 10 mg, to prevent shivering.
- Start a cold IV/IO saline bolus at 30 mL/kg, up to a maximum of 2 L, if available.
- If systolic blood pressure drops to < 90 mm Hg, start a dopamine drip at 10 mcg/kg/min. Maintain systolic blood pressure > 110 mm Hg to ensure adequate perfusion.
- Continually monitor and reassess the patient.
- If at any time the patient has a loss of spontaneous circulation, discontinue cooling and refer to the appropriate protocol.

ALS Level 2

None.

Note

(a) Intranasal administration of benzodiazepines requires the use of a mucosal atomization device.

2.4 Other Adult Cardiac Emergencies

The paramedic should use these protocols to guide him/her through the treatment of patients with other cardiac-related emergencies who are exhibiting signs and symptoms. In addition to these protocols, the paramedic may need to refer to additional protocols for continued treatment (e.g., adult cardiac dysrhythmias protocols).

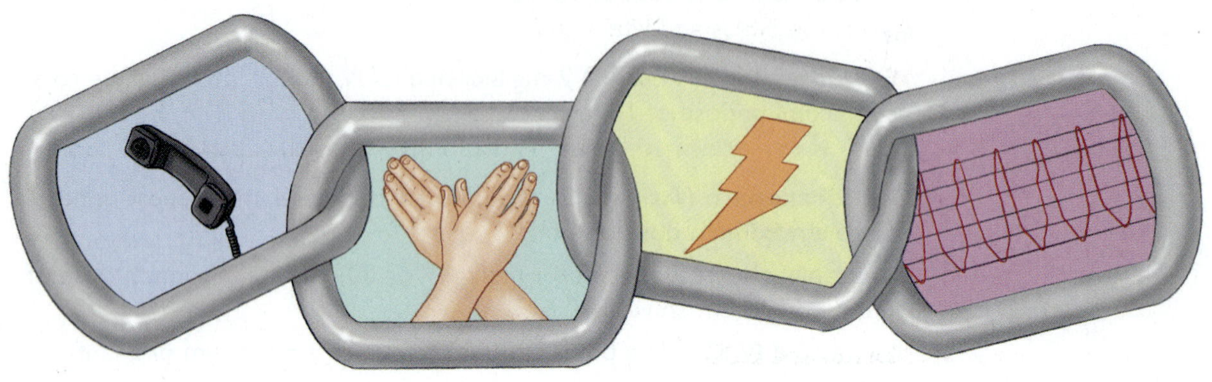

The chain of survival.
Source: American Heart Association.

2.4.1 Cardiogenic Shock

This protocol is used for the patient who is hypotensive (systolic BP < 90 mm Hg) with signs and/or symptoms that are cardiac in origin (see Adult Protocol 2.2.4, Pulmonary Edema–CHF; Adult Protocol 2.3, Adult Cardiac Dysrhythmias; and Adult Protocol 2.4.2, Chest Pain–Suspected AMI).

Supportive Care

- Assess the ABCs and vital signs.
- Perform a SAMPLE history.
- Administer oxygen via non-rebreather mask (10–15 L/min). If the patient's airway is compromised, assist ventilations by using the appropriate airway adjunct.
- Consider possible causes (i.e., the H's and T's).

ALS Level 1

- Monitor the ECG.
- Perform a 12-lead ECG, and initiate a Cardiac Alert if AMI is present.
- Start IV/IO normal saline. If time permits, establish a second IV/IO line if possible.
- If the patient is not experiencing pulmonary edema, administer a fluid challenge of 500 mL normal saline. If this measure does not improve the patient's systolic blood pressure, the fluid challenge may be repeated once (a).
- If the patient has an anterior wall MI or if the fluid challenge does not improve blood pressure, start a dopamine infusion at 5–20 mcg/kg/min (b).
- Titrate dopamine to maintain a minimum SBP of 90 mm Hg and a maximum SBP of 120 mm Hg.
- If the heart rate is slow (< 60/min), see Adult Protocol 2.3.2, Bradycardia.
- If the heart rate is fast (> 100/min), see Adult Protocol 2.3.3, Narrow Complex Tachycardia, or Adult Protocol 2.3.6, Wide Complex Tachycardia with a Pulse, as appropriate.

ALS Level 2

None.

NOTE

(a) Avoid giving fluids if an anterior wall MI is suspected (evidenced by ST elevations in leads I, AVL, V1 through V6).

(b) 1600 mcg/mL infusion concentration = 15–60 gtts/min with a 60-gtt set. The maximum dose is 20 mcg/kg/min.

2: adult protocols

2.4.2 Chest Pain/Suspected AMI

This protocol is used for the patient who is experiencing **chest pain or discomfort.** Other signs and/or symptoms associated with acute coronary syndrome include dyspnea, diapheresis, nausea/vomiting, and weakness/fatigue. If these additional signs and symptoms are present in the absence of chest pain or discomfort, AMI may still be present. This protocol should be followed when an AMI is suspected.

Nontraumatic chest pain should first be assessed as a possible AMI. Other potential causes of nontraumatic chest pain include angina pectoris, dissecting aortic aneurysm, pericarditis, spontaneous pneumothorax, pulmonary embolism, pneumonia, pleurisy, costochondritis, hiatal hernia, esophageal spasm, peptic ulcer, cholecystitis, pancreatitis, and cervical disk problem (see Appendix 7.5, Chest Pain Differential).

Supportive Care

- Assess the ABCs and vital signs.
- Perform a SAMPLE history.
- Perform an OPQRRRST evaluation.
- Administer oxygen via nasal cannula at 4 L/min.
  - If $SpO_2 < 92\%$ and the patient is in respiratory distress, administer oxygen via a non-rebreather mask at 15 L/min.
- Perform a focused physical exam.
- EMTs should:
  - Assist the patient in self-administration of previously prescribed aspirin.
  - Assist the patient in self-administration of previously prescribed nitroglycerin. The total dose should not exceed three doses (tablets or spray), including doses that the patient may have taken prior to your arrival.
- Do not administer nitroglycerin if:
  - SBP < 90 mm Hg.
  - The patient has taken erectile dysfunction medications within the last 24 hours (Viagra) or within the last 48 hours (Levitra or Cialis).

ALS Level I

- Monitor the ECG.
- Establish IV access; give normal saline KVO.
- Give aspirin 162 mg, up to 324 mg PO (chewable), unless contraindicated (a).
- Perform a 12-lead ECG and transmit the results to the destination hospital, if possible.
- If an inferior wall MI is identified, perform an additional 12-lead ECG with V4R to confirm/rule out concurrent right ventricular MI (b).
- If the patient is hypotensive (SBP < 90 mm Hg), see Adult Protocol 2.4.1, Cardiogenic Shock.

2.4.2 Chest Pain/Suspected AMI

- If the patient is experiencing chest pain or discomfort and systolic BP ≥ 90 mm Hg, administer nitroglycerin (Nitrostat® or Nitrolingual® Spray) 0.4 mg SL; repeat every 3–5 minutes (maximum dose = 1.2 mg).
- **Do not administer nitroglycerin if:**
  - SBP < 90 mm Hg.
  - The patient has taken erectile dysfunction medications within the last 24 hours (Viagra) or within the last 48 hours (Levitra or Cialis).
- If pain is reduced or relieved with nitroglycerin SL, apply 1–2 inches of nitropaste (Nitro-Bid® ointment) to the patient's chest (spread nitropaste on the chest to an area the size of the patient's palm), if available.
- If pain continues and the patient is normotensive (systolic BP > 90 mm Hg), administer morphine sulfate via slow IV in 2-mg increments every 3–5 minutes, titrated to pain and BP ≥ 90 mm Hg, up to a maximum of 10 mg.
- Treat dysrhythmia per specific protocol.
- Perform fibrinolytic screening (see Medical Procedure 4.38).
- **If AMI is probable (c), initiate a Cardiac Alert and transport the patient to the appropriate cardiac interventional facility.**
- If an ST-elevation MI (STEMI) is identified (c) with signs, symptoms, and history suggestive of AMI, and the patient has a heart rate > 80 beats/min with SBP > 110 mm Hg, administer Lopressor 5 mg via slow IVP. Consider repeating once in 5 minutes if heart rate > 80 beats/min and SBP > 110 mm Hg.

ALS Level 2

- If there is a delay in transport and heart rate > 80 beats/min with SBP > 110 mm Hg, administer a third dose of Lopressor 5 mg via slow IVP.
- Administer a nitroglycerin (Tridil®) infusion at 5 mcg/min, if available. Titrate to effect, with the maximum dose being 20 mcg/min.

Note

(a) Allergies to ASA should be suspected in patients with anaphylaxis signs and symptoms (e.g., flushed itchy skin, increased heart rate, dyspnea, urticaria).

(b) Bradycardia with hypotension may be due to an inferior wall MI associated with right ventricular MI (confirmed on 12-lead ECG by ST elevation in lead V4R); see Adult Protocol 2.3.2, Bradycardia. When an inferior wall MI is associated with right ventricular MI, avoid the use of nitrates (nitroglycerin). If bradycardia and hypotension exist, pacing and IV fluids may improve the patient's hemodynamic status.

(c) AMI is probable when there is:

1. A minimum of 1-mm ST elevation in two or more related leads on the 12-lead ECG with a history suggestive of AMI.
2. A left bundle branch block (LBBB) on the ECG with signs/symptoms and history suggestive of AMI.

2.4.3 Hypertensive Emergencies

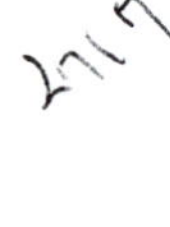

This protocol should be applied to patients who have a systolic BP > 220 mm Hg and/or a diastolic BP > 120 mm Hg and who are experiencing symptoms (headache and/or neck pain, epistaxis). Do not delay transport. Eclampsia should be considered with female patients in their third trimester of pregnancy or postpartum who are hypertensive and/or seizing (see Adult Protocol 2.7.4).

Supportive Care

- Medical Supportive Care Protocol 2.1.3: Administer oxygen via nasal cannula at 4 L/min (use a non-rebreather mask at 15 L/min if $SpO_2 < 92\%$). If the patient is asymptomatic, contact medical control.

ALS Level 1

- If the patient has pulmonary edema, see Adult Protocol 2.2.4.
- If the patient has signs of CVA (altered mental status or focal deficit), see Adult Protocol 2.5.4.
- If the patient is experiencing pain or is agitated, treat the underlying cause (e.g., alcohol withdrawal, musculoskeletal injury, amphetamine or cocaine use).

ALS Level 2

- Give labetolol (Normodyne® or Trandate®) 20 mg IV over 2 minutes for hypertension not associated with CVA (a); this treatment may be repeated in 20 minutes.
- Give nitrostat 0.4 mg SL; this treatment may be repeated two times (a)(b).

Note

(a) **In the presence of acute stroke (CVA), hypertension may be lowered in special circumstances only with a physician order (Level 2).**

(b) If available, a nitroglycerin (Tridil®) infusion may be given at 5–20 mcg/min, for hypertension not associated with CVA.

2.5 Adult Neurologic Emergencies

The paramedic should use these protocols to guide him/her through the treatment of atraumatic patients with signs and symptoms that are suggestive of neurological impairment or when the cause of the patient's altered mental status is unknown. In addition to these protocols, the paramedic may need to refer to other protocols for continued treatment (e.g., adult cardiac dysrhythmias protocols).

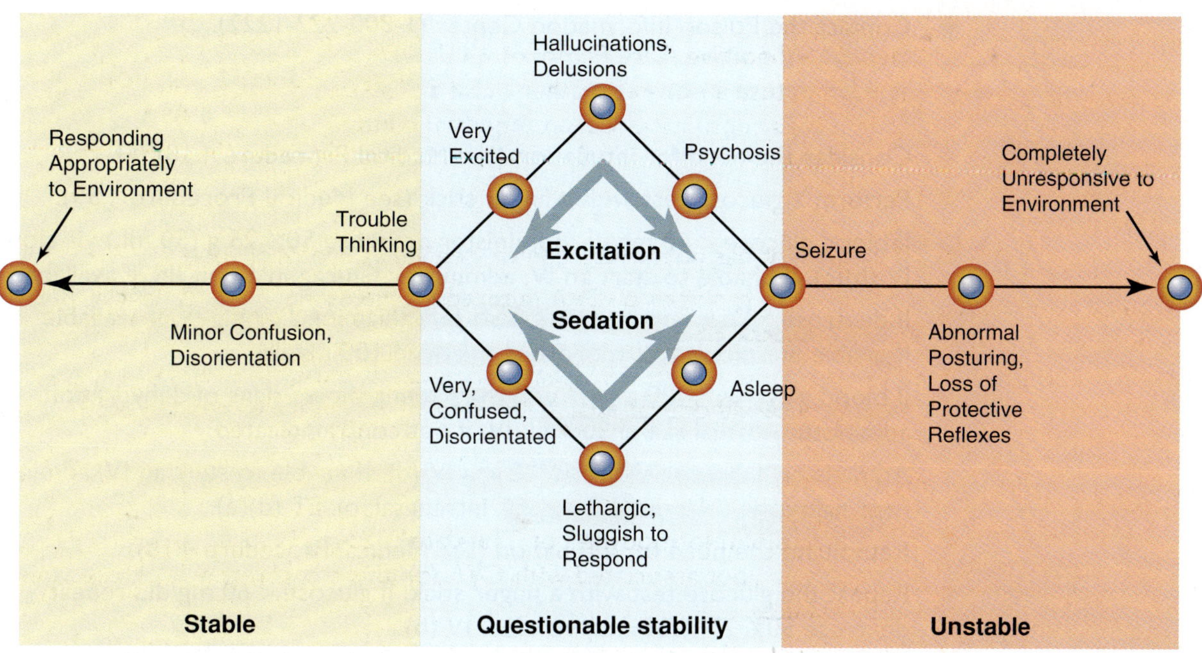

Level of consciousness continuum.

2.5.1 Altered Mental Status Unknown Etiology

This protocol is used for patients with altered mental status where the etiology is unknown (e.g., patients with a history of diabetes; see Adult Protocol 2.8.2).

Supportive Care

- Medical Supportive Care Protocol 2.1.3: Consider the need for cervical spine immobilization.
- Contact the Poison Information Center (1-800-222-1222).

ALS Level 1

- Consider the need for intubation (see Medical Procedure 4.18) (a).
- Perform a glucose test with a finger stick (see Medical Procedure 4.39).
- If blood glucose < 60 mg/dL, administer dextrose 50% 25 g (50 mL) via slow IV (b)(c). If unable to start an IV, administer Glucagon 1 unit IM, if available.
- If dextrose 50% is administered, also give thiamine 100 mg IV, if available. If unable to start an IV, administer thiamine 100 mg IM.
- If blood glucose > 300 mg/dL and the patient shows signs of dehydration, administer normal saline 500 mL IV, if not contraindicated.
- Administer naloxone (Narcan®) 2 mg IV (d). If unable to start an IV, administer naloxone (Narcan®) 2 mg IM, intranasal, or ET (d)(e).
- Reevaluate the need for intubation (see Medical Procedure 4.18).
- Repeat the glucose test with a finger stick. If glucose < 60 mg/dL, repeat dextrose 50% 25 g (50 mL) via slow IV (b).
- Repeat naloxone (Narcan®) 2 mg IV *as needed.*

ALS Level 2

None.

NOTE

(a) Use appropriate discretion regarding immediate intubation of patients who may quickly regain consciousness, such as hypoglycemics after administration of D_{50} or opiate overdose cases after administration of Narcan.

(b) To avoid infiltration and resultant tissue necrosis, dextrose 50% should be given via slow IV with intermittent aspiration of the IV line to confirm IV patency, followed by saline flush.

(c) If the patient is conscious with control of the airway, oral glucose may be given.

(d) Narcan should be administered slowly (e.g., 0.4 mg/min) when the patient's history is unknown or there is a possibility of chronic use of narcotics. Administration of Narcan to patients with chronic use of narcotics may induce withdrawal, seizures, and/or violent behavior. In these instances, the therapeutic goal is to restore adequate ventilatory effort. Consider restraining the patient (see Medical Procedure 4.41, Physical Restraints).

(e) Intranasal administration of Narcan requires the use of a mucosal atomization device.

2: adult protocols

2.5.2 Violent and/or Impaired Patient

This treatment protocol is used in conjunction with General Protocol 2.1, Behavioral Emergencies. If the patient is violent and poses an immediate threat to self, the EMS crew, or bystanders, restraints should be used to prevent the patient from harming himself/herself or others. If the patient is not violent, be observant for the possibility of violence and avoid provoking the patient. **Particular caution should be exercised when any "nonlethal" law enforcement device (e.g., pepper spray, Taser) has been employed.**

Supportive Care

- Have the patient placed under the Baker Act via the police when appropriate, and refer to the Impaired/Incapacitated Persons Act (see General Protocol 2.1).
- Follow Medical Supportive Care Protocol 2.1.3 (a).
- Rule out non-psychiatric causes (e.g., drug overdose, CVA, ETOH, hypoxia, hypoglycemia).
- Physically restrain the patient **only** when appropriate (see Medical Procedure 4.41).

ALS Level 1

- Administer one of the following benzodiazepines:
  - **Diazepam (Valium®)** 5 mg IV or intranasal; may repeat once *as needed,* up to a maximum dose of 10 mg (b).

  or

  - **Midazolam (Versed®)** 2 mg IV or intranasal; may repeat once *as needed,* up to a maximum dose of 4 mg (b).

  or

  - **Lorazepam (Ativan®)** 2 mg IV, IM, or intranasal; may repeat once *as needed,* up to a maximum dose of 4 mg (a)(b).
- Administer diphenhydramine HCl (Benadryl®) 50 mg IM or IV (a).

ALS Level 2

- Administer haloperidol (Haldol®) 5 mg IM or IV. If not already given, administer diphenhydramine HCl (Benadryl®) 50 mg IM or 25 mg IV (a)(c)(d).
- Repeat haloperidol (Haldol®) 5 mg IM or IV (a)(c)(d).

Note

(a) In some instances, IV administration may present a safety concern; in these case, IM administration of sedatives may be the more desirable route.

(b) Intranasal administration of benzodiazepines requires the use of a mucosal atomization device.

(c) Haloperidol (Haldol®) may result in a dystonic reaction if it is administered alone. This effect can be avoided or reversed with Benadryl.

(d) **Haloperidol should be used with caution in cases of suspected overdose, especially cocaine, and its use should be preceded by benzodiazepine administration.**

2: adult protocols

2.5.3 Seizure Disorders

This protocol should be used when the patient has witnessed, continuous convulsions (generalized tonic–clonic seizure or grand mal) or repeating episodes without regaining consciousness or sufficient respiratory decompensation. Consider the underlying etiology, such as hypoglycemia, drug overdose, head injury, or fever. Other types of seizures include absence (petit mal), simple partial (focal motor and Jacksonian), complex partial (psychomotor or temporal lobe), atonic (drop attacks), and myoclonic. When the patient is continuously showing signs of these other types of seizures, Medical Supportive Care Protocol 2.1.3 should be initiated and the paramedic should contact medical control for further direction.

Supportive Care

- Medical Supportive Care 2.1.3.

ALS Level 1

- If the patient is an eclamptic female, administer magnesium sulfate 4 g IV (mixed in 50 mL of D_5W given over 5–10 minutes). See Adult Protocol 2.7.4, Toxemia of Pregnancy (a).
- Administer one of the following benzodiazepines:
  - **Diazepam (Valium®)** 5 mg IV or intranasal; may repeat once *as needed,* up to a maximum dose of 10 mg (b)(c).

  or

  - **Midazolam (Versed®)** 2 mg IV or intranasal; may repeat once *as needed,* up to a maximum dose of 4 mg (b).

  or

  - **Lorazepam (Ativan®)** 2 mg IV, IM, or intranasal; may repeat once *as needed,* up to a maximum dose of 4 mg (b).
- Administer diphenhydramine HCl (Benadryl®) 50 mg IM or IV.
- Perform a glucose test with a finger stick (see Medical Procedure 4.39).
- If glucose < 60 mg/dL, administer dextrose 50% 25 g (50 mL) via slow IV (d). If unable to start an IV, administer Glucagon 1 unit IM if available.
- If dextrose 50% is administered, also give thiamine 100 mg IV, if available. If unable to start an IV, administer thiamine 100 mg IM.

ALS Level 2

None.

2.5.3 Seizure Disorders

NOTE

(a) Females in their second or third trimester of pregnancy (≥ 20 weeks gestation) who are seizing should be assumed to have eclampsia. It should also be noted that eclampsia can occur postpartum (≤ 1 week after giving birth).

(b) Intranasal administration of benzodiazepines requires the use of a mucosal atomization device.

(c) Valium may be given *as needed* for seizures as a Level 1 order up to a total dose of 10 mg IV or PR. Additional Valium (more than 10 mg total dose) is Level 2 care only. Use a lubricated 3–5 mL syringe **without the needle** to administer diazepam (Valium®). Position the patient in a decubitus knee position or supine with the legs held apart, and insert lubricated syringe approximately 5 cm (approximately 2 inches) into the rectum. Inject Valium, remove the syringe, and tape the buttocks closed.

(d) To avoid infiltration and resultant tissue necrosis, D_{50} should be given via slow IV with intermittent aspiration of the IV line to confirm IV patency, followed by saline flush.

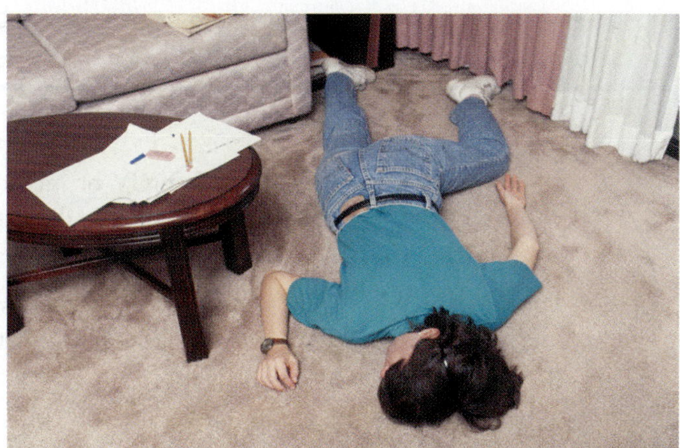

A patient who has had a seizure may be found in the postictal state when you arrive. If this is the case, be sure to ask family members or bystanders to verify that a seizure has occurred and how the seizure developed.

2.5.4 Suspected Stroke (CVA)

This protocol is used for those patients exhibiting signs consistent with acute stroke/cerebrovascular accident (CVA)/"brain attack," such as altered mental status, slurred speech, loss of function of any body part, hemiplegia, loss of vision, weakness of facial muscles, loss of sensation, and drooling. Other causes should be ruled out (e.g., hypoglycemia, drug overdose, hypoxia).

History	Signs and Symptoms	Differential Diagnosis
Previous stroke/TIA Previous neurological deficit Hypertension Heart disease Diabetes Anticoagulant medications Family history Smoking	Impaired understanding of speech Aphasia/dysarthria Weakness/hemiparesis Facial droop Poor coordination/balance Loss of peripheral vision Syncope, dizziness/vertigo Headache, vomiting, stiff neck, seizures	TIA Seizure Hypoglycemia Drug ingestion Tumor Trauma **Stroke:** ◆ Ischemic ◆ Hemorrhagic

Stroke Alert Criteria

- Time of onset < 5 hours.
- *Any* "abnormal" findings on Cincinnati Prehospital Stroke Scale (CPSS) or on expanded neurological examination.
- Deficit not likely due to head trauma or stroke mimic.
- Blood glucose > 60 mg/dL.

Supportive Care

- Assess the ABCs and vital signs.
- Perform a SAMPLE history.
- Position the patient supine, with head elevation of 30 degrees, unless the patient cannot tolerate this position.
- Administer oxygen according to following criteria:
  - $SpO_2 \geq 92\%$: Do not administer O_2.
  - $SpO_2 < 92\%$: Administer O_2 by nasal cannula at 2 L/min.
- If SpO_2 cannot be maintained at 92% with nasal cannula at 2 L/min and/or the patient is in respiratory distress, administer high-flow O_2 and assist ventilations with a bag-valve mask if indicated.
- **Determine and document the time of onset of stroke symptoms,** defined as "the last time the patient was seen without symptoms."

2.5.4 Suspected Stroke (CVA)

ALS Level 1

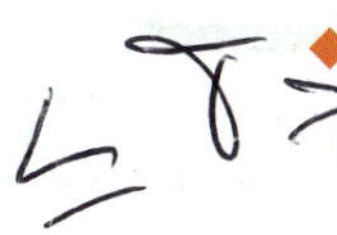

- If the patient has a decreased level of consciousness and does not have an intact gag reflex, intubate the patient (see Medical Procedure 4.18), confirm tube placement and oxygenation, and monitor ventilations with $EtCO_2$.
- Establish IV access; give normal saline KVO.
- Perform a glucose test with a finger stick (see Medical Procedure 4.39). If glucose < 60 mg/dL, administer D_{50} 25 g (50 mL) IVP. Recheck glucose in 5 minutes, and reevaluate the patient.
- If drug overdose is suspected, refer to Adult Protocol 2.6, Adult Toxicologic Emergencies.
- Perform a neurological exam, including assessment of the patient's level of consciousness, Glasgow Coma Scale score, and **Cincinnati Prehospital Stroke Scale (CPSS) score.**
- If CVA is suspected, complete the "Stroke Alert" checklist (see the Online Forms). **If the patient meets the Stoke Alert criteria and symptom onset occurred ≤ 5 hours previously, initiate a Stroke Alert** (a)(b).
- If a Stroke Alert is initiated, perform fibrinolytic screening (see Medical Procedure 4.38).
- Urgently transport the patient to the closest appropriate stroke center.
- Contact the stroke center, and advise its personnel of the time of symptom onset, baseline neurological examination findings, and any changes found in reassessment.

ALS Level 2

- Elevated blood pressure is commonly present with stroke. Severely elevated blood pressure may be lowered with a physician order.

NOTE

(a) Minimize the Stroke Alert on-scene time to 10 minutes or less.
(b) If your findings do not indicate the patient has experienced an ischemic or hemorrhagic stroke, see the appropriate protocol.
(c) Continually reassess the patient to determine if his/her symptoms are worsening or improving, and advise the stroke center of any changes.

2.5.5 Syncopal Episode

This protocol should be used for patients with a chief complaint of syncopal episode. **Consider the patient's history and the possibility of medication side effects, glucose imbalance, inner ear disorders, CVA, TIA, and MI.**

Supportive Care

- Medical Supportive Care 2.1.3 (refer to other protocols as appropriate): Treat the underlying cause, if it can be determined.
- All patients with a known syncopal episode, or a syncopal episode that was witnessed by a reliable source, should be transported to the hospital via ambulance.

ALS Level 1

- Perform a 12-lead ECG. If an inferior wall MI is identified, perform an additional 12-lead ECG with V4R to confirm/rule out concurrent right ventricular MI. Transmit the 12-lead ECG results to the destination hospital, if possible (a). If acute coronary syndrome is suspected, see Adult Protocol 2.4.2.

ALS Level 2

None.

Note

(a) Bradycardia with hypotension may be due to inferior wall MI associated with right ventricular MI (confirmed on the 12-lead ECG by ST elevation in lead V4R); see Adult Protocol 2.3.2, Bradycardia. When an inferior wall MI is associated with right ventricular MI, avoid the use of nitrates (nitroglycerin). If bradycardia and hypotension exist, pacing and IV fluid may improve the patient's hemodynamic status.

2.6 Adult Toxicologic Emergencies

This protocol is to be used for those patients suspected of exposure to toxic substances via any route of exposure (e.g., drug overdose, snake bite). The protocols give specific considerations for each type of exposure as well as general treatment guidelines. Additional assistance may be necessary in certain cases (e.g., hazardous materials team for toxic exposure or police for scene control, including management of a violent and/or impaired patient; see Adult Protocol 2.5.2). **If the toxic substance is unknown or cannot be readily determined, see Adult Protocol 2.6.7, Unknown Toxicity.**

A history of the events leading to the illness or injury should be obtained from the patient and bystanders:

1. To which drugs, poisons, or other substances was the patient exposed? Consider exposure to multiple substances, especially on overdoses.
2. What was the route of exposure?
3. When did the exposure occur, and how much exposure was there?
4. What is the duration of symptoms?
5. Is the patient depressed or suicidal? Does he/she have a history of previous overdose (if applicable)?
6. Was the exposure accidental? What was the nature of the accident?
7. What was the duration of exposure (if applicable)?

Collect all pill bottles, empty or full, and check for "suicide notes" (if applicable). Transport any/all information or items that may assist in the treatment of the patient to the emergency department.

Contact the Poison Information Center (1-800-222-1222) for consultation regarding specific therapy.

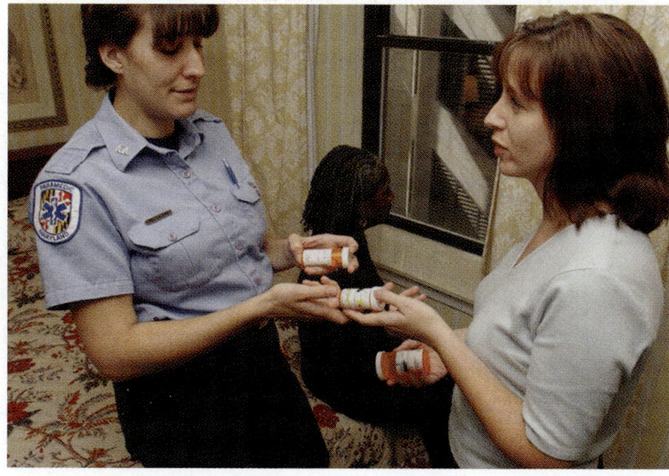

Collect all pill bottles, empty or full.

2.6.1 Bites and Stings

This protocol includes the treatment for snake bites, dog and cat bites, insect stings, and marine animal envenomations and stings. All bite victims should be transported to the hospital. **Contact the Poison Information Center (1-800-222-1222) for treatment and transport decision and consultation in all cases involving bites and stings.**

Snake Bites

Supportive Care

- Trauma Supportive Care Protocol 2.1.4.
- Consider the need for Adult Protocol 2.8.1, Allergic Reactions/Anaphylaxis.
- Contact the Poison Information Center (1-800-222-1222).
- Splint the affected area. Place the patient supine, with extremities kept at a neutral level. Keep patient quiet. Remove and secure all jewelry.
- Wash the area of the bite with copious amounts of water.
- Attempt to identify the snake, if it is safe to do so.
- Check the patient's temperature and pulse distal to the bite on an extremity, and mark the level of swelling and time with pen every 15 minutes.

ALS Level 1

- Refer to Adult Protocol 2.1.5 for pain management guidelines.

ALS Level 2

None.

Dog, Cat, and Wild Animal Bites

Supportive Care

- Trauma Supportive Care Protocol 2.1.4 (see Appendix 7.19, Infectious Exposure Reference Sheet).
- Wound care: BLS (do not use hydrogen peroxide on deep puncture wounds or wounds exposing fat). Clean the wound area with soap and water.
- Advise dispatch to contact animal control and the police department for identification and quarantine of the animal.
- Contact the Poison Information Center (1-800-222-1222).

ALS Level 1

- Refer to Adult Protocol 2.1.5 for pain management guidelines.

ALS Level 2

None.

2.6.1 Bites and Stings

Insect Stings (Including Centipedes, Scorpions, and Spiders)

Supportive Care

- Trauma Supportive Care Protocol 2.1.4.
- Consider the need for Adult Protocol 2.8.1, Allergic Reactions/Anaphylaxis.
- Remove the stinger by scraping the patient's skin with the edge of a flat surface (e.g., a credit card). Do not attempt to pull the stinger out, as this action may release more venom.
- Clean the wound area with soap and water.
- Contact the Poison Information Center (1-800-222-1222).

ALS Level 1

- Refer to Adult Protocol 2.1.5 for pain management guidelines.

ALS Level 2

None.

Marine Animal Envenomations: Stingray, Scorpionfish (Lionfish, Zebrafish, Stonefish), Catfish, Weeverfish, Starfish, Sea Urchin

Supportive Care

- Trauma Supportive Care Protocol 2.1.4.
- Consider the need for Adult Protocol 2.8.1, Allergic Reactions/Anaphylaxis.
- Immerse the punctures in nonscalding hot water to tolerance (110–113°F) to achieve pain relief (30–90 minutes). Transport should not be delayed for this measure; immersion in nonscalding hot water may be continued during transport.
- Remove any visible pieces of the spine(s) or sheath. Gently wash the wound with soap and water, and then irrigate it vigorously with fresh water (avoid scrubbing).
- Contact the Poison Information Center (1-800-222-1222).

ALS Level 1

- Refer to Adult Protocol 2.1.5 for pain management guidelines.

ALS Level 2

None.

2.6.1 Bites and Stings

Marine Animal Stings: Jellyfish, Man-of-War, Sea Nettle, Irukandji, Anemone, Hydroid, Fire Coral

Supportive Care

- Trauma Supportive Care Protocol 2.1.4.
- Consider the need for Adult Protocol 2.8.1, Allergic Reactions/Anaphylaxis.
- Rinse the skin with sea water. (Do not use fresh water; do not apply ice; do not rub the skin.)
- Apply soaks of acetic acid 5% (vinegar) until the pain is relieved. If vinegar is not available, use a paste of baking soda or unseasoned meat tenderizer.
- Remove large tentacle fragments using forceps (use gloves to avoid contact with your bare hands).
- Apply a lather of shaving cream or a paste of baking soda, and shave the affected area with the edge of a flat surface (e.g., a credit card).
- Contact the Poison Information Center (1-800-222-1222).

ALS Level 1

- Refer to Adult Protocol 2.1.5 for pain management guidelines.

ALS Level 2

None.

Human Bites

Supportive Care

- Trauma Supportive Care Protocol 2.1.4 (see General Protocol 1.12, Personal Exposure to Infectious Diseases).
- Wound care: BLS (do not use hydrogen peroxide on deep puncture wounds or wounds exposing fat). Clean the wound area with soap and water.
- Consider contacting the police department for investigation.

ALS Level 1

- Refer to Adult Protocol 2.1.5 for pain management guidelines.

ALS Level 2

None.

2.6.2 CNS Depressant Overdose

Signs and symptoms of CNS depressant overdose include altered mental status, respiratory depression, hypotension, bradycardia, pulmonary edema, coma, and constricted pupils (opioids only). The following is a partial list of CNS depressants.

Barbiturates: Generic Name (Trade Name)

butabarbital sodium (Butisol Sodium)
mephobarbital (Mebaral)
pentobarbital sodium (Nembutal Sodium)
phenobarbital
secobarbital sodium (Seconal Sodium)

Benzodiazepines: Generic Name (Trade Name)

alprazolam (Xanax)
chlordiazepoxide (Librium)
clonazepam (Klonopin)
clorazepate (Tranxene)
diazepam (Valium)
flunitrazepam (Rohypnol)
flurazepam (Dalmane)
halazepam (Paxipam)
lorazepam (Ativan)
midazolam (Versed)
oxazepam (Serax)
prazepam (Centrax)
quazepam (Doral)
temazepam (Restoril)
triazolam (Halcion)

Designer Drugs

Blue Nitro, GHB

2.6.2 CNS Depressant Overdose

Opioids, Narcotics, Synthetics, and Combinations: Generic Name (Trade Name)

acetaminophen and codeine phosphate (Tylenol #3, Tylenol #4)
alfentanil HCl (Alfenta)
alfentanyl (Alfenta)
alphaprodine (Nisentil)
aspirin and codeine phosphate (Empirin with Codeine #3 and #4)
belladonna and opium (B & O Supprettes)
buprenophine (Buprenex)
butalbital, aspirin, caffeine, codeine phosphate (Fiorinol or Fioricet with Codeine)
butorphanol (Stadol)
codeine
dextromethorphan
diacetylmorphine (heroin)
diamorphine (heroin)
difenoxin HCl with atropine sulfate (Motofin)
dihydrocodeine bitartrate, acetaminophen, and caffeine (DHCplus)
diphenoxylate HCl and atropine sulfate (Lomotil)—no miosis
fentanyl citrate (Sublimaze)
fentanyl citrate and droperidol (Innovar)
fentanyl transdermal (Duragesic)
hydrocodone bitartrate (Loratab, Hycodan, Anexsia)
hydrocodone bitartrate and acetaminophen (Hydrocet, Loracet, Vicodin)
hydromorphone HCl (Dilaudid, Hydrostat)
levorphanol tartrate (Levo-Dromoran)
loperamide HCl (Imodium, Imodium A-D)
meperidine HCl (Demerol)—no miosis
meperidine HCl and promethazine HCl (Mepergan)—no miosis
methodone HCl (Dolophine)
morphine sulfate (Astramorph/PF, Duramorph, Infumorph 200, Infumorph 500, MS Contin, MSIR, Oramorph, Rescudose, Roxanol)
nalbuphine HCl (Nubain)
napsylate (Darvocet-N)
oxycodone (Percodan, Percocet, Tylox, Roxicodone)
oxymorphone HCl (Numorphan)
pentazocine HCl (Talwin, Talacen)
propoxyphene HCl (Darvon-N)
propoxyphene HCl and acetaminophen (Wygesic)
sufentanil (Sufenta)

2.6.2 CNS Depressant Overdose

Sedative Hypnotics: Generic Name (Trade Name)

Compoz
estazolam (Prosom)
ethchlorvynol (Placidyl)
etomidate (Amidate)
propofol (Diprivan)
Sleep-Eze
Sominex
zolpidem tartrate (Ambien)

Selective Serotonin Reuptake Inhibitors (SSRIs): Generic Name (Trade Name)

citalopram (Celexa)
fluoxetine (Prozac)
fluvoxamine (Luvox)
paroxetine (Paxil)
sertraline (Zoloft)

Supportive Care

- Medical Supportive Care 2.1.3.
- Contact the Poison Information Center (1-800-222-1222).

ALS Level 1

- Consider the need for intubation (see Medical Procedure 4.18) (a).
- Perform a glucose test with a finger stick (see Medical Procedure 4.39). If glucose < 60 mg/dL, see Adult Protocol 2.8.2, Diabetic Emergencies.
- If ECG QRS complex is wide (> 0.10), administer sodium bicarbonate 1 mEq/kg IV (see Adult Protocol 2.6.6).
- If respiration is depressed, administer naloxone (Narcan®) 2 mg IV (b).
- If no response, repeat naloxone (Narcan®) 2 mg IV *as needed.*
- If the patient is experiencing chest pain, see Adult Protocol 2.4.2, Chest Pain/Suspected AMI.

2.6.2 CNS Depressant Overdose

- If the patient is seizing, administer one of the following benzodiazepines:
  - **Diazepam (Valium®)** 5 mg IV. If unable to start an IV, administer diazepam 5 mg intranasal or 10 mg per rectum. May repeat *as needed,* up to a maximum dose of 20 mg (c)(d).

  or

  - **Lorazepam (Ativan®)** 2 mg IV. If unable to start an IV, administer lorazepam 2 mg IM. May repeat once *as needed,* up to a maximum dose of 4 mg.

  or

  - **Midazolam (Versed®)** 2 mg IV. If unable to start an IV, administer midazolam 2 mg intranasal. May repeat once *as needed,* up to a maximum dose of 4 mg (c).
- If the patient is hypotensive (systolic BP < 90 mm Hg), administer a fluid challenge of 500 mL.
- If the patient is combative, consider the need for physical and chemical restraints (see Adult Protocol 2.5.2, Violent and/or Impaired Patient, and Medical Procedure 4.41, Physical Restraints).

ALS Level 2

- Treat tachydysrhythmias as per physician order.
- Consider additional fluid challenge if the patient is still hypotensive.

NOTE

(a) Use appropriate discretion regarding immediate intubation of patients who may quickly regain consciousness, such as hypoglycemics after D_{50} administration or opiate overdose patients after Narcan administration.

(b) If the patient is a suspected opioid addict, the administration of Narcan should be titrated (e.g., 0.4 mg/min) to increase respirations to normal levels without fully awakening the patient, so as to prevent hostile and confrontational episodes. Consider restraining the patient (see Medical Procedure 4.41, Physical Restraints). Naloxone (Narcan®) may need to be repeated in 20–30 minutes to maintain effect.

(c) Intranasal administration of benzodiazepines requires the use of a mucosal atomization device.

(d) Use a lubricated 3–5 mL syringe **without the needle** to administer diazepam (Valium®). Position the patient in a decubitus knee position or supine with the legs held apart, and insert the lubricated syringe approximately 5 cm (approximately 2 inches) into the rectum. Inject the Valium, remove the syringe, and tape the buttocks closed.

2.6.3 CNS Stimulant Overdose

Signs and symptoms of CNS stimulant overdose include dilated pupils, agitation, paranoia, bizarre behavior, PVC, tachycardia, hypertension, hyperthermia, and seizures. The following is a partial list of CNS stimulants.

COCAINE

Cocaine, crack (a)

AMPHETAMINES

Amphetamine variants (DMA, PMA, STP, MDA, MMDA, TMA, DOM, DOB)

DESIGNER DRUGS

Ecstasy

Supportive Care

- Medical Supportive Care 2.1.3.
- Contact the Poison Information Center (1-800-222-1222).

ALS Level I

- If the patient is experiencing chest pain, see Adult Protocol 2.4.2, Chest Pain/Suspected AMI.
- Establish IV access; give normal saline.
- If the patient is seizing, administer one of the following benzodiazepines:
  - **Diazepam (Valium®)** 5 mg IV. If unable to start an IV, administer diazepam 5 mg intranasal or 10 mg per rectum. May repeat *as needed*, up to a maximum dose of 20 mg (b)(c).

    or
  - **Lorazepam (Ativan®)** 2 mg IV. If unable to start an IV, administer lorazepam 2 mg IM. May repeat once *as needed*, up to a maximum dose of 4 mg.

    or
  - **Midazolam (Versed®)** 2 mg IV. If unable to start an IV, administer midazolam 2 mg intranasal (b). May repeat once *as needed*, up to a maximum dose of 4 mg.
- If the patient is hyperthermic (hot to the touch), aggressively cool the patient.
- If the patient is combative, consider the need for physical and chemical restraints (see Adult Protocol 2.5.2, Violent and/or Impaired Patient, and Medical Procedure 4.41, Physical Restraints).

2.6.3 CNS Stimulant Overdose

ALS Level 2

- Treat tachydysrhythmias as per physician order.

NOTE

(a) Beta blockers are contraindicated in cocaine overdose.

(b) Intranasal administration of benzodiazepines requires the use of a mucosal atomization device.

(c) Use a lubricated 3–5 mL syringe **without the needle** to administer diazepam (Valium®). Position the patient in a decubitus knee position or supine with the legs held apart, and insert the lubricated syringe approximately 5 cm (approximately 2 inches) into the rectum. Inject the Valium, remove the syringe, and tape the buttocks closed.

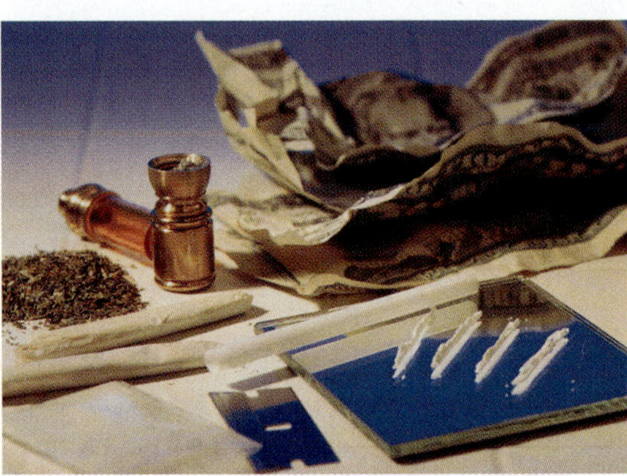

2.6.4 Digitalis Toxicity

Digitalis toxicity should be suspected in patients who are taking digitalis and have signs and symptoms associated with digitalis toxicity—for example, bradycardia, AV blocks with rapid ventricular response, supraventricular tachycardias, ventricular ectopy, and other ECG changes: wide PR interval > 0.20, short QT interval (rate dependent), spoon-shaped ST segment, peaked T wave. Contact with the oleander tree can also cause a digitalis-type toxicity, which will cause the same type of dysrhythmias and requires the same treatment.

Digitalis: Generic Name (Trade Name)

digoxin (Lanoxicaps, Lanoxin, Digoxin)
digitoxin (Crystodigin)

Supportive Care

- Medical Supportive Care 2.1.3.
- Contact the Poison Information Center (1-800-222-1222).

ALS Level 1

- Treat tachydysrhythmias with medication per specific protocol (see Adult Protocol 2.3). Avoid the use of calcium chloride.
- If unstable tachycardia (heart rate > 150 beats/min), synchronize and cardiovert. Energy settings for synchronized cardioversion should be in the range of 5–20 joules.
- If the patient has unstable bradycardia with wide QRS (> 0.10 second), administer sodium bicarbonate 1 mEq/kg IV.

ALS Level 2

None.

2.6.5 Hallucinogen Overdose

This protocol includes the hallucinogenic drugs: LSD (acid, microdot), mescaline and peyote (mesc, buttons, cactus), and similar agents (e.g., DET, EMT, psilocybin). Signs and symptoms of hallucinogen overdose include illusions and hallucinations, poor perception of time and distance, possible paranoia, anxiety, panic, unpredictable behavior, emotional instability, possible flashbacks, dilated pupils, and rambling speech.

Supportive Care

- Medical Supportive Care 2.1.3: "Talk down" the patient.
- Contact the Poison Information Center (1-800-222-1222).

ALS Level I

- Consider the need for intubation (see Medical Procedure 4.18) (a).
- Perform a glucose test with a finger stick. If glucose < 60 mg/dL, see Adult Protocol 2.8.2, Diabetic Emergencies.
- If respiration is depressed, administer naloxone (Narcan®) 2 mg IV (b). If there is no response, repeat naloxone (Narcan®) 2 mg IV *as needed.*
- If the patient is experiencing chest pain, see Adult Protocol 2.4.2, Chest Pain/Suspected AMI.
- If the patient is seizing, administer one of the following benzodiazepines:
  - **Diazepam (Valium®)** 5 mg IV. If unable to start an IV, administer diazepam 5 mg intranasal or 10 mg per rectum. May repeat *as needed,* up to a maximum dose of 20 mg (c)(d).

  or
  - **Lorazepam (Ativan®)** 2 mg IV. If unable to start an IV, administer lorazepam 2 mg IM. May repeat once *as needed,* up to a maximum dose of 4 mg.

  or
  - **Midazolam (Versed®)** 2 mg IV. If unable to start an IV, administer midazolam 2 mg intranasal. May repeat once *as needed,* up to a maximum dose of 4 mg (c).
- If the patient is combative, consider the need for physical and chemical restraints (see Adult Protocol 2.5.2, Violent and/or Impaired Patient, and Medical Procedure 4.41, Physical Restraints).

2: adult protocols

2.6.5 Hallucinogen Overdose

ALS Level 2

- Treat tachydysrhythmias as per physician order.

NOTE

(a) Use appropriate discretion regarding immediate intubation of patients who may quickly regain consciousness, such as hypoglycemics after D_{50} administration or opiate overdose patients after Narcan administration.

(b) If the patient is a suspected opioid addict, the administration of Narcan should be titrated (e.g., 0.4 mg/min) to increase respiration to normal levels without fully awakening the patient, so as to prevent hostile and confrontational episodes. Consider restraining the patient (see Medical Procedure 4.41, Physical Restraints). Naloxone (Narcan®) may need to be repeated in 20–30 minutes to maintain effect.

(c) Intranasal administration of benzodiazepines requires the use of a mucosal atomization device.

(d) Use a lubricated 3–5 mL syringe **without the needle** to administer diazepam (Valium®). Position the patient in a decubitus knee position or supine with the legs held apart, and insert the lubricated syringe approximately 5 cm (approximately 2 inches) into the rectum. Inject the Valium, remove the syringe, and tape the buttocks closed.

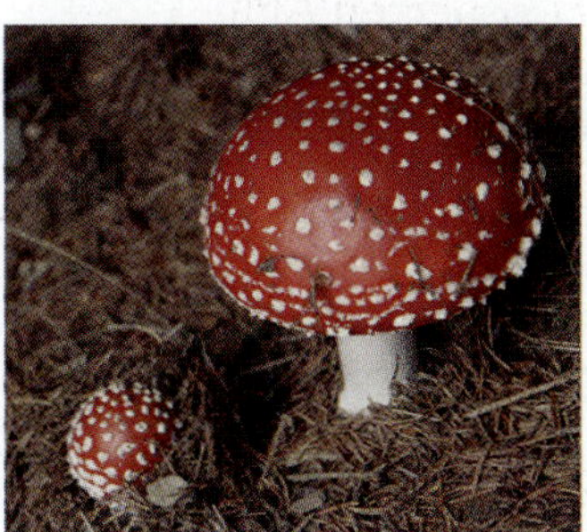

Certain mushrooms are hallucinogenic if ingested.

2.6.6 Tricyclic Antidepressant Overdose

Signs and symptoms of TCA overdose include CNS depression, tachycardia, dilated pupils, respiratory depression, slurred speech, twitching and jerking, seizures, ST-segment and T-wave changes, wide QRS complex, R waves in lead avR, S waves in lead avL and lead I, and shock.

Tricyclic Antidepressants: Generic Name (Trade Name)

amitriptyline HCl (Elavil, Endep)
amoxapine (Asendin)
chlordiazepoxide and amitriptyline HCl (Limbitrol)
clomipramin HCl (Anafranil)
desipramine HCl (Norpramin)
doxepin HCl (Adapin, Sinequan)
imipramine pamoate (Tofranil)
nortriptyline HCl (Pamelor)
perphenazine and amitriptyline HCl (Etrafon, Triavil)
protriptyline HCl (Vivactil)
trimipramine maleate (Surmontil)

Cyclic Antidepressants: Generic Name (Trade Name)

venlafaxine (Effexor)

Supportive Care

- Medical Supportive Care Protocol 2.1.3(a).
- Contact the Poison Information Center (1-800-222-1222).

2.6.6 Tricyclic Antidepressant Overdose

ALS Level 1

- Consider the need for intubation (see Medical Procedure 4.18).
- If QRS > 0.10 second, administer sodium bicarbonate 1 mEq/kg IV.
- If the patient is seizing, administer one of the following benzodiazepines:
  - **Diazepam (Valium®)** 5 mg IV. If unable to start an IV, administer diazepam 5 mg intranasal or 10 mg per rectum. May repeat *as needed*, up to a maximum dose of 20 mg (b)(c).

  or

  - **Lorazepam (Ativan®)** 2 mg IV. If unable to start an IV, administer lorazepam 2 mg IM. May repeat once *as needed*, up to a maximum dose of 4 mg.

  or

  - **Midazolam (Versed®)** 2 mg IV. If unable to start an IV, administer midazolam 2 mg intranasal. May repeat once *as needed*, up to a maximum dose of 4 mg (b).
- Perform a 12-lead ECG (see Medical Procedure 4.33).
- Treat dysrhythmias per specific protocol (see Adult Protocol 2.3).

ALS Level 2

None.

Note

(a) Romazicon, procainamide, and labetalol are contraindicated in tricyclic antidepressant overdose.

(b) Intranasal administration of benzodiazepines requires the use of a mucosal atomization device.

(c) Use a lubricated 3–5 mL syringe **without the needle** to administer diazepam (Valium®). Position the patient in a decubitus knee position or supine with the legs held apart, and insert the lubricated syringe approximately 5 cm (approximately 2 inches) into the rectum. Inject the Valium, remove the syringe, and tape the buttocks closed.

2.6.7 Unknown Toxicity

This protocol is to be used for those patients suspected of exposure to toxic substances via any route of exposure, where the toxic substance is unknown or cannot be readily determined.

Supportive Care

- Medical Supportive Care Protocol 2.1.3. If the patient has an altered mental status, dyspnea, or $SpO_2 < 92\%$, administer high-flow oxygen.
- Contact the Poison Information Center (1-800-222-1222).

ALS Level I

- If the patient has an altered mental status, see Adult Protocol 2.5.1.
- If bronchospasm is present, administer albuterol (Ventolin®): one nebulizer treatment containing 2.5 mg of albuterol premixed with 2.5 mL normal saline (see Medical Procedure 4.27). This treatment may be repeated twice as needed (a).
- If albuterol is administered, may add ipratropium bromide (Atrovent®) 0.5 mg (0.5 mL) to the albuterol nebulizer treatment **for the first nebulizer treatment only.**
- Treat dysrhythmias with medication per specific protocol (see Adult Protocol 2.3).
- If the patient has unstable bradycardia with wide QRS (> 0.10 second), administer sodium bicarbonate 1 mEq/kg IV (see Adult Protocol 2.6.6).
- If the patient is hypotensive and not in pulmonary edema, administer a fluid challenge of normal saline 500 mL IV (see Adult Protocol 2.4.1).
- If the patient is seizing, administer one of the following benzodiazepines:
    - **Diazepam (Valium®)** 5 mg IV. If unable to start an IV, administer diazepam 5 mg intranasal or 10 mg per rectum. May repeat *as needed,* up to a maximum dose of 20 mg (b)(c).

    or

    - **Lorazepam (Ativan®)** 2 mg IV. If unable to start an IV, administer lorazepam 2 mg IM. May repeat once *as needed,* up to a maximum dose of 4 mg.

    or

    - **Midazolam (Versed®)** 2 mg IV. If unable to start an IV, administer midazolam 2 mg intranasal. May repeat once *as needed,* up to a maximum dose of 4 mg (b).

2: adult protocols

2.6.7 Unknown Toxicity

ALS Level 2

- If the patient's heart rate ≥ 140, contact medical control for bronchodilator orders.

NOTE

(a) **Do not give albuterol or ipratropium bromide if the heart rate ≥ 140.**

(b) Intranasal administration of benzodiazepines requires the use of a mucosal atomization device.

(c) Use a lubricated 3–5 mL syringe **without the needle** to administer diazepam (Valium®). Position the patient in a decubitus knee position or supine with the legs held apart, and insert the lubricated syringe approximately 5 cm (approximately 2 inches) into the rectum. Inject the Valium, remove the syringe, and tape the buttocks closed.

2.7 Adult OB/GYN Emergencies

The paramedic should use these protocols to guide him/her through the treatment of patients who are pregnant. These protocols cover complications of pregnancy and normal and abnormal labor delivery. In addition to these protocols, the paramedic may need to refer to other protocols (e.g., protocols for seizures). The assessment of these patients should follow the normal approach to patient assessment as well as ask specific questions related to the history of the pregnancy. Questions for pregnancy history include:

1. Number of previous pregnancies (*gravida*).
   a. Miscarriages.
2. Number of previous live births (*para*).
3. Expected date of delivery or due date.
4. When did contractions begin?
5. Any history of labor complications?
   a. Premature births?
   b. C-section?
   c. Multiple births?
6. What are the duration and frequency of contractions?
   a. *Duration* is timed from when the contraction starts to when the contraction stops (e.g., 45 seconds, 1 minute).
   b. *Frequency* is timed from the beginning of one contraction to the beginning of the next contraction (e.g., 2 minutes apart, 4 minutes apart).
7. Evidence of blood show or spotting?
8. Did the water break?
   a. When?
   b. What was the color (e.g., clear, greenish, brownish)?
   c. Did it have an unusual odor?
9. Does the patient have an urge to push?
10. Does the patient feel like she has to move her bowels?

If the patient complains of uterine contractions, an external visual examination for crowning should be done to determine if the delivery is imminent.

2.7.1 Complications of Labor and Delivery

This protocol outlines the specific treatment for complications of labor and delivery. All care outlined is supportive care, with care for each specific problem starting with Trauma Supportive Care Protocol 2.1.4.

Supportive Care

- Trauma Supportive Care Protocol 2.1.4. Notify the nearest appropriate OB–capable hospital early and prepare for transport to an OB–capable hospital.

Prolapsed Cord

- Place the mother in a knee-chest position or supine position with pillows under the buttocks.
- Do not attempt to push the cord back. Wrap the cord in a warm, sterile-saline-soaked dressing.
- With a gloved hand, palpate the cord for a pulse.
- If a pulse is absent in the umbilical cord, and positioning of the mother does not restore the pulse, insert a gloved hand into the vagina and lift the fetal head, or other presenting part, off of the umbilical cord while gently pushing the fetus into the uterus. With the other hand, press on the lower abdomen in an upward or cephalic direction. Push the fetus back only far enough to regain a pulse in the umbilical cord.
- Transport immediately, while maintaining fetal position so as to maintain umbilical pulse.

Breech Birth

- **Do not pull on the newborn.** Allow the delivery to proceed normally, supporting the newborn with the palm of your hand and arm, and allowing the head to deliver.
- If the head does not deliver within 3 minutes, place a gloved hand in the vagina with your palm toward the newborn's face. Form a "V" with your index and middle fingers on either side of the newborn's nose, and push the vaginal wall away from the newborn's face to create an airspace for the newborn until delivery of the head. Suction may be provided *as needed.*
- Transport immediately, while maintaining the airspace for the newborn.

Limb Presentation

- Place the mother in either a knee-chest position or a supine position with pillows under the buttocks.
- Transport immediately.

2.7.1 Complications of Labor and Delivery

Shoulder Dystocia

- Determine the presence of shoulder dystocia as follows: The newborn's head will deliver normally, and then it will retract back into the perineum because the shoulders are trapped between the symphysis pubis and the sacrum (the "turtle sign").
- If this occurs, **do not pull on the newborn's head.**
- Have the mother drop her buttocks off the end of the bed and flex her thighs upward to facilitate delivery.
- Apply firm pressure with an open hand immediately above the symphysis pubis.
- If delivery does not occur, transport immediately.

ALS Level 1

None.

ALS Level 2

None.

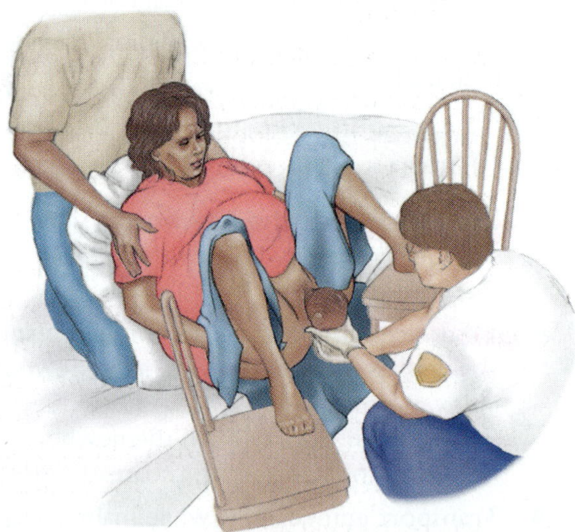

Have the mother drop her buttocks off the end of the bed and flex her thighs upward.

2.7.2 Normal Labor and Delivery

This protocol should be used when the paramedic encounters an imminent delivery prior to arrival at the hospital. Imminent delivery is evidenced by crowning at the vaginal opening.

Supportive Care

- Trauma Supportive Care Protocol 2.1.4. Notify the nearest appropriate OB–capable hospital early and prepare for transport.
- Place the mother in a comfortable, supine position.
- Prepare the OB kit. (Also have a pediatric kit on standby.)
- Gently and carefully assist expulsion of the newborn from the birth canal in its natural descent. **Do not pull or push the newborn.**
- Upon complete presentation of newborn's head:
  - Instruct the mother to stop pushing.
  - Clear the airway by gentle suction of the newborn's mouth, and then nose, with a bulb syringe.
  - Inspect and palpate the newborn's neck for the umbilical cord. If it is present, carefully unwrap the cord from the neck. If unable to remove the cord, apply two umbilical clamps and cut between the clamps to release the cord.
  - Once the newborn's airway is clear and the cord is free from around its neck, instruct the mother to push on her next contraction to complete delivery.
- Upon complete delivery of the newborn:
  - Keep the newborn at the level of the vagina to prevent over- or under-transfusion of blood from the cord.
  - Never "milk" the cord. Apply two umbilical cord clamps (2 inches apart and at least 8 inches from the navel), and then cut the cord between the clamps.
  - Avoid holding the newborn by the legs, allowing the head to hang below the body, as this may cause cerebral hemorrhage to occur.
  - Gently suction the newborn's mouth and nose with the bulb syringe.
  - If meconium is noted in the airway, see Pediatric Protocol 3.4.1, Newborn Resuscitation.
  - Dry and wrap the newborn in a blanket to preserve body heat. Be sure to cover the newborn's head, as this is a major area of heat loss.
- Evaluate the newborn:
  - If the newborn is not breathing, see Pediatric Protocol 3.4.1, Newborn Resuscitation.
  - Evaluate the Apgar scores at 1 and 5 minutes (see Appendix 7.2).
  - If Apgar score < 7, see Pediatric Protocol 3.4.1, Newborn Resuscitation.

2.7.2 Normal Labor and Delivery

- Following delivery of the newborn, the mother's vagina should continue to ooze blood. **Do not pull on the umbilical cord.**
- If active hemorrhage is noted from the vagina, apply firm continuous massage manually to the uterine fundus. If the mother wants to breastfeed, encourage her to do so; this will aid in the contraction of the uterus, which will help stop the bleeding and facilitate delivery of the placenta. (Do not attempt to examine the patient internally. Never pack the vagina to stop bleeding.) Apply a sanitary napkin to the vaginal opening.
- If the placenta does deliver, preserve it in a plastic bag and transport it with the mother. It is not necessary to delay transport to wait for the placenta to deliver.
- After delivery of the placenta, clean the perineal area and remove soiled drop sheets from under the mother's buttocks. Visually inspect the perineal area for tears. If active bleeding is present, apply direct pressure with sterile gauze. Apply a sanitary napkin to vaginal opening.

ALS Level 1

None.

ALS Level 2

- Administer Nitronox for pain control during a normal, uncomplicated delivery (see Medical Procedure 4.28).
- Consider oxytocin (Pitocin®) 10 units (1 mL) in 100 mL of normal saline, IV infusion at 1–2 mL/min. Titrate to effect according to the mother's uterine response.

2.7.3 Nontraumatic Vaginal Bleeding

This protocol should be used for female patients who may or may not be pregnant and who present with nontraumatic vaginal bleeding. Examples of causes include antepartum hemorrhage (abruption placenta, placenta previa, and uterine rupture), postpartum hemorrhage, ruptured ectopic pregnancy, ruptured ovarian cyst, and spontaneous abortion.

Supportive Care

- Trauma Supportive Care Protocol 2.1.4.
- Place all products of delivery (e.g., undeveloped fetus, placenta) in a plastic bag and transport with the patient to the hospital.

ALS Level 1

- If the patient is hypotensive (systolic BP < 100 mm Hg), administer a fluid challenge of 250–500 mL.

ALS Level 2

- Consider oxytocin (Piotocin®) 10 units (1 mL) in 100 mL of normal saline, IV infusion at 1–2 mL/min. Titrate to effect according to the mother's uterine response.

2.7.4 Toxemia of Pregnancy

This protocol should be used for the patient in her third trimester of pregnancy (≥ 20 weeks gestation) who is exhibiting signs of pre-eclampsia or eclampsia. The signs of toxemia include proteinuria (dark-colored urine), excessive weight gain, and hypertension. The presence of two of these signs constitutes pre-eclampsia; the presence of all three constitutes eclampsia. The seizing patient in her third trimester of pregnancy should be assumed to be eclamptic and treated as specified below. However, consideration of another underlying etiology, such as hypoglycemia, drug overdose, head injury, or fever, should also be considered. **Eclamptic seizures can also occur postpartum (≤ 1 week after giving birth).** Witnessed continuous convulsions (generalized tonic–clonic seizure or grand mal) or repeating episodes without regaining consciousness or sufficient respiratory decompensation demonstrate a need for immediate treatment.

Supportive Care

- Trauma Supportive Care 2.1.4.

ALS Level I

- If the patient is seizing, administer magnesium sulfate 4 g IV (mixed in 50 mL of D_5W given over 5–10 minutes). May repeat once at 2 g IV (mixed in 50 mL of D_5W given over 5–10 minutes) *as needed.*
- If the patient continues to seize, administer one of the following benzodiazepines:
  - **Diazepam (Valium®)** 5 mg IV. If unable to start an IV, administer diazepam 5 mg intranasal or 10 mg per rectum. May repeat *as needed,* up to a maximum dose of 20 mg (a)(b).

  or

  - **Lorazepam (Ativan®)** 2 mg IV. If unable to start an IV, administer lorazepam 2 mg IM. May repeat once *as needed,* up to a maximum dose of 4 mg.

  or

  - **Midazolam (Versed®)** 2 mg IV. If unable to start an IV, administer midazolam 2 mg intranasal. May repeat once *as needed,* up to a maximum dose of 4 mg (a).
- Perform a glucose test with a finger stick (see Medical Procedure 4.39).
- If glucose < 60 mg/dL, administer dextrose 50% 25 g (50 mL) via slow IV (c).
- If glucose is given, administer thiamine (if available) 100 mg IV or IM.

2.7.4 Toxemia of Pregnancy

ALS Level 2

- If the patient is hypertensive, administer labetalol (Normadyne®) 20 mg via slow (over 2 minutes) IV.

Note

(a) Intranasal administration of benzodiazepines requires the use of a mucosal atomization device.

(b) Use a lubricated 3–5 mL syringe **without the needle** to administer diazepam (Valium®). Position the patient in a decubitus knee position or supine with the legs held apart, and insert the lubricated syringe approximately 5 cm (approximately 2 inches) into the rectum. Inject the Valium, remove the syringe, and tape the buttocks closed.

(c) To avoid infiltration and resultant tissue necrosis, dextrose 50% should be given slow IV with intermittent aspiration of the IV line to confirm IV patency, followed by saline flush.

2.8 Other Adult Medical Emergencies

The paramedic should use these protocols to guide him/her through the treatment of patients with other medical emergencies who are exhibiting signs and symptoms. In addition to these protocols, the paramedic may need to refer to other protocols for continued treatment.

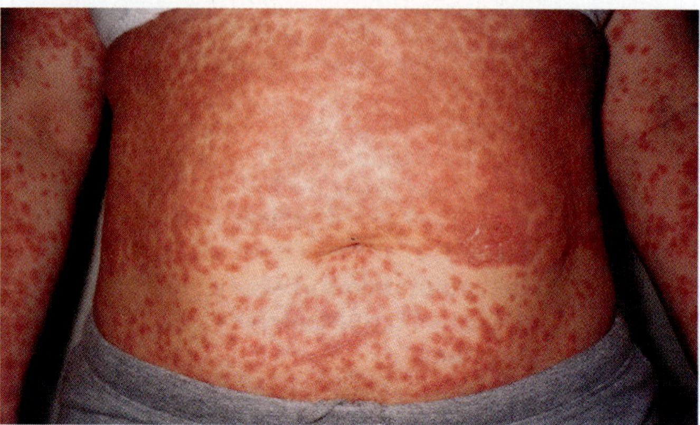

A severe allergic reaction to medication.

2.8.1 Allergic Reactions/Anaphylaxis

This protocol should be used for patients exhibiting signs and symptoms consistent with allergic reaction, as follows:

- **Skin:** flushing, itching, hives, swelling, cyanosis.
- **Respiratory:** dyspnea, sneezing, coughing, wheezing, stridor, laryngeal edema, laryngospasm, bronchospasm.
- **Cardiovascular:** vasodilation, increased heart rate, decreased blood pressure.
- **Gastrointestinal:** nausea/vomiting, abdominal cramping, diarrhea.
- **CNS:** dizziness, headache, convulsions, tearing.

Treatment is outlined here according to the severity of the allergic reaction (mild, moderate, and severe or anaphylaxis).

Mild Reactions

These reactions consist of redness and/or itching, stable vital signs with a systolic BP > 110 mm Hg without dyspnea.

Supportive Care

- Trauma Supportive Care Protocol 2.1.4.

ALS Level 1

- Diphenhydramine HCl (Benadryl®) 50 mg IM or 25 mg IV.

ALS Level 2

None.

2.8.1 Allergic Reactions/Anaphylaxis

Moderate Reactions

These reactions are evidenced by edema, hives, dyspnea, wheezing, "lump in throat" feeling, difficulty swallowing, facial swelling, and stable vital signs with a systolic BP > 90 mm Hg.

Supportive Care

- Trauma Supportive Care Protocol 2.1.4.

ALS Level 1

- Diphenhydramine HCl (Benadryl®) 50 mg IM or IV.
- Epinephrine (1:1000) 0.3 mg SQ (a)(b).
- If bronchospasm is present, administer albuterol (Ventolin®): one nebulizer treatment containing 2.5 mg of albuterol premixed with 2.5 mL normal saline (see Medical Procedure 4.27). May be repeated twice *as needed* (a)(c).
- If albuterol is administered, may add ipratropium bromide (Atrovent®) 0.5 mg (0.5 mL) to the albuterol nebulizer treatment **for the first nebulizer treatment only.**
- If the patient has respiratory distress, choose one of the following steroids:
  - Methylprednisolone sodium succinate (Solu-Medrol®) 125 mg IV, if available.

  or

  - Dexamethasone (Decadron®) 10 mg IV, if available.
- May repeat epinephrine (1:1000) 0.3 mg SQ (a)(b).

ALS Level 2

- If the patient's heart rate ≥ 140, contact medical control for bronchodilator orders.

2.8.1 Allergic Reactions/Anaphylaxis

Severe Reactions

Signs and symptoms include edema, hives, severe dyspnea and wheezing, unstable vital signs with a systolic BP < 100 mm Hg, and possibly cyanosis and laryngeal edema.

Supportive Care

- Trauma Supportive Care Protocol 2.1.4.

ALS Level 1

- Diphenhydramine HCl (Benadryl®) 50 mg IM or IV.
- Epinephrine (1:1000) 0.3 mg SQ (a)(b).
- If the patient remains in respiratory distress, administer albuterol (Ventolin®): one nebulizer treatment containing 2.5 mg of albuterol premixed with 2.5 mL normal saline (see Medical Procedure 4.27). May be repeated twice *as needed* (a)(c).
- If albuterol is administered, may add ipratropium bromide (Atrovent®) 0.5 mg (0.5 mL) to the albuterol nebulizer treatment **for the first nebulizer treatment only.**
- Consider the need for intubation (see Medical Procedure 4.18).
- If the patient has respiratory distress, choose one of the following steroids:
  - Methylprednisolone sodium succinate (Solu-Medrol®) 125 mg IV, if available.

  or

  - Dexamethasone (Decadron®) 10 mg IV, if available.
- May repeat epinephrine (1:1000) 0.3 mg SQ (a)(b).

ALS Level 2

- Epinephrine (1:10,000) 0.3 mg via slow IV in 0.1-mg increments over 2 minutes (a)(b).
- If the patient's heart rate ≥ 140, contact medical control for bronchodilator orders.

Note

(a) Caution should be used with administration of epinephrine when the patient has a history of hypertension or heart disease.

(b) The EpiPen® may be used if other means of epinephrine administration are not available (see Medical Procedure 4.53).

(c) Do not give albuterol or ipratropium bromide if the patient's heart rate ≥ 140.

2: adult protocols

2.8.2 Diabetic Emergencies

This protocol is to be used for those patients whose blood glucose is less than 60 mg/dL or more than 300 mg/dL.

Supportive Care

- Medical Supportive Care Protocol 2.1.3.

ALS Level 1

- Perform a glucose test with a finger stick (see Medical Procedure 4.39).
- **If glucose < 60 mg/dL:**
  - If the patient is conscious and has an intact gag reflex, assist with self-administration of oral glucose, if possible.
  - If available, administer thiamine 100 mg IV. If unable to start an IV, administer thiamine 100 mg IM.
  - If the patient is stuporous or unconscious, administer D_{50} 50 mL via slow IV (a).
  - If unable to start an IV, administer Glucagon 1 unit dose IM, if available.
  - Perform a second glucose test with a finger stick. If glucose remains less than 60 mg/dL, administer D_{50} 50 mL IV (a).
- **If blood glucose > 300 mg/dL:**
  - Administer normal saline 500 mL IV, unless contraindicated.

ALS Level 2

None.

Note

(a) To avoid infiltration and resultant tissue necrosis, D_{50} should be given via slow IV with intermittent aspiration of the IV line to confirm IV patency, followed by saline flush.

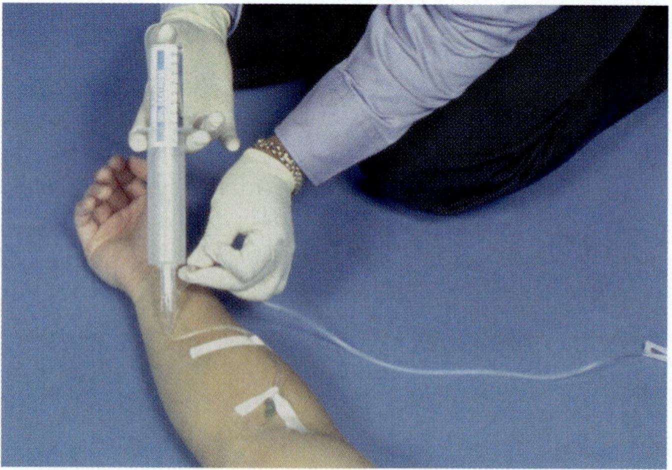

50% glucose solution for IV administration.

2.8.3 Nontraumatic Abdominal Pain

This protocol should be used for patients who complain of abdominal pain without a history of trauma.

Assessment should include specific questions pertaining to the GI/GU systems.

Abdominal physical assessment:

- Ask the patient to point to the area of pain (palpate this area last).
- Gently palpate for tenderness, rebound tenderness, distention, rigidity, guarding, and pulsatile masses. Also palpate the flank for CVA tenderness.

Abdominal history:

- History of pain (OPQRST)
- History of nausea/vomiting (color, bloody, coffee grounds)
- History of bowel movement (last BM, diarrhea, bloody, tarry)
- History of urine output (painful, dark, bloody)
- History of abdominal surgery
- History of acute onset of back pain
- SAMPLE history (attention to last meal)

Additional questions should be asked of the female patient regarding OB/GYN history (see Adult Protocol 2.7, Adult OB/GYN Emergencies). **All female patients of childbearing age who complain of abdominal pain should be considered to have an ectopic pregnancy (even if vaginal bleeding is absent) until proven otherwise.**

An acute abdomen can be caused by appendicitis, cholecystitis, duodenal ulcer perforation, diverticulitis, abdominal aortic aneurysm, kidney infection, urinary tract infection (UTI), kidney stone, pelvic inflammatory disease (PID—female), or pancreatitis (see Appendix 7.1, Abdominal Pain Differential).

Supportive Care

- Trauma Supportive Care Protocol 2.1.4.

ALS Level 1

- If the patient is hypotensive (systolic BP < 90 mm Hg), administer a fluid challenge of normal saline 500 mL.

ALS Level 2

None.

2.8.4 Sickle Cell Anemia

Sickle cell anemia is a chronic hemolytic anemia occurring almost exclusively in African Americans; it is characterized by the presence of sickle-shaped red blood cells. Sickle cell crisis results from the occlusion of a blood vessel by masses of these misshapen blood cells. Pain is the principal manifestation and represents the most common type of crisis. Typical pain occurs in the joints and back. Hepatic, pulmonary, or central nervous system involvement can occur, with each type being associated with its own group of symptoms. Keep in mind that patients with sickle cell disorder have a high incidence of life-threatening disorders at a very young age.

Supportive Care

- Medical Supportive Care Protocol 2.1.3. Administer 100% oxygen via non-rebreather mask at 15 L/min.
- Provide emotional support.

ALS Level 1

- Fluid challenge of normal saline 500–1000 mL IV.
- If pain persists and systolic BP > 90 mm Hg, morphine sulfate may be given via slow IV in 2-mg increments every 3–5 minutes, titrated to pain and BP ≥ 90 mm Hg, up to a maximum of 10 mg (a).

ALS Level 2

None.

Note

(a) Extreme caution should be used with administering narcotic analgesics to a patient with an $SpO_2 < 92\%$.

2.9 Adult Environmental Emergencies

The following protocols cover a range of problems attributable to the environment, including trauma due to changes in atmospheric pressure, exposure to heat and cold extremes, water submersion, and exposure to electricity. Initial efforts should focus on removing the patient from the harmful environment.

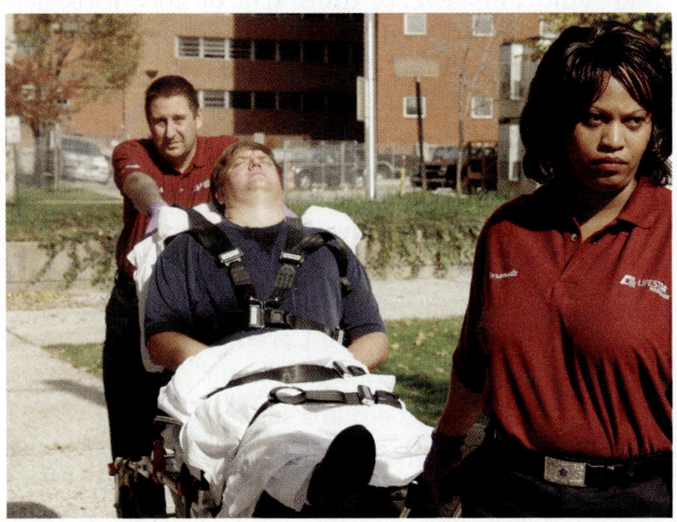

Remove the patient from the harmful environment.

2.9.1 Barotrauma/Decompression Illness: Dive Injuries

Barotrauma and decompression illness are caused by changes in the surrounding atmospheric pressure beyond the body's capacity to compensate for excess gas load. These injuries are most commonly associated with the use of SCUBA (Self-Contained Underwater Breathing Apparatus). SCUBA diving emergencies can occur at any depth, with the most serious injuries manifesting symptoms after a dive. If a patient took a breath underwater, from any source of compressed gas (e.g., submerged vehicle, SCUBA) while greater than three (3) feet in depth, the patient may be a victim of barotrauma. Barotrauma may cause several injuries to occur, including arterial gas embolism (AGE), pneumothorax, pneumomediastinum, subcutaneous emphysema, and the "squeeze." Decompression illnesses may also include decompression sickness ("bends").

Supportive Care

- Trauma Supportive Care Protocol 2.1.4. Administer 100% oxygen via non-rebreather mask at 15 L/min.
- Place the patient in a supine position.
- Complete the Dive Accident Signs and Symptoms checklist (see Appendix 7.6).
- Obtain a Dive History Profile, if possible (the patient's dive buddy may be helpful in answering many of these questions).
- Whenever possible, have the legal authority in charge (e.g., police, Florida Marine Patrol, U.S. Coast Guard) secure all of the victim's dive gear and maintain the proper chain of custody for testing, analysis, and other measures.
- Manage the patient according to the appropriate protocol(s).
- Transport the patient to the closest emergency department or trauma center with a helipad (air transport of diving accident victims must remain at an altitude of less than 1000 feet).
- Contact the Diver's Alert Network (DAN) at Duke University Medical Center, by calling collect at 919-684-4326, for further assistance (a).
- Bring the dive computer to the hospital if available.

ALS Level 1

None.

ALS Level 2

None.

Note

(a) DAN may be contacted while on scene or after arrival at the hospital. If the contact is made at the hospital, provide DAN with the name of the ED physician and the ED phone number.

2.9.2 Cold-Related Emergencies

Factors that predispose and/or cause a patient to develop hypothermia include geriatric and pediatric age, poor nutrition, diabetes, hypothyroidism, brain tumors or head trauma, sepsis, use of alcohol and certain drugs, and prolonged exposure to water or low atmospheric temperature. Patients can be classified into three categories based on their degree of hypothermia: mild (temperature = 94–97°F), moderate (temperature = 86–94°F), and severe (temperature < 86°F). Most oral thermometers will not register below 96°F. However, some tympanic thermometers (Braun Thermoscan™ Pro-1 and Pro 3000) will register in the range of 68–108°F.

Mild to moderate hypothermia patients will generally present with shivering, lethargy, and stiff, uncoordinated muscles.

Severe hypothermia patients may be disoriented and confused to the point of stupor and coma. Shivering will usually stop and physical activity will be uncoordinated. In addition, severe hypothermia will frequently produce an Osborn wave or J wave on the ECG, as well as dysrhythmias (bradycardia, ventricular fibrillation).

Supportive Care

- Trauma Supportive Care Protocol 2.1.4 (a).
- Remove all wet clothes and dry the patient.
- Protect the patient from heat loss and wind chill.
- Maintain the patient in a horizontal position.
- Avoid rough movement and excess activity.
- Monitor the patient's temperature.
- Add heat to the patient's head, neck, chest, and groin.
- For severe hypothermia, warm IV fluids.

For severe hypothermic cardiac arrest:

- Start CPR.
- For VF or pulseless VT, see Adult Protocol 2.3.7 (the EMT should apply an AED; see Medical Procedure 4.1).

2.9.2 Cold-Related Emergencies

ALS Level 1

- Intubate and hyperventilate the patient with warm humidified oxygen, if possible (see Medical Procedure 4.18).
- Establish an IV with warm normal saline.

If temperature > 86°F:

- Follow the appropriate dysrhythmia treatment (see Adult Protocol 2.3).

If temperature < 86°F:

- Continue CPR and transport immediately. Do not treat dysrhythmias in patients with severe hypothermia (warm the patient prior to treatment).

ALS Level 2

None.

Note

(a) Cases of frostbite should be bandaged with dry sterile dressings and transported without attempting rewarming in the prehospital setting.

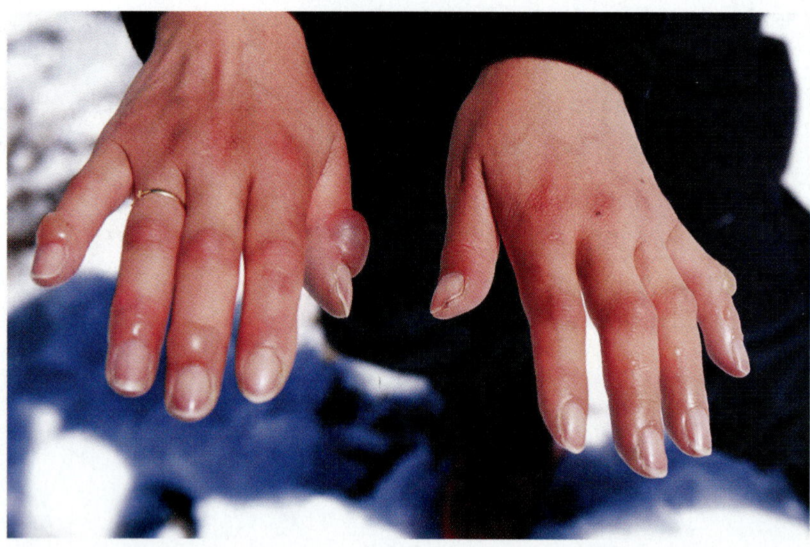

Frostbitten parts are hard and usually waxy to the touch.

2.9.3 Heat-Related Emergencies

Hyperthermia occurs when the patient is exposed to increased environmental temperature and can manifest as heat cramps, heat exhaustion, or heat stroke. Certain drugs may cause an increase in temperature (e.g., cocaine, Ecstasy)

Some tympanic thermometers (Braun Thermoscan™ Pro-1 and Pro 3000) will register in the range of 68–108°F.

- **Heat cramps:** Signs and symptoms include muscle cramps of the fingers, arms, legs, or abdomen; hot, sweaty skin; weakness; dizziness; tachycardia; normal BP; and normal temperature.
- **Heat exhaustion:** Signs and symptoms include cold and clammy skin, profuse sweating, nausea/vomiting, diarrhea, tachycardia, weakness, dizziness, transient syncope, muscle cramps, headache, positive orthostatic vital signs, and normal or slightly elevated temperature.
- **Heat stroke:** Signs and symptoms include hot dry skin (sweating may be present), confusion and disorientation, rapid bounding pulse followed by slow weak pulse, hypotension with low or absent diastolic reading, rapid and shallow respirations (which may later slow), seizures, coma, and elevated temperature > 105°F.

Heat Cramps and Heat Exhaustion

Supportive Care

- Trauma Supportive Care Protocol 2.1.4.
- Remove the patient from the warm environment; cool the patient.
- Monitor the patient's temperature.
- For mild to moderate heat cramps and heat exhaustion, **if the patient is conscious and alert,** encourage the patient to drink salt-containing fluids (e.g., half-strength Gatorade®).

ALS Level I

- If heat cramps are severe or if the patient's level of consciousness is diminished, administer a fluid challenge of normal saline 500 mL IV.

2.9.3 Heat-Related Emergencies

Heat Stroke

Supportive Care

- Trauma Supportive Care Protocol 2.1.4.
- Remove the patient from the warm environment; aggressively cool the patient. Remove the patient's clothing, and wet the patient directly with ice water. Also, turn air-conditioning units and fans on high, and apply ice packs to the patient's head, neck, chest, and groin.
- Monitor the patient's temperature. Cool the patient to 102°F, then dry the patient, remove any ice packs, and turn off fans (avoid lowering the patient's temperature too much).

ALS Level 1

- Treat hypotension (systolic BP < 90 mm Hg) with IV fluids. Avoid using vasopressors and anticholinergic drugs; they may potentiate heat stroke by inhibiting sweating. Administer a fluid challenge of normal saline 500 mL IV.

ALS Level 2

None.

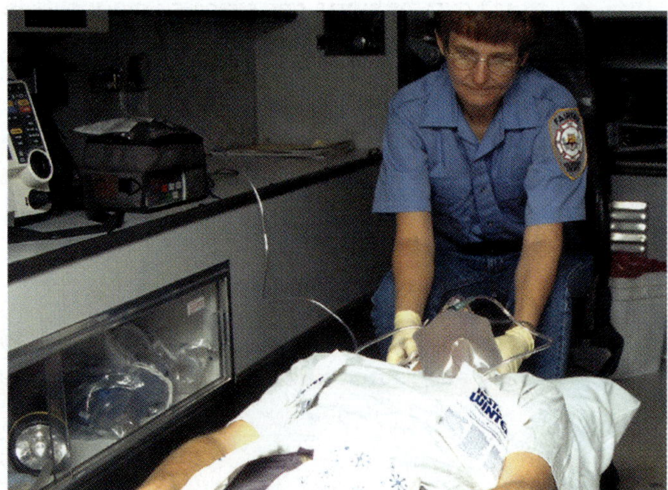

Apply cool packs to the patient's neck, groin, and armpits.

2.9.4 Near Drowning

Near-drowning patients are those persons who have been submerged in fresh or salt water and may or may not be conscious. If the patient is still in the water upon arrival of EMS, a Dive Rescue Team should be used to remove the patient from the water whenever possible. Additional protocols may be needed for treatment decisions (e.g., Adult Protocol 2.9.1, Barotrauma/Decompression Illness: Dive Injuries). **Drownings are *not* Trauma Alerts, unless there is a specific traumatic component associated with the event.**

Supportive Care

- Trauma Supportive Care Protocol 2.1.4 (protect the c-spine).
- Determine any pertinent history (e.g., duration of submersion, depth, water temperature, possible seizure, drug and/or alcohol use).
- Maintain the patient's body temperature; dry and warm the patient.
- **All near-drowning patients should be transported to the hospital,** regardless of how well they may seem to have recovered. Delayed death or complications due to pulmonary edema or aspiration pneumonia are not uncommon.
- Consider contacting the police department for investigation.

ALS Level 1

- Treat dysrhythmias per specific protocol (see Adult Protocol 2.3).

ALS Level 2

None.

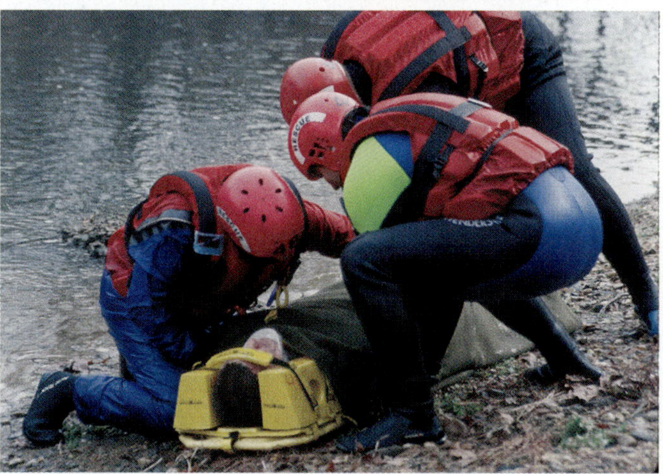

Dry and warm the patient before and during transport.

2.9.5 Electrical Emergencies

A wide range of injuries can be caused by a lightning strike or contact with electricity. Electrical injury can occur from direct contact, an arc, or a flash of the electricity, and from a direct hit or a splash from lightning. The movement of electrical current through the body can cause violent muscle contractions that can lead to fractures; as a consequence, the patient's c-spine should be protected. The thermal energy can cause external burns, but in many cases the majority of thermal damage is internal, with few external signs of injury. Dysrhythmias are also common (e.g., ventricular fibrillation). **The rescuer should be sure that the patient is no longer in contact with the electrical current before initiating treatment.**

Supportive Care

- Trauma Supportive Care Protocol 2.1.4 (protect the c-spine) (a).
- Treat burns per Adult Protocol 2.10.8.
- Try to determine the amps, volts, and duration of contact with the electricity, if possible.
- Consider the need to transport the patient to a trauma center (see General Protocol 1.10).

ALS Level 1

- Treat dysrhythmias per specific protocol (see Adult Protocol 2.3).

ALS Level 2

None.

Note

(a) Asystole is a common presentation with lightning strikes. These patients should be aggressively resuscitated unless their injuries are incompatible with life.

2.9.6 Taser Deployments

This protocol outlines and defines the steps that EMS personnel should carry out when they encounter a patient who has been subdued with a Taser. Typically it is not the "Taser event" itself that leads to the need for transport to the hospital, but rather the events that led to the individual being Tasered, such as "excited delirium," or the events following the Taser event, such as a sudden fall to the ground.

Excited delirium is a state in which a person is in a psychotic and extremely agitated state. Mentally, the subject is unable to focus and process any rational thought or to focus his/her attention on any one thing. Physically, the organs within the subject are functioning at such an excited rate that they begin to shut down. When these two factors occur at the same time, they cause a person to act erratically enough that he/she becomes a danger to self and to the public. It is typically at this point that law enforcement comes into contact with the person.

Essentially three things bring on excited delirium:

- Overdose on stimulant or hallucinogenic drugs
- Drug withdrawal
- Mental subject who is off of medication for a significant amount of time

Some of the symptoms of excited delirium are as follows:

- Bizarre and aggressive behavior
- Dilated pupils
- High body temperature
- Incoherent speech
- Inconsistent breathing patterns
- Fear and panic
- Profuse sweating
- Shivering
- Nudity

Another key symptom that occurs prior to the onset of death while experiencing excited delirium is "instant tranquility." It is noted when a patient who has been very violent and vocal suddenly becomes quiet and docile.

2.9.6 Taser Deployments

The following is a systematic, seven-step approach to responding to and evaluating patients who have been subdued with a Taser:

1. Find out what happened before the patient was Tasered; this history will provide you with information regarding the patient's mental status prior to being Tasered and suggest the potential for future decompensation. Consider any report of extreme behavior prior to the Taser event as significant, regardless of the patient's current presentation.
2. Approach the patient with caution. The Taser event can dramatically change a patient's outward presentation. Assume that any patient who has been Tasered was violent and dangerous.
3. Complete a thorough physical exam and history. The exam should include a basic neurological exam, skin signs, pupil assessment, a complete set of vital signs, and a close look for traumatic injuries. All Tasered patients are considered to have experienced a fall until proven otherwise. It is not uncommon to find minor first-degree burns located between the Taser probe sites on the patient's body. Anything that looks worse than minor sunburn should be considered abnormal. Incontinence should be considered abnormal. Chest pain, shortness of breath, vomiting, and headaches should all be treated according to the appropriate medical treatment protocol.
4. Consider the potential for sudden unexpected death syndrome. The vast majority of patients who have died following a Taser event have shown signs of excited delirium.
5. During transport, be very conscientious of patients whom exhibit one or more of the following signs and symptoms:
   a. Evidence of excited delirium prior to being Tasered
   b. Persistent abnormal vital signs
   c. History or physical findings consistent with amphetamine or hallucinogenic drug use
   d. Cardiac history
   e. Altered level of consciousness or aggressive, violent behavior, including resistance to evaluation
   f. Evidence of hyperthermia
   g. Abnormal subjective complaints, including chest pain, shortness of breath, nausea, or headaches
6. Removal of the Taser probes will not be performed by EMS personnel. To transport the patient, the wires to the probes will likely need to be removed. This can be done by simply cutting the wires with a pair of trauma sheers.
7. In the event that the probes are removed by the police officer, the probes should be treated as a contaminated sharp. The probes can be stored in the Taser cartridge in the absence of a sharps container.

2.9.6 Taser Deployments

All EMS personnel will treat and transport any patient who has been Tasered and requests treatment and transport. This treatment will be guided by the signs and symptoms that the patient is exhibiting, as well as possible occult injuries that may have occurred while the individual was being subdued. At minimum, all Taser-event patients will receive the supportive and ALS Level 1 care outlined next.

In the event that a patient resists the delivery of care, these actions will be carried out with the safety of the crew in mind. If a patient is violent, a police officer will be required to accompany the patient in the rescue unit during transport and appropriate chemical restraints will be utilized according to Adult Protocol 2.5.2, Violent and/or Impaired Patient.

Supportive Care

- Establish that the scene has been secured and determine which events led up to the individual being subdued with a Taser.
- Determine whether the patient wants to be treated. If the patient refuses treatment, see General Protocol 1.8 (a).
- Perform a complete physical examination (including glucose and temperature). See Initial Assessment Protocol 2.1.1 (a).
- Provide general supportive care, including:
  - C-spine precautions, unless a cervical spine injury can be definitively ruled out.
  - Oxygen as needed.
- Determine how many 5-second cycles of energy the individual was exposed to, and document this information in the Patient Care Report.

ALS Level 1

- Initiate cardiac monitoring.
- Establish an IV; give normal saline KVO. If patient is exhibiting signs of excited delirium, use "cool" normal saline.
- Treat dysrhythmias per specific protocol (see Adult Protocol 2.3).
- Monitor the patient's glucose.
- Evaluate the patient's temperature; cool the patient as necessary.

2.9.6 Taser Deployments

ALS Level 2

None.

NOTE

(a) Determine whether the patient will consent to be medically evaluated by Fire/Rescue personnel and/or transported to a medical facility (per General Protocol 1.1). In the event that the patient refuses treatment/transport, refer to General Protocol 1.8. Keep in mind that it is the patient's right to accept or refuse treatment. The only exceptions would involve a patient who is a minor or a patient who has an altered mental status, in which case implied consent would be initiated, or a patient who refuses treatment/transport in an attempt to cause harm to self, in which case invocation of the Baker Act would be appropriate. At no time should Fire/Rescue or Police Department personnel advise a patient that he/she does not need to be transported to a hospital. That decision is at the sole discretion of the patient based on the information that EMS personnel provide the patient during the physical exam.

(b) In the majority of Taser incidents, it will not be possible for EMS personnel to determine the extent of injuries that the patient has sustained. While it is unlikely that the Taser itself will have caused an injury, there is a high likelihood of an occult injury secondary to the event. Examples would include fall injuries as a result of the incapacitation, pathological fractures secondary to muscle contraction, and impending demise secondary to a state of excited delirium.

References

Whitehead S, NREMT-P: *After Shock: A Rational Response to Taser Strikes*, JEMS, Vol. 30, No. 5, May 2005.

Glendale Police Department: *Excited Delirium*, November 2003.

DGG Taser, X-26 Taser Specifications, 2005.

2.10 Adult Trauma Emergencies

These protocols cover specific types of injuries and their treatment. The initial assessment of the trauma patient should include determination of trauma alert criteria (see General Protocol 1.10, Trauma Transport). When the situation demands it (e.g., when Trauma Alert criteria are met), scene time should be limited as much as possible (e.g., 10 minutes) and the patient should be expeditiously transported to a trauma center. Do not delay transport to establish vascular access or bandage and splint every injury. Priority should be given to airway management and rapid preparation for transport (e.g., full immobilization on a backboard) and control of gross hemorrhage.

If a vascular access is obtained and hypovolemia is suspected (e.g., the patient shows signs and symptoms of shock, such as systolic BP < 90 mm Hg), a fluid challenge of 1–2 L (20 mL/kg) may be administered until a systolic BP of 90 mm Hg is maintained. If the patient is still in shock after receiving 2 L of fluid, an additional 1 L of fluid may be administered (maximum total fluid administration = 3 L). However, administration of large volumes of IV fluids has been found to be deleterious to the survival of patients with uncontrolled hemorrhage, internally or externally. Studies (*NEJM,* 1994) have shown that maximal fluid resuscitation may increase the bleeding, thereby preventing the formation of a protective thrombus or dislodging it once the intraluminal pressure exceeds the tamponading pressure of the thrombus. For this reason, **consult with the physician should be made prior to the administration of large volumes of IV fluids when the transport time is relatively short (e.g., less than 20 minutes).**

A female in her third trimester of pregnancy should be placed on her left side for transport. If the injuries require the use of a backboard, following full immobilization to the backboard, the backboard should be tilted to the left. Failure to follow this practice may cause hypotension due to decreased venous return.

2.10.1 Head and Spine Injuries

If history, symptoms, or signs of head or spinal injuries are present, manually immobilize the patient's head and neck while maintaining a patent airway using a modified jaw-thrust method. Immobilization of the entire spine is indicated following initial stabilization. **Cases involving hangings that do not meet Trauma Alert criteria <u>are not</u> considered Trauma Alert patients (e.g., a "suffocation type" patient without c-spine deformity).**

Supportive Care

- Trauma Supportive Care Protocol 2.1.4 (see the Spinal Immobilization flowchart in Medical Procedure 4.52).
- If the patient is not hypotensive (systolic BP > 100 mm Hg), elevate the head of the backboard to 30 degrees (12–18 inches).

ALS Level 1

- If signs of brain stem herniation exist (e.g., pupillary dilation, asymmetric pupillary reactivity, or motor posturing), consider intubation and hyperventilate the patient to achieve an optimal $EtCO_2$ of 30–40 mm Hg (see Medical Procedure 4.18 and Medical Procedure 4.4).
- If the patient is seizing, see Adult Protocol 2.5.3; avoid administration of glucose-containing solutions and medications.

ALS Level 2

None.

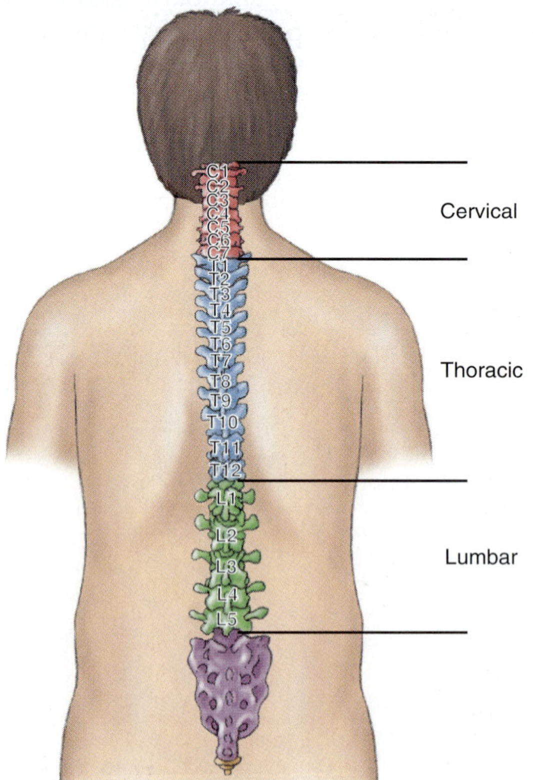

The spinal column.

2.10.2 Eye Injuries

This protocol covers a variety of injuries to the eye. If other injuries to the body exist, priority of care should be given as appropriate.

Supportive Care

- Trauma Supportive Care Protocol 2.1.4 (establish an IV *as needed*).
- Remove, or ask to the patient to remove, contact lenses, if still in the affected eye(s).
- For a penetrating object, stabilize the object and cover the affected eye with an ocular shield or similar rigid device. Cover both eyes to minimize eye movement. Avoid direct pressure on either the eye or the penetrating object.
- If the eyeball has been forced out of the socket, cover the entire eye area with a rigid container, such as a disposable drinking cup. Avoid contact with the exposed globe. If bleeding is present, control it by administering direct pressure with a sterile dry dressing.
- If there are signs and symptoms or suspicion of ocular exposure to chemicals or foreign body, without obvious or suspected penetrating injury or laceration of the cornea or globe, irrigate the eye with a normal saline IV solution (see Medical Procedure 4.45, Morgan Lens).

ALS Level 1

- If the patient is experiencing eye pain, administer tetracaine, 1 drop in each affected eye. Tetracaine may be given in penetrating eye injuries or in patients with allergies to lidocaine.

ALS Level 2

None.

2.10.3 Chest Injuries

This protocol covers both blunt and penetrating chest trauma and should be part of initial resuscitation if the patient's breathing is compromised.

Supportive Care

- Trauma Supportive Care Protocol 2.1.4.
- Penetrating injuries to the chest or upper back should be covered immediately with an occlusive dressing (e.g., Vaseline gauze).
- Do not attempt to remove an impaled object; instead, stabilize it with a bulky dressing or other means. If the impaled object is very large or unwieldy, attempt to cut object to no less than 6 inches from the chest.

ALS Level 1

- For tension pneumothorax, decompress the chest **on the affected side** (see Medical Procedure 4.14).
- For massive flail chest with severe respiratory compromise, intubate the patient and assist ventilations (see Medical Procedures 4.18 and 4.4). If flail chest does not cause severe respiratory compromise, stabilize the chest externally by placing the patient's ipsilateral arm in a sling and swathe.
- For traumatic asphyxia, establish two large-bore IVs. If the crushing object is still on the patient, infuse a minimum of 1 L of fluid before attempting to lift the object off the patient.
- For traumatic asphyxia, administer sodium bicarbonate 1 mEq/kg IV.

ALS Level 2

None.

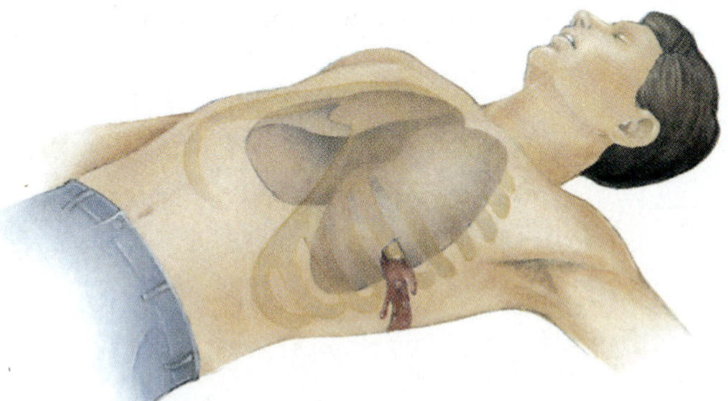

Open injuries occur when the chest wall is penetrated by some object or the broken end of a fractured rib.

2.10.4 Traumatic Chest Pain

Chest pain due to blunt trauma may be an indication of underlying injury. Blunt injuries such as pulmonary contusion and cardiac contusion may cause respiratory insufficiency and/or myocardial infarction.

Supportive Care

- Trauma Supportive Care Protocol 2.1.4.

ALS Level 1

- Treat dysrhythmias per specific protocol (see Adult Protocol 2.3).
- Consider the need for other protocols (see Adult Protocol 2.4.2).

ALS Level 2

None.

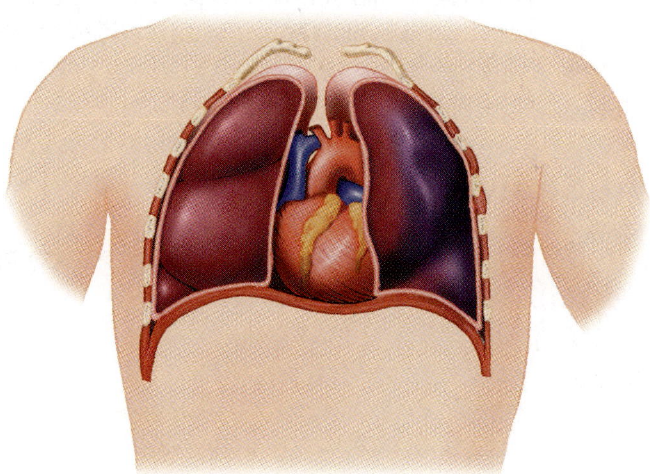

Blunt trauma injury to the chest.

2.10.5 Abdomino-Pelvic Injuries

This protocol covers blunt and penetrating abdomino-pelvic trauma. Penetrating injuries may also include the chest (see Adult Protocol 2.10.3, Chest Injuries).

Supportive Care

- Trauma Supportive Care Protocol 2.1.4.
- For penetrating injuries, apply an occlusive dressing (e.g., Vaseline gauze).
- For evisceration, cover the organs with a saline-soaked sterile dressing and then cover it with an occlusive dressing (e.g., foil). Do not attempt to put the organs back into the abdomen.
- Do not log-roll any patient with a suspected pelvic fracture (may use scoop stretcher).
- If a pelvic fracture is suspected, stabilize the patient with a "sheet sling" or "scoop and run"; do not waste time by applying a commercial device or PASG.

ALS Level 1

None.

ALS Level 2

None.

2.10.6 Extremity Injuries

This protocol covers open and closed injuries to the extremities, including amputation.

Supportive Care

- Trauma Supportive Care Protocol 2.1.4 (establish an IV *as needed*).
- Any fracture or suspected fracture should be splinted appropriately, with ice being applied to the affected area. Remove and secure all jewelry. Check pulse sensation and movement before and after splinting.
- Closed angulated fractures should be aligned using proximal and distal traction during splinting, except in fractures that involve joints, which should be splinted in the position in which they are found.
- Traction splints should be used in cases of closed femur fractures, unless a pelvic fracture is suspected.
- Amputations should be dressed with bulky dressings. The amputated part should be placed in a plastic bag and then the bag placed on ice for transportation to the hospital.
- Apply direct pressure for hemorrhage control.

ALS Level 1

- See Adult Protocol 2.1.5 for pain management guidelines.

ALS Level 2

None.

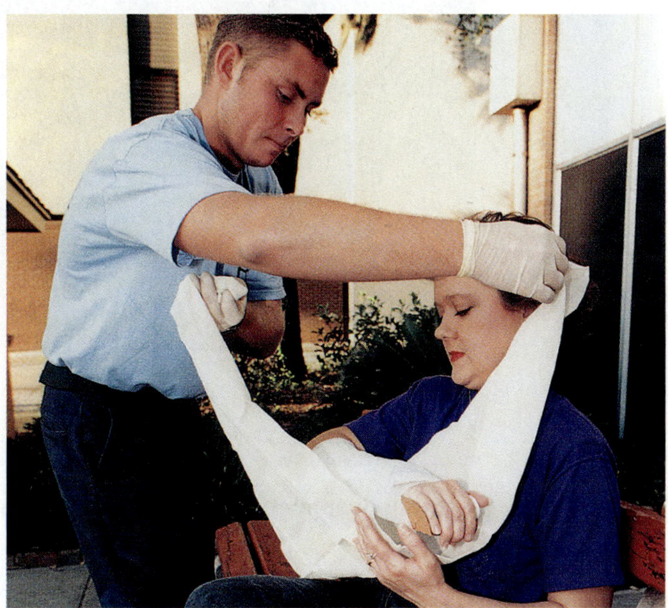

Splinting reduces pain and prevents additional damage to the extremity.

2.10.7 Traumatic Arrest

The decision to attempt resuscitation of a traumatic arrest should be based on the paramedic's judgment as to the possibility of survival and/or the possibility of organ harvest. There are instances where resuscitation of a traumatic arrest is not warranted (see General Protocol 1.4, Death in the Field).

Supportive Care

- Trauma Supportive Care Protocol 2.1.4.
- Rapidly prepare the patient for transport and then expeditiously transport the patient to the trauma center.

ALS Level 1

- If IV(s) can be established, infuse up to 3 L of fluid.
- Avoid use of vasopressors in cases of suspected hypovolemia.

ALS Level 2

None.

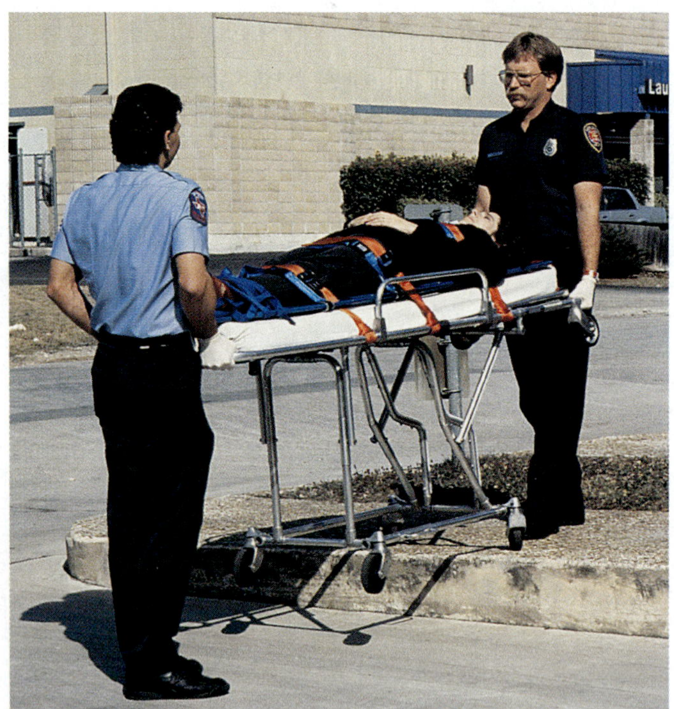

Rapidly prepare the patient for transport.

2.10.8 Burn Injuries

Burns can be caused by thermal, chemical, and electrical sources. If an electrical burn is suspected, also see Adult Protocol 2.9.5, Electrical Emergencies. Remember that burn patients are volume depleted. However, burns do not bleed, so you should look for other sources of bleeding. Many burn injuries are associated with inhalation injury. The signs and symptoms of inhalation injury include nasal and oropharyngeal burns, charring of the tongue or teeth, sooty (blackened) sputum, singed nasal and facial hair, abnormal breath sounds (e.g., stridor, rhonchi, wheezing), and respiratory distress.

In cases of inhalation injury, attention should be given to the patency of the airway. Acute swelling can cause an airway obstruction. The paramedic should consider the need for early intubation to avoid a complete airway obstruction that requires a cricothyroidotomy.

Supportive Care

- Trauma Supportive Care Protocol 2.1.4.
- Stop the burning process:
  - **Thermal turns:** Lavage the burned area with tepid water (sterile, if possible) to cool the skin. Do not attempt to wipe off semisolids (e.g., grease, tar, wax).
  - **Dry chemical burns:** Brush off dry powder, then lavage with copious amounts of tepid water (sterile, if possible) for 15 minutes.
  - **Liquid chemical burns:** Lavage the burned area with copious amounts of tepid water (sterile, if possible) for 15 minutes. (When *phenol* has caused the burn, also see HAZMAT Protocol 8.1.20, Phenol.)
- Remove clothing from around the burned area, but do not remove/peel off skin or tissue.
- Remove and secure all jewelry and tight-fitting clothing.
- Assess the extent of the burn using the Rule of Nines and the degree of burn severity (see Appendix 7.4, Burn Severity Categorization, and Appendix 7.15, Rule of Nines).

2.10.8 Burn Injuries

- Apply a dressing to the burned area as follows:
  - If there is **greater than or equal to** 20% second-degree burns or 5% third-degree burns, cover the burned area with dry sterile dressings or Water Gel™ wraps.
  - If there is **less than** 20% second-degree burns or 5% third-degree burns, apply wet sterile dressings to the burned areas for 15 minutes to aid in pain control. Alternatively, Burn Free™ gel pads or Water Gel™ wraps may be applied continuously to aid in pain control.
- Prevent hypothermia by keeping the patient warm and ensuring that all outer layers of dressings are dry.

ALS Level 1

- Pain Management Protocol (see Adult Protocol 2.1.5).

ALS Level 2

None.

2.11 Adults with Special Healthcare Needs

These protocols cover specific types of special healthcare needs in adult patients. Adults with special healthcare needs are those who have or are at risk for chronic physical, developmental, behavioral, and emotional conditions that necessitate use of health and related services of a type or amount not usually required by typical adults.

The general approach to adults with special healthcare needs includes the following:

1. Priority is given to the ABCs.
2. Do not be overwhelmed by the machines.
3. Listen to the caregiver.
4. If a nurse is present, rely on his/her judgment.
5. Remember that the patient's cognitive level of function may be altered.
6. Assume that the patient can understand exactly what you say.
7. Bring all medications and equipment to the hospital.

Obtaining a history includes asking the parent/caregiver about the following issues:

1. The patient's normal vital signs.
2. The patient's actual weight.
3. Developmental level of the patient.
4. The patient's allergies, including to latex.
5. Pertinent medications/therapies.

2.11.1 Home Mechanical Ventilator

Home mechanical ventilators may be indicated for chronically ill adults with abnormal respiratory drive, severe chronic lung disease, or severe neuromuscular weakness. Some patients require continuous mechanical ventilations, whereas others require only intermittent support during sleep or acute illness. Home ventilators may either be volume limited or pressure limited. All are equipped with alarms.

Types of Ventilator Alarms

- **Low pressure or apnea**—may be caused by a loose or disconnected circuit or an air leak in the circuit or at the tracheostomy, resulting in inadequate ventilation.
- **Low power**—caused by a depleted battery.
- **High pressure**—can be caused by a plugged or obstructed airway or circuit tubing, by coughing, or by bronchospasm.
- **Setting error**—caused by ventilator settings outside the capacity of the equipment.
- **Power switchover**—occurs when the unit switches from alternating-current power to the battery.

Supportive Care

- Medical Supportive Care Protocol 2.1.3.
- If a ventilator-dependent patient is in respiratory distress and the cause is not easily ascertained and corrected, remove the ventilator and provide assisted manual ventilations with a bag-valve device. Suction *as needed.*
- Consider the need for other protocols (e.g., Adult Protocol 2.2, Adult Respiratory Emergencies).

ALS Level 1

None.

ALS Level 2

None.

2.11.2 Tracheostomy

Tracheostomies are indicated for long-term ventilatory support to bypass an upper airway obstruction and to aid in the removal of secretions. Tracheostomies come in a variety of sizes and can either be single lumen or double lumen. Special attachments include a tracheostomy nose (filtration device), tracheostomy collar (for oxygen or humidification), and Passy-Muir valve (speaker valve).

Signs of Tracheostomy Obstruction

- Excess secretions.
- No chest wall movement.
- Cyanosis.
- Accessory muscle use.
- No chest wall rise with bag-valve ventilations.

Supportive Care

- Medical Supportive Care Protocol 2.1.3.
- If an obstruction is present, inject 1–3 mL of normal saline into the tracheostomy tube and suction *as needed.*
- If unable to clear the obstruction by suctioning, remove the tracheostomy tube and insert a new tube (either of the same size or one size smaller). **Do not force the tube.**
- If unable to insert a new tracheostomy tube, or if one is unavailable, insert an endotracheal tube of similar size into the stoma and ventilate with a bag-valve device *as needed.*
- If unable to insert an endotracheal tube, ventilate with a bag-valve mask over the stoma or over the patient's mouth while covering the stoma *as needed.*
- Consider the need for other protocols (e.g., Adult Protocol 2.2, Adult Respiratory Emergencies).

ALS Level 1

None.

ALS Level 2

None.

2.11.3 Central Venous Lines

Central venous lines are indicated for administration of medications, delivery of chemotherapy, nutritional support, infusion of blood products, and blood draws. Types of central venous lines include Broviac/Hickman, Port-a-Cath/Med-a-Port, and percutaneous intravenous catheters (PIC). Central venous line emergencies include the catheter coming completely out, bleeding at the site, the catheter broken in half, blood embolus, thrombus, air embolus, and internal bleeding. **Use of SQ ports requires special training; these ports should *not* be used for IV access.**

Signs of blood embolus, thrombus, air embolus, and internal bleeding are as follows:

- Chest pain.
- Cyanosis.
- Dyspnea.
- Shock.

Supportive Care

- Medical Supportive Care Protocol 2.1.3. CVP and PIC lines may be used for emergency IV access under sterile conditions.
- If the catheter has come completely out, apply direct pressure to the site.
- If there is bleeding at the site, apply direct pressure.
- If the catheter is broken in half, clamp the end of the remaining tube.
- If blood embolus, thrombus, or internal bleeding is suspected, clamp the line.
- If air embolus is suspected, clamp the line and place the patient on his/her left side.
- Consider the need for other protocols (e.g., Adult Protocol 2.2, Adult Respiratory Emergencies).

ALS Level 1

None.

ALS Level 2

None.

2.11.4 Feeding Tubes

Feeding tubes are indicated for administration of nutritional supplements and in patients who have an inability to swallow. Types of feeding tubes include nasogastric tubes (temporary) and gastrostomy tubes (G tube). Types of G tubes include those that are surgically placed, percutaneous endoscopic gastrostomy tubes (PEG tubes), and jejunal tubes (J tube). Potential complications include leaks, bleeding around the site, and displacement of the tube.

Supportive Care

- Medical Supportive Care Protocol 2.1.3.
- If the catheter has come completely out, cover the site with Vasoline gauze and apply direct pressure to the site.
- If there is bleeding at the site, apply direct pressure.

ALS Level 1

None.

ALS Level 2

None.

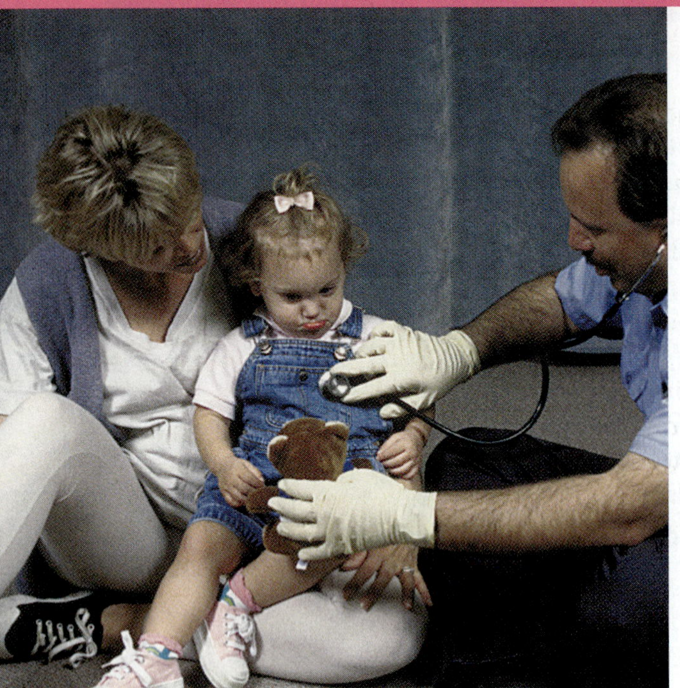

chapter **3**

Pediatric Protocols

3.1 Pediatric Initial Assessment and Management

The protocols in Section 3.1 are designed to guide the EMT or paramedic in his or her initial approach to assessment and management of pediatric patients. The Level 1 care is specified as either *EMT and Paramedic* (BLS) or *Paramedic Only* (ALS).

Protocol 3.1.1 should be used on all pediatric patients for initial assessment. During this assessment, if the paramedic determines that there is a need for airway management, Protocol 3.1.2 should be used for the management of the pediatric airway. These protocols are frequently referred to by other protocols, which may or may not override them in recommending more specific therapy.

Protocol 3.1.3 presents the basic components of preparation for transport of medical patients. Due to the significant differences in priorities and packaging in the prehospital care of trauma and hypovolemia cases, a separate Trauma Supportive Care protocol has been developed. After following Protocol 3.1.1, this Medical Supportive Care protocol may be the only protocol used in medical emergency situations where a specific diagnostic impression and choice of additional protocol(s) cannot be made. Judgment must be used in determining whether patients require ALS- or BLS-level care. Protocol 3.1.3 is frequently referred to by other protocols, which may or may not override it in recommending more specific therapy.

Protocol 3.1.4 presents the basic components of preparation for transport of trauma patients. Due to the significant differences in priorities and packaging in the prehospital care of medical cases, a separate Medical Supportive Care protocol has been developed. After following Protocol 3.1.1, this Trauma Supportive Care protocol may be the only protocol used in trauma or hypovolemia situations where a specific diagnostic impression and choice of additional protocol(s) cannot be made. Judgment must be used in determining whether patients require ALS- or BLS-level care. This protocol is frequently referred to by other protocols, which may or may not override it in recommending more specific therapy.

Paramedics only should use Protocol 3.1.5 for pain management.

3.1.1 Pediatric Assessment

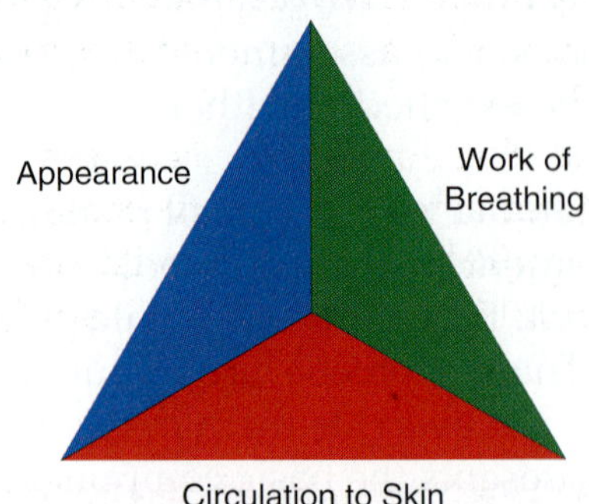

Pediatric Assessment Triangle.

The initial assessment of the pediatric patient will vary with the age of the patient. Nevertheless, some initial components of assessment remain consistent for all patients, regardless of their age. The paramedic or EMT should follow the appropriate approach to patient assessment with respect to the patient's age. In addition to addressing the patient, the responder may need to interview the parents or caregiver to gain information needed for a complete assessment of the patient.

A five-step, systematic approach should be used when assessing the child:

1. Scene size-up
2. General assessment (pediatric assessment triangle [PAT]).
    a. Appearance
    b. Work of breathing
    c. Circulation
3. Primary assessment
    a. ABCDE
    b. Cardiopulmonary function
    c. Neurological function
    d. Vital signs
4. Secondary assessment
    a. SAMPLE
    b. Head-to-toe survey
5. Ongoing assessment

EMT and Paramedic

I. **Scene Size-up.**
    A. Review the dispatch information.
    B. Assess the need for body substance isolation.
    C. Assess scene safety.
    D. Determine the mechanism of injury.
    E. Determine the number and location of patients.
    F. Determine the need for additional resources.
    G. Observe the environment of the pediatric patient.

3.1.1 Pediatric Assessment

II. **Pediatric Assessment Triangle: Rapid Cardiopulmonary Assessment.** The PAT has three major components: appearance, work of breathing, and circulation to the skin.

A. **Appearance.** The appearance is assessed by considering the following clinical signs: tone, interactiveness, consolability, look or gaze, and speech or cry (Table 3-1). This particular component is influenced by developmental issues and must be applied with knowledge of normal childhood development.

Table 3-1 Characteristic of Appearance: The "Tickles" (TICLS) Mnemonic

Characteristic	Features to Look For
Tone	Is the infant/child moving or resisting examination vigorously? (*Normal*) Does the infant/child have good muscle tone? (*Normal*) Or is the infant/child limp, listless, or flaccid? (*Abnormal*)
Interactiveness	How alert is the infant/child? (*Alert is normal*) How readily does a person, object, or sound distract/draw the infant/child's attention? (*Distract or draw attention is normal*) Will the infant/child reach for, grasp, and play with a toy or exam instrument, such as a penlight or tongue blade? (*Reaching is normal*) Or is the infant/child uninterested in playing or interacting with the caregiver or prehospital professional? (*Abnormal*)
Consolability	Can the infant/child be consoled or comforted by the caregiver or by the prehospital professional? (*Normal*) Or is the infant/child's crying or agitation unrelieved by gentle reassurance? (*Abnormal*)
Look/gaze	Does the infant/child make eye contact with you? (*Normal*) Or is there a "nobody home," glassy-eyed stare? (*Abnormal*)
Speech/cry	Is the infant/child's cry strong and spontaneous? (*Normal*) Or is the cry weak or high-pitched? (*Abnormal*) Is the content of speech age appropriate? (*Normal*) Or is the content confused or garbled? (*Abnormal*)

3.1.1 Pediatric Assessment

B. **Work of Breathing.** The work of breathing reflects a child's respiratory status—specifically, the degree of respiratory effort needed to oxygenate and ventilate the child's body. As work of breathing increases, physical signs appear to alert the prehospital provider to an underlying illness or injury. Table 3-2 outlines the clinical signs associated with increased work of breathing. The presence of any of these features indicates abnormal work of breathing; the presence of specific signs may further delineate the category of disease process as upper or lower airway obstruction, disease of the lungs, or disorders of breathing.

Table 3-2 Characteristics of Work of Breathing

Characteristic	Abnormal Features to Look For
Abnormal airway sounds	Snoring, muffled or hoarse speech, stridor, grunting, wheezing
Abnormal positioning	Sniffing position, tripoding, refusing to lie down
Retractions	Supraclavicular, intercostal, or substernal retractions of the chest wall; head bobbing in infants
Flaring	Flaring of the nares on inspiration

C. **Circulation to Skin.** Circulation to the skin is assessed by looking at the overall skin color and color pattern. A child's appearance will reflect inadequacies in brain perfusion, but altered appearance may be caused by a number of other conditions, including overdose/intoxication, metabolic disease, primary injury, and hypoxia. As a consequence, the addition of skin and mucous membrane color/perfusion changes to the PAT adds to the evaluation of core perfusion (Table 3-3). When faced with fluid or blood loss or changes in venous capacitance, the body will preserve perfusion to vital organs (heart and brain) through increased systemic vascular resistance (decreasing skin perfusion) and increases in heart rate; thus changes in skin color and skin perfusion are important early signs of shock in children.

Table 3-3 Characteristics of Circulation to Skin

Characteristic	Abnormal Features to Look For
Pallor	White or pale skin or mucous membrane coloration from inadequate blood flow
Mottling	Patchy skin discoloration due to vasoconstriction/vasodilation
Cyanosis	Bluish discoloration of skin and mucous membranes

3.1.1 Pediatric Assessment

D. Each component of the PAT is evaluated separately, utilizing specific predefined physical findings as outlined in Tables 3-1, 3-2, and 3-3. If an abnormal physical finding is noted, the corresponding component is, by definition, abnormal. Abnormalities in the three components can then be combined to form a general impression (Table 3-4).

Table 3-4 Components of the PAT and the General Impression

Component	Stable	Respiratory Distress	Respiratory Failure	Shock	CNS/ Metabolic	Cardiopulmonary Failure
Appearance	Normal	Normal	Abnormal	Normal/ Abnormal	Abnormal	Abnormal
Work of breathing	Normal	Abnormal	Abnormal	Normal	Normal	Abnormal
Circulation to the skin	Normal	Normal	Normal/ Abnormal	Abnormal	Normal	Abnormal

III. **Primary Assessment.**

A. Assess airway, c-spine, and initial level of consciousness (AVPU: **A**lert, responds to **V**erbal stimuli, responds to **P**ain, **U**nresponsive).

B. Assess breathing.

C. Assess circulation and presence of hemorrhage.

D. Assess disability—movement of extremities.

E. Expose and examine the patient's head, neck, chest, abdomen, and pelvis (check the back when the patient is rolled on his/her side).

F. Identify priority patients.

G. Assess the vital signs:

1. Blood pressure
2. ECG
3. SpO_2

IV. **Initial Management.** (See Pediatric Protocol 3.1.3, Medical Supportive Care, or Pediatric Protocol 3.1.4, Trauma Supportive Care.)

A. Life-threatening (urgent)

B. Non-life-threatening (not urgent)

V. **Secondary Assessment.**

A. Conduct a toe-to-head survey.

B. Neurological assessment.

1. Pupillary response.
2. Pediatric Glasgow Coma Scale score.

C. Repeat–PAT and rapid cardiopulmonary assessment.

3.1.1 Pediatric Assessment

D. Obtain a medical history.
   1. **S**—Symptoms; assessment of chief complaint.
   2. **A**—Allergies.
   3. **M**—Medications.
   4. **P**—Past medical history.
   5. **L**—Last oral intake.
   6. **E**—Events leading to illness or injury.

VI. **Ongoing Assessment.** Reassess the patient every fifteen (15) minutes, or for critical patients every five (5) minutes.
   A. Continually monitor:
      1. Respiratory effort
      2. Skin color
      3. Mental status
      4. Temperature
      5. Pulse oximetry
   B. Reevaluate vital signs and compare with baseline vital signs.

VII. **Other Assessment Techniques.**
   A. Glucose determination (see Medical Procedure 4.39).
   B. Capnography (see Medical Procedure 4.22).
   C. Dealing with the autistic patient (see Medical Procedure 4.42).

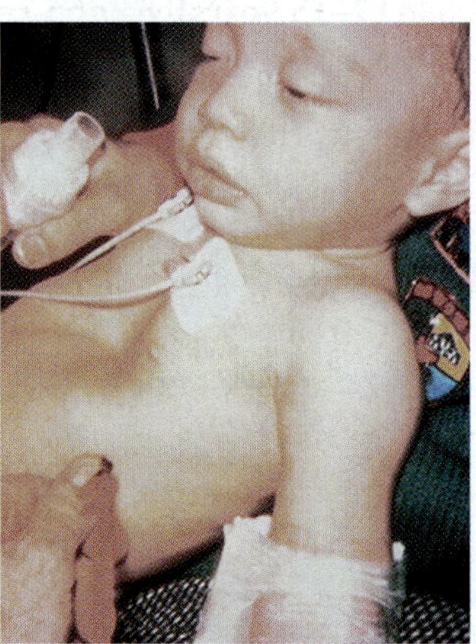

A limp, pale child unable to make eye contact or a child with retractions may be critically ill or injured.

3.1.2 Airway Management

Supportive Care

EMT and Paramedic

- Initial Assessment Protocol 3.1.1.

If spontaneous breathing is present without compromise:

- Monitor breathing during transport.
- Administer oxygen as needed (a).
  - Infants via infant mask at 2–4 L/min.
  - Small child (1–8 years) via pediatric mask at 6–8 L/min.
  - Older child (9–15 years) via non-rebreather mask at 10–15 L/min.
  - If the mask is not tolerated, administer oxygen via blow-by method.

If spontaneous breathing is present with compromise:

- Maintain the patient's airway (e.g., modified jaw-thrust procedure) (see Medical Procedure 4.6).
- Suction as needed (see Medical Procedure 4.9, Flexible Suctioning, and Medical Procedure 4.10, Rigid Suctioning).
- Administer oxygen.
  - Infants via infant mask at 2–4 L/min.
  - Small child (1–8 years) via pediatric mask at 6–8 L/min.
  - Older child (9–15 years) via non-rebreather mask at 10–15 L/min.
  - If the mask is not tolerated, administer oxygen via blow-by method.
- If unable to maintain the patient's airway, insert an oropharyngeal, nasopharyngeal, or supraglottic airway (e.g., King tube or LMA) as needed (see Medical Procedure 4.13, King Supraglottic Airway).
- Assist ventilations with bag-valve mask as needed (see Medical Procedure 4.4, Rescue Breathing).
- Apply and monitor a pulse oximeter and capnography monitoring device, as soon as possible (see Medical Procedures 4.29 and 4.22).

If spontaneous breathing is absent or markedly compromised:

- Maintain the patient's airway (e.g., modified jaw-thrust procedure) (see Medical Procedure 4.6).
- Suction as needed (see Medical Procedure 4.9, Flexible Suctioning, and Medical Procedure 4.10, Rigid Suctioning).
- If unable to maintain the patient's airway, insert an oropharyngeal, nasopharyngeal, or supraglottic airway (e.g., King tube or LMA) (see Medical Procedure 4.13, King Supraglottic Airway).
- Ventilate with a bag-valve mask (see Medical Procedure 4.4, Rescue Breathing).

3.1.2 Airway Management

ALS Level 1

Paramedic Only

- Perform endotracheal intubation as a procedure of last resort if previous supraglottic/bag-valve mask support is ineffective (a)(b)(c) (see Medical Procedure 4.18, Intubation).
  - Attach an end-tidal CO_2 monitoring device.
  - Confirm ETT placement via auscultation and capnography.
  - Secure the ETT with tape or an ETT-stabilizing device.
  - Monitor SpO_2 with the pulse oximeter.
- Insert a nasogastric tube and decompress the patient's stomach. *Do not delay transport to place the NG tube.* (See Medical Procedure 4.18, Intubation.)
- If unable to intubate and the patient cannot be adequately ventilated by other means, perform a needle cricothyroidotomy (see Medical Procedure 4.15, Needle Cricothyroidotomy for Pediatrics) and transport the patient rapidly to the hospital.

ALS Level 2

None.

Note

(a) Ineffective ventilations may be evident by poor chest rise, poor lung sounds, and capnography readings failing to improve with ventilations.

(b) **The bag-valve mask should be initially used for ventilatory support.** Endotracheal intubation should be used only when the BVM is ineffective or prolonged ventilatory support is necessary.

(c) Follow the Universal Airway Algorithm on all intubations.

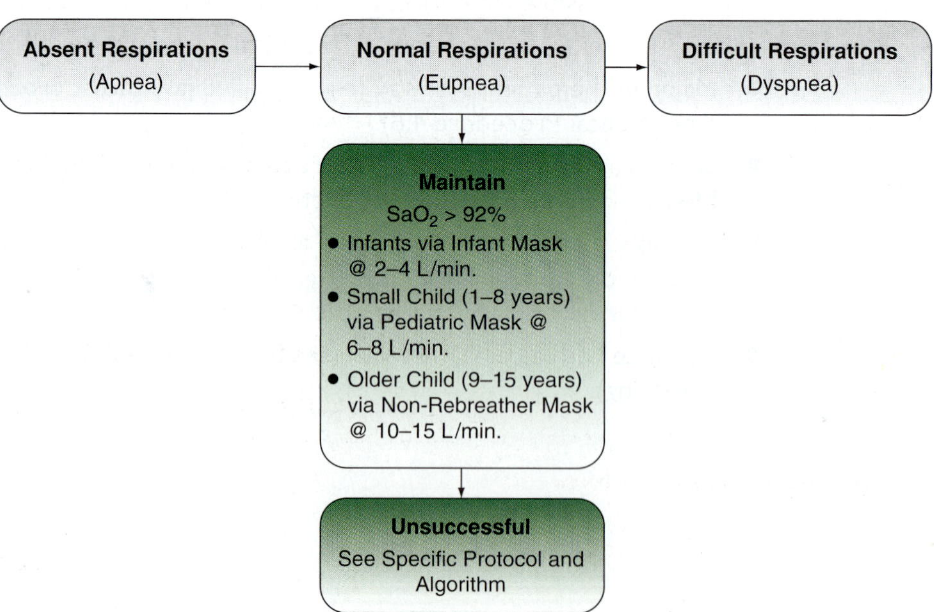

Eupnea Airway Algorithm.

3.1.2 Airway Management

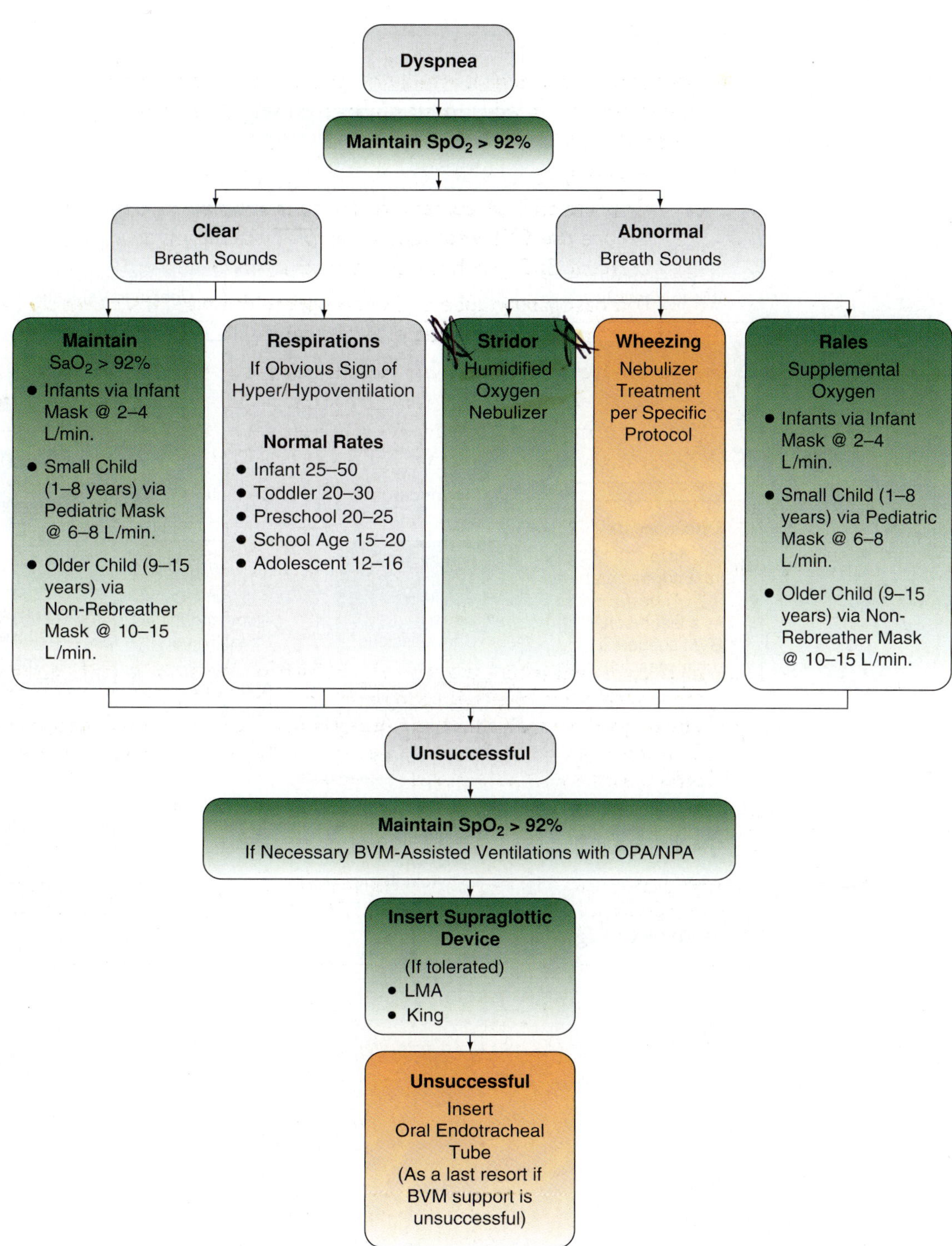

Dyspnea Airway Algorithm.

3.1.2 Airway Management

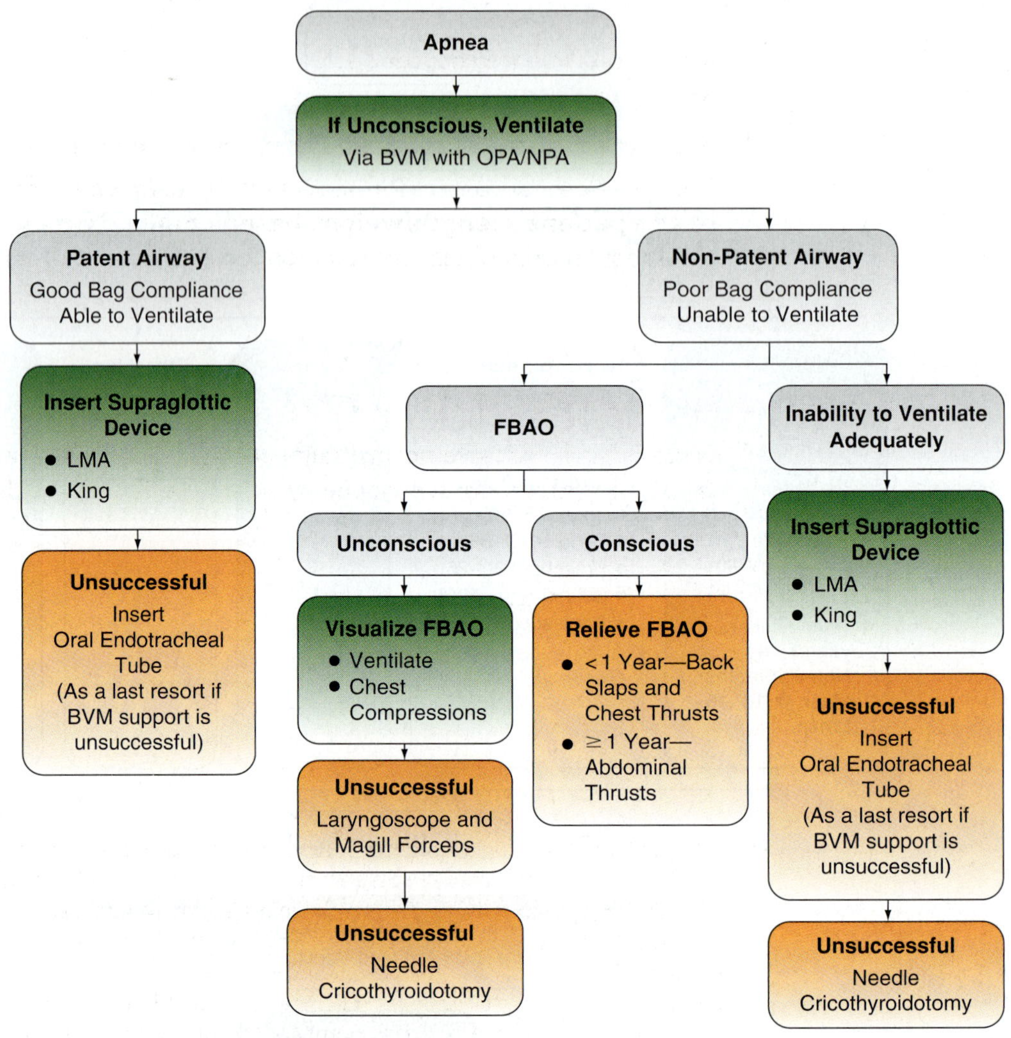

Apnea Airway Algorithm.

3.1.3 Medical Supportive Care

Supportive Care

EMT and Paramedic

- Initial Assessment Protocol 3.1.1.
- Airway Management Protocol 3.1.2.
- Attempt to maintain or restore normal body temperature.
- Establish hospital contact for notification of an incoming patient and **advise of the patient's length/weight-based color category.** In addition, the paramedic should obtain consultation for ALS Level 2 orders.

ALS Level 1

Paramedic and Authorized EMT

- Establish an IV/IO; give normal saline with a regular infusion set as needed (a)(b)(c)(d)(e), unless overridden by other specific protocols.

Paramedic Only

- Monitor the ECG as needed.

ALS Level 2

None.

Note

(a) Authorized IV routes include all peripheral venous sites. External jugular veins may be utilized when other peripheral site attempts have been unsuccessful or would be inappropriate. A large-bore intracath should be used for unstable patients; avoid establishing access sites below the diaphragm.

(b) A Buretrol, Volutrol, or Soluset should be used in lieu of a regular infusion set when starting an IV on patients who are 8 years old or younger.

(c) An IV lock or medication access point (MAP) may be used in lieu of an IV bag in some patients with intravenous lines, when appropriate.

(d) An EMT who has been authorized by his/her Medical Director may establish an IV.

(e) When unable to establish an IV in a pediatric patient who needs to be resuscitated, an intraosseous line may be used by the *Paramedic Only* (see Medical Procedures 4.56, 4.57, and 4.59).

3.1.4 Trauma Supportive Care

Supportive Care

EMT and Paramedic

- Initial Assessment Protocol 3.1.1. Initiate a Trauma Alert, if applicable (see General Protocol 1.10, Trauma Transport).
- Airway Management Protocol 3.1.2. Manually stabilize the patient's c-spine as needed.
- Correct any open wound/sucking chest wound (occlusive dressing).

Paramedic Only

- Correct any massive flail segment that causes respiratory compromise (intubate).
- Correct any tension pneumothorax (see Medical Procedure 4.14, Chest Decompression).

EMT and Paramedic

- Control any hemorrhage.
- Immobilize the c-spine and secure the patient to a backboard or pediatric immobilizer as needed (see Medical Procedure 4.52, Spinal Immobilization) (a).
- Keep the patient warm.
- Expedite transport.

The following steps should not delay transport:

- Complete bandaging, splinting, and packaging as needed.
- Contact online medical control for notification of an incoming patient and obtain consultation for ALS Level 2 orders.

ALS Level 1

Paramedic and Authorized EMT

- Establish an IV; give normal saline with a regular infusion set as needed (b)(c)(d), unless overridden by other specific protocol.
- Monitor the ECG.

Paramedic Only

- Monitor the ECG.

3.1.4 Trauma Supportive Care

ALS Level 2

None.

NOTE

(a) Infants and small children in car seats may be immobilized without removing them from the car seat, as long as it will not interfere with patient assessment and other needed procedures and the car seat is intact. If the patient is not in a car seat on your arrival, do not put the patient back into the car seat to immobilize him/her; use a backboard or pediatric immobilizer instead.

(b) Authorized IV routes include all peripheral venous sites. The external jugular vein may be utilized when other peripheral site attempts have been unsuccessful or would be inappropriate. Two IVs, using large-bore intracaths, should be used for unstable patients; avoid establishing access sites below the diaphragm. **Rapid transport should not be delayed to establish an IV.**

(c) A Buretrol, Volutrol, or Soluset should be used in lieu of a regular infusion set when starting an IV on patients who are younger than 8 years old.

(d) When unable to establish an IV in the pediatric patient who needs to be resuscitated, an intraosseous line may be used by the *Paramedic Only* (see Medical Procedures 4.56, 4.57, and 4.59).

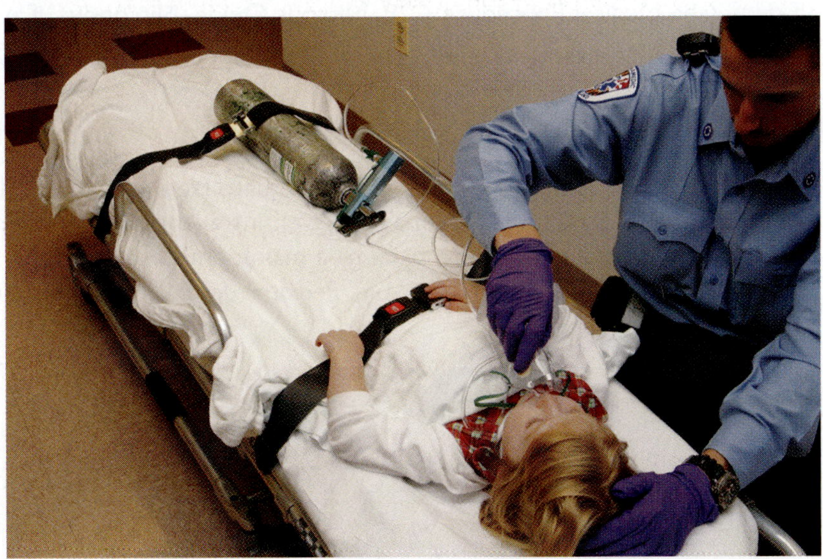

Rapid transport should not be delayed to establish an IV.

3.1.5 Pain Management

Paramedic Only

This entire protocol is ALS/Paramedic Only.

Isolated Extremity Fracture

The purpose of this procedure is to manage pain associated with isolated extremity fractures that are not associated with multisystem trauma or hemodynamic instability.

ALS Level 1

- Patients should be asked to quantify their pain on an analog pain scale (from 0 = least severe to 10 = most severe) or Wong-Baker Faces Scale; for infants, an infant behavior score may be used (a)(b). This score should be documented and used to measure the effectiveness of analgesia.
- Distal circulation, sensation, and movement in the injured extremity should be noted and recorded.
- The extremity should be immobilized as described in Pediatric Protocol 3.9.5, Extremity Injuries. **Self-administered** analgesia with nitrous oxide should be given special consideration for pain management during this procedure (see Medical Procedure 4.28, Nitrous Oxide–Nitronox), if available.
- Extremity fractures should be elevated, if possible, and cold applied.

ALS Level 2

- If pain persists and systolic BP is adequate (see Appendix 7.11, Pediatric Vital Signs), morphine sulfate may be given intravenously in increments every 3–5 minutes, titrated to pain, to a maximum dose of 10 mg. Administer at a rate not to exceed 1 mg/min. *Pediatric dose:* 0.1 mg/kg IV. *Infant dose:* 0.05 mg/kg IV (c).

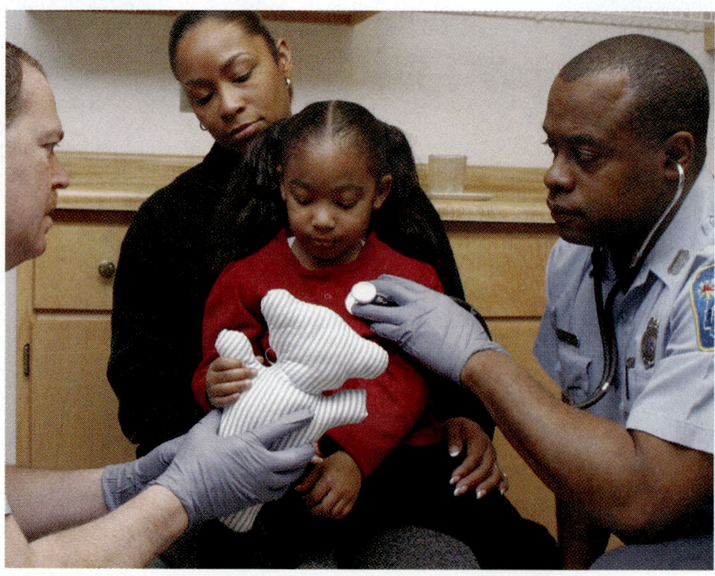

Use distraction techniques to help reduce the child's pain.

3.1.5 Pain Management

Acute Back Strain

This procedure should be used in the isolated back strain where an acute abdominal process is not suspected (see Appendix 7.1, Abdominal Pain Differential).

ALS Level 1

- Patients should be asked to quantify their pain on an analog pain scale (from 0 = least severe to 10 = most severe) or Wong-Baker Faces Scale; for infants, an infant behavior score may be used (a)(b). This score should be documented and used to measure the effectiveness of analgesia.
- **Self-administered** nitrous oxide may be given (see Medical Procedure 4.28, Nitrous Oxide–Nitronox), if available.
- Secure the patient to a backboard as needed.

ALS Level 2

- If pain persists and systolic BP is adequate (see Appendix 7.11, Pediatric Vital Signs), morphine sulfate may be given intravenously in increments, titrated to pain, to a maximum dose of 5 mg. Administer at a rate not to exceed 1 mg/min. *Pediatric dose:* 0.1 mg/kg IV. *Infant dose:* 0.05 mg/kg IV.
- For patients > 2 years of age: If pain persists and systolic BP is adequate (see Appendix 7.11, Pediatric Vital Signs), ketorolac tromethamine (Toradol®) may be given as 1 mg/kg (maximum 30 mg) IV or 2 mg/kg (maximum 60 mg) IM, if available (d).

3.1.5 Pain Management

Soft-Tissue Injuries, Burns, Bites, and Stings

This procedure is used for pain associated with soft-tissue injuries, burns, bites, and stings that are not associated with multisystem trauma or hemodynamic instability.

ALS Level 1

- Patients should be asked to quantify their pain on an analog pain scale (from 0 = least severe to 10 = most severe) or Wong-Baker Faces Scale; for infants, an infant behavior score may be used (a)(b). This score should be documented and used to measure the effectiveness of analgesia.
- **Self-administered** nitrous oxide may be given (see Medical Procedure 4.28, Nitrous Oxide–Nitronox), if available.

ALS Level 2

- If pain persists and systolic BP is adequate (see Appendix 7.10, Pediatric Vital Signs), morphine sulfate may be given intravenously in increments, titrated to pain, to a maximum dose of 5 mg. Administer at a rate not to exceed 1 mg/min. *Pediatric dose:* 0.1 mg/kg IV. *Infant dose:* 0.05 mg/kg IV.
- For patients > 2 years of age: If pain persists and systolic BP is adequate (see Appendix 7.10, Pediatric Vital Signs), ketorolac tromethamine (Toradol®) may be given as 1 mg/kg (maximum 30 mg) IV or 2 mg/kg (maximum 60 mg) IM, if available (d).

Note

(a) Wong-Baker Faces Scale.

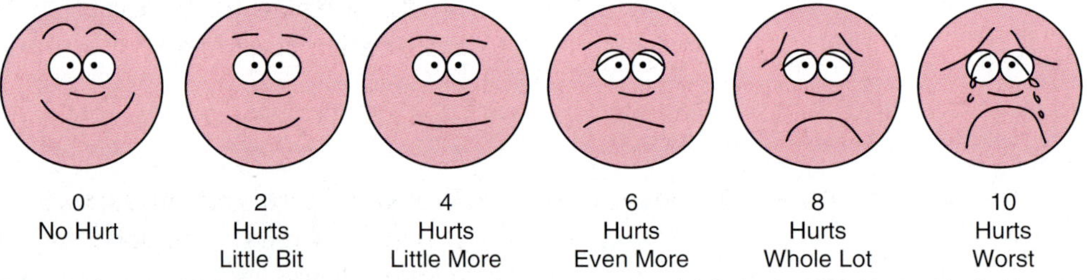

From Hockenberry MJ, Wilson D. *Wong's essentials of pediatric nursing, ed. 8,* St. Louis, 2009, Mosby. Used with permission. Copyright Mosby.

(b) Infant Behavior Score.

3: pediatric protocols

3.1.5 Pain Management

Assessment of Score

0	"Relaxed": infant comfortable, not distressed.
1–2	Some transitory distress caused: returns immediately to "relaxed."
3–4	Transitory distress; likely to respond to consolation.
5	Infant experiences pain; if no response to consolation, **may require analgesia.**
6	"Anguished" and "exaggerated": infant experiencing acute pain; is unlikely to respond to consolation, **will probably benefit from analgesia.**
7–8	"Inert": no response to traumatic procedure; infant is habituated to pain; will not respond to consolation; **systematic pain control by analgesia should be considered.**

Facial Expression

0	Relaxed	Smooth muscled; relaxed expression; either in deep sleep or quietly alert.
1	Anxious	Anxious expression; frown; REM behind closed lids; wandering gaze; eyes narrowed; lips parted; pursed lips as if "oo" is pronounced.
2	Anguished	Anguished expression/crumpled face; brow bulge; eye squeeze; nasolabial furrow pronounced; square-stretched mouth; cupped tongue; "silent cry."
3	Inert	No response to trauma; no crying; rigidity; gaze avoidance; fixed/staring gaze; apathy; diminished alertness (only during or immediately after traumatic procedure).

Body Movement

0	Relaxed	Relaxed trunk and limbs; body in tucked position; hands in cupped position or willing to grasp a finger.
1	Restless	Moro reflex; startles; jerky or uncoordinated movement of limbs; flexion/extension of limbs; attempt to withdraw limb from site of injury.
2	Exaggerated	Abnormal position of limbs; limb/neck extension; splaying of fingers and/or toes; flailing or thrashing of limbs; arching of back; side swiping/guarding site of injury.
3	Inert	No response to trauma; inertia; limpness/rigidity; immobility (only during or immediately after traumatic procedure).

3.1.5 Pain Management

Color

0	Normal skin color.
1	Redness; congestion.
2	Pallor; mottling; gray.

(c) Extreme caution should be used with administering morphine to a patient with an $SpO_2 < 95\%$.

(d) Toradol is contraindicated with the following:

- Potential surgical candidate (e.g., trauma patient)
- Known allergies to nonsteroidal anti-inflammatory drugs (e.g., aspirin, ibuprofen)
- History of nasal polyps
- Angioedema
- Bronchospastic reactivity (e.g., asthma)
- Bleeding disorders (e.g., ulcers)
- Kidney dysfunction

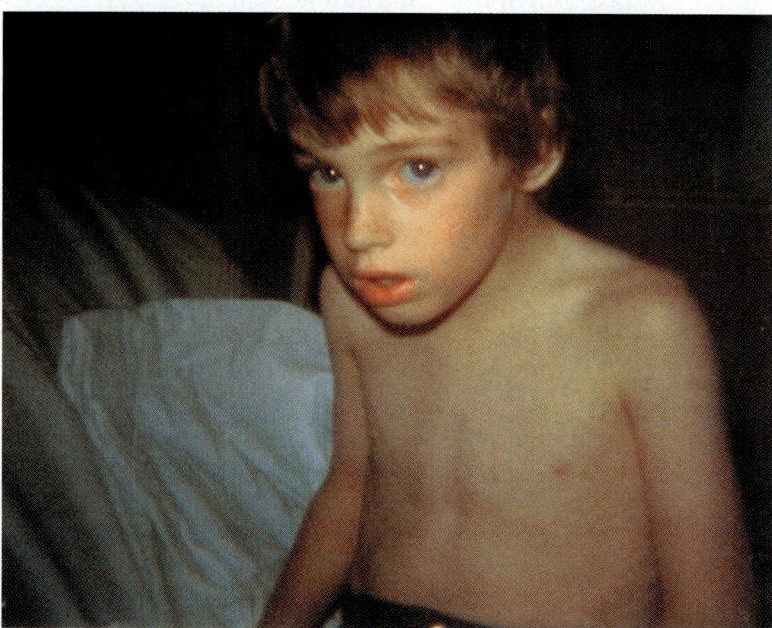

Assess the patient for facial expression, body movement, and color.

3.2 Pediatric Respiratory Emergencies

Most children requiring urgent intervention have primary respiratory problems. Approximately 80–90% of all pediatric cardiac arrests originate in the respiratory system. When the child who is in respiratory distress can no longer compensate, respiratory failure will be followed by cardiac failure. It is crucial to recognize respiratory distress and dysfunction early, so that cardiopulmonary failure may be prevented. Note that the respiratory system also attempts to compensate for the hypoxia and acidosis found in primary circulatory failure. Assessment of the pediatric respiratory system should focus not on clinical status, as reflected by general appearance (adequacy of cerebral oxygenation and ventilation) and work of breathing.

Components of Appearance

1.	**Alertness**	How responsive and interactive is the child with a stranger or other changes in the environment? Is the patient restless, agitated or lethargic?
2.	**Distractibility**	How readily does a person, object, or sound draw the child's interest or attention? Will the patient play with a toy or new object?
3.	**Consolability**	Can the patient be comforted by the caregiver or by the paramedic?
4.	**Eye contact**	Does the child maintain eye contact with objects or people? Will the patient fix his/her gaze on a face?
5.	**Speech/cry**	Is the speech/cry strong and spontaneous? Weak and muffled? Hoarse?
6.	**Spontaneous motor activity**	Is the patient moving and resisting vigorously and spontaneously? Is there good muscle tone and responsiveness?
7.	**Color**	Is the patient pink? Or is the patient pale, ashen, blue, or mottled? Does the skin coloring of the trunk differ from that of the extremities?

Signs of Work of Breathing

1.	**Use of accessory muscles**	Pediatric patients will use accessory muscles early to compensate for deficiencies in perfusion. Intercostal and supraclavicular retractions, as well as diaphragmatic breathing (see-saw), may be very apparent.
2.	**Respiratory rate**	Significant finding if > 60/min or < 10–20/min.
3.	**Tidal volume**	Inspection of chest wall movement may not be adequate for assessment of tidal volume. It is imperative to auscultate bilateral lung sounds to determine the adequacy of tidal volume.
4.	**Nasal flaring**	Flaring of the external nares indicates respiratory distress.

3.2 Pediatric Respiratory Emergencies

5.	**Grunting**	Grunting is an ominous sign associated with severe distress. It is caused by a premature closure of the glottis on exhalation due to atelectasis. The patient is attempting to maintain a positive end-expiratory pressure (PEEP) to allow for better lung inflation.
6.	**Cyanosis**	Cyanosis is usually a late finding and will initially be visible around the mouth and gums (perioral) and nail beds.
7.	**Pulse oximeter**	$SpO_2 < 90\%$ is suggestive of respiratory insufficiency.
8.	**Lung sounds**	Auscultation of bilateral lung sounds not only assesses tidal volume, but may also uncover abnormal sounds (e.g., wheezing, stridor, rales).

Specific treatments for the different causes of respiratory distress are outlined in the following protocols. When the paramedic is unsure as to which protocol to follow, he/she should follow the protocols in Section 3.1 and contact medical control for further direction.

References

American Academy of Pediatrics, Pediatric Education for Prehospital Professionals, Boston, 2006.

American Heart Association/American Academy of Pediatrics, *Textbook of Pediatric Advanced Life Support*, Dallas, 2006.

American Heart Association, "2005 Guidelines for CPR and ECC," *Supplement to Circulation*, 112:24, 2005.

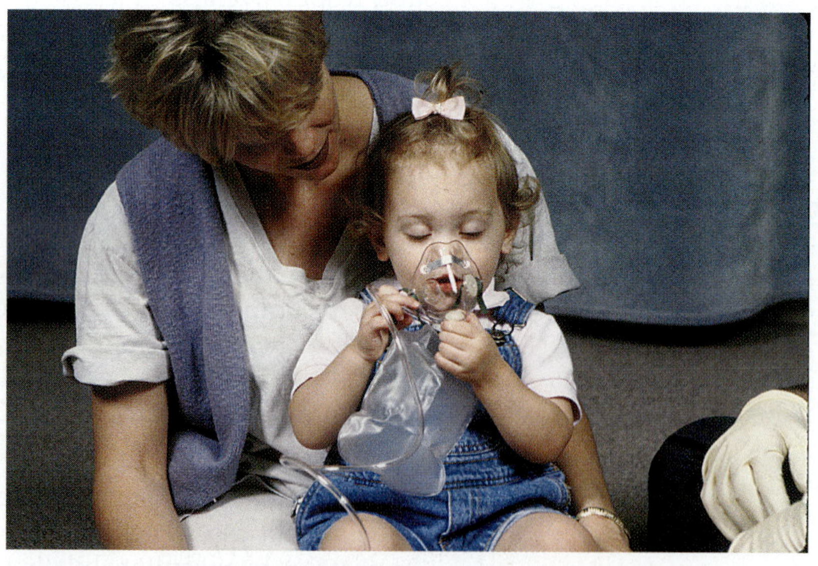

3.2.1 Airway Obstruction

Causes of upper airway obstruction include the tongue, foreign bodies, swelling of the upper airway due to angio-neurotic edema (see Pediatric Protocol 3.7.1, Allergic Reactions/Anaphylaxis), trauma to the airway, and infections (see Pediatric Protocol 3.2.2, Upper Airway [Stridor–Croup/Epiglottitis]). Differentiation of the cause of upper airway obstruction is essential to determine the proper treatment.

Supportive Care

- Medical Supportive Care Protocol 3.1.3.
- If air exchange is inadequate and there is a reasonable suspicion of foreign body airway obstruction (FBAO), apply abdominal thrusts (see Medical Procedure 4.3, Suspected Foreign Body Airway Obstruction [FBAO 4.3]) (a).

ALS Level 1

- If unable to relieve the FBAO, visualize it with a laryngoscope and extract the foreign body with Magill forceps.
- If the obstruction is due to trauma and/or edema, or if uncontrollable bleeding into the airway causes life-threatening ventilatory impairment, proceed directly to endotracheal intubation (see Medical Procedure 4.18, Pediatric Intubation).
- If unable to intubate and the patient cannot be adequately ventilated by other means, perform a needle cricothyroidotomy (see Medical Procedure 4.15, Needle Cricothyroidotomy for Pediatrics).

ALS Level 2

None.

Note

(a) If air exchange is adequate with a partial airway obstruction, do not interfere, but rather encourage the patient to cough up the obstruction. Continue to monitor for adequacy of air exchange. If air exchange becomes inadequate, continue with the protocol.

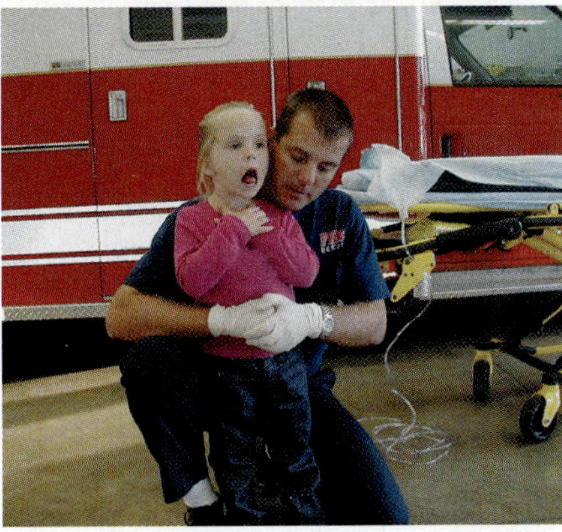

Use abdominal thrusts to treat complete airway obstruction in the conscious child.

3.2.2 Upper Airway (Stridor–Croup/Epiglottitis)

Stridor is a high-pitched "crowing" sound caused by restriction of the upper airway (usually heard on inspiration). In addition to FBAO (see Pediatric Protocol 3.2.1), stridor can be caused by croup and epiglottitis.

Croup (laryngotracheobronchitis) is a viral infection of the upper airway, which causes edema/inflammation below the larynx and glottis with a resultant narrowing of the lumen of the airway. Croup most often occurs in children 6 months to 4 years of age. The child with croup will have stridor, a distinctive barking cough, and cold symptoms (low-grade fever [100–101°F]), with a gradual onset of respiratory distress.

Epiglottitis is an acute infection and inflammation of the epiglottis that potentially is life-threatening. Since the *Haemophilus influenzae*, type B (Hib) vaccine became available, the incidence of epiglottitis has markedly decreased, yet it may still occur from other bacterial pathogens. Epiglottitis usually occurs in children 4 years of age and older. The child with epiglottitis will present with stridor, acute respiratory distress, sore throat, pain upon swallowing that causes the distinctive drooling, and high-grade fever (102–104°F). The patient may assume the classic tripod position.

Supportive Care

- Medical Supportive Care Protocol 3.1.3, including use of a pulse oximeter (see Medical Procedure 4.29, Pulse Oximeter). Avoid IVs in these patients (a).
- Avoid agitating the child with suspected epiglottitis. Keep the patient in a position of comfort (he/she may be held by a parent to avoid agitation). Never examine the epiglottis (a).
- Administer humidified oxygen. If humidified oxygen is unavailable, use nebulized saline. Do not force an oxygen mask on a pediatric patient; use the blow-by technique if necessary (a).

ALS Level 1

None.

ALS Level 2

None.

Note

(a) Avoid any procedure that will agitate the pediatric patient.

3.2.3 Lower Airway (Wheezing–Asthma/Bronchiolitis)

Wheezing is a whistling-type breath sound associated with narrowing or spasm of the smaller airways (usually heard on expiration, but may also be heard on inspiration).

Wheezing in the child younger than 1 year of age is usually the result of **bronchiolitis,** a viral infection of the bronchioles that causes prominent expiratory wheezing, clinically resembling asthma.

Asthma is a chronic inflammatory disease that is triggered by many different factors (e.g., environmental allergens, cold air, exercise, foods, irritants, certain medications). Asthma is characterized by a two-phase response. The first phase is associated with a histamine release, which causes bronchoconstriction and bronchial edema. Early treatment with bronchodilators may reverse the bronchospasm. The second phase consists of inflammation of the bronchioles and additional edema. The second phase will usually not respond to bronchodilators; instead, an anti-inflammatory medication (e.g., a corticosteroid) is typically required.

Assessment of the asthma patient usually includes a history of asthma with associated medications. The patient will be tachypneic and may have an unproductive cough. Use of accessory muscles is evident and wheezing may be heard, most commonly on expiration. In a severe asthma attack, the patient may not wheeze at all due to a lack of air flow.

Supportive Care

- Medical Supportive Care Protocol 3.1.3, including use of a pulse oximeter (see Medical Procedure 4.29, Pulse Oximeter).

ALS Level I

- Use the following bronchodilator:
  - Albuterol (Ventolin®): one nebulizer treatment. If patient < 1 year or < 10 kg, mix 1.25 mg in 1.5 mL of normal saline (0.083%); if patient > 1 year or > 10 kg, mix 2.5 mg in 3 mL of normal saline (0.083%) (see Medical Procedure 4.27, Nebulizer). May repeat twice as needed.
- If a bronchodilator is administered, add ipratropium bromide (Atrovent®) 0.5 mg (0.5 mL) to albuterol nebulizer treatment.
- Consider the need for assisted ventilation and intubation (see Medical Procedure 4.18, Intubation).
- If respiratory distress is severe, administer epinephrine (1:1000) 0.01 mg/kg SQ (if < 8 years, give 0.15 mg up to a maximum dose of 0.3 mg ; if > 8 years, maximum dose is 0.3–0.5 mg).

3.2.3 Lower Airway (Wheezing–Asthma/Bronchiolitis)

- If respiratory distress is severe, administer one of the following steroids:
  - Methylprednisolone sodium succinate (Solu-Medrol®) 2 mg/kg IV (maximum dose = 125 mg), if available.

  or

  - Dexamethasone (Decadron®) 0.5 mg/kg IV (maximum dose = 10 mg), if available.

ALS Level 2

- For severe dyspnea, administer magnesium sulfate 40 mg/kg (maximum dose = 2 g) IV (mixed in 50 mL of D_5W given over 15–20 minutes), as needed.
- Repeat epinephrine (1:1000) 0.01 mg/kg SQ (if < 8 years, 0.15 mg up to a maximum dose of 0.3 mg; if > 8 years, maximum dose is 0.3–0.5 mg).

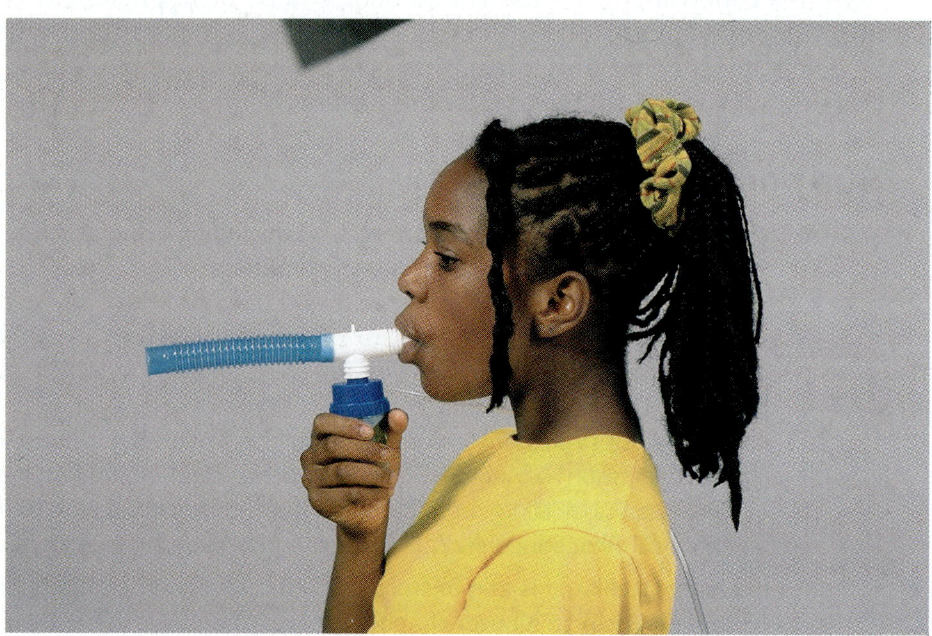

Oxygen-powered nebulizer.

3.3 Pediatric Cardiac Dysrhythmias

Cardiac dysrhythmias in pediatric patients are uncommon and are usually due to noncardiac problems, unless the patient is known to have congenital or acquired cardiac disease. Cardiac arrest is usually the end result of hypoxemia and acidosis resulting from respiratory insufficiency or shock. Therefore, attention should be given initially to support of the respiratory system. Pediatric dysrhythmias can be classified into three categories: slow rhythms, fast rhythms, or no rhythm. The most common dysrhythmia is bradycardia, which is the result of hypoxia or acidosis. Tachycardia can be a compensatory mechanism or a result of a reentry mechanism. Ventricular fibrillation, although rare in pediatric patients, is usually the result of hypoxia. Asystole is a terminal event, following prolonged, untreated bradycardia.

In July 2003, the Pediatric Advanced Life Support (PALS) Task Force of the International Liaison Committee on Resuscitation (ILCOR) made the following recommendation regarding use of AEDs in children:

> Automated external defibrillators (AEDs) may be used for children 1 to 8 years of age who have no signs of circulation. Ideally the device should deliver a pediatric dose. The arrhythmia detection algorithm used in the device should demonstrate high specificity for pediatric shockable rhythms; i.e., it will not recommend delivery of a shock for non-shockable rhythms (Class IIb).[1]

The protocols in Section 3.3 follow the PALS guidelines. The paramedic should use these protocols to guide him/her through the treatment of cardiac patients with specific dysrhythmias and accompanying signs and symptoms. After stabilization of the patient, the paramedic may need to refer to additional protocols for continued treatment (e.g., other cardiac protocols).

In cardiac arrest, a major component of the primary and secondary survey is to consider the secondary *differential diagnosis* and to think carefully about what could be causing the arrest. The "H's and T's" chart will assist in the recognition of a possible underlying cause.

[1]American Heart Association, National ECC Training Memo, August 15, 2003.

3.3 Pediatric Cardiac Dysrhythmias

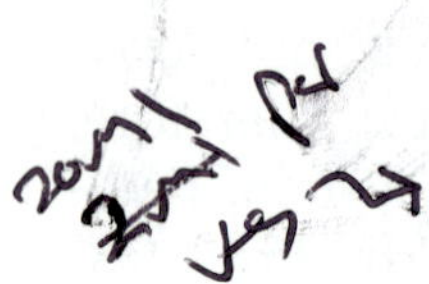

H's

Cause	Treatment	Protocol
Hypovolemia	Fluid challenge with normal saline 500 mL IV/IO	Shock Protocol
Hypoxia	Airway management	Protocol 3.1.2
Hydrogen ion–acidosis	Airway management, ventilate, consider sodium bicarbonate	Protocol 3.1.2 Drug Summary 5.45
Hyperkalemia	Consider calcium chloride; Consider sodium bicarbonate 1 mEq/kg	Drug Summary 5.9 Drug Summary 5.45
Hypothermia	Cold-related emergencies	Protocol 3.8.3
Hypoglycemia	If glucose < 60 mg/dl, consider D_{50} or Glucagon	Protocol 3.7.2 Drug Summary 5.13 and 5.22
Hypocalcemia	Consider calcium chloride	Drug Summary 5.9

T's

Cause	Treatment	Protocol
Tablets		Protocol 3.6
Tamponade, cardiac	Consider fluid challenge, dopamine drip	Protocol 3.4.1
Tension pneumothorax	Consider chest decompression	Procedure 4.14
Thrombosis, coronary	Consider AMI, cardiogenic shock	Protocol 3.4
Thrombosis, pulmonary		Protocol 3.4
Trauma		Protocol 3.9

3.3.1 Asystole

Supportive Care

- Medical Supportive Care Protocol 3.1.3.
- Determine the patient's (un)responsiveness and check the ABCs.
- Oxygenate with 15–25 L/min via bag-valve mask with an appropriate airway adjunct device at 8–10 BPM (see Airway Protocol 3.1.2) (a).
- Begin immediate chest compressions at a rate of 100/min for 2 minutes while the monitor is being attached.
- **Do not interrupt CPR to check the heart rhythm. Continuous uninterrupted compressions are paramount to patient survival.**
- Check the heart rhythm; confirm asystole in two leads.
- Resume 2 minutes of continuous compressions at 100/min; check the heart rhythm.
- If available, attach an impedance threshold device (ITD).
- Obtain a SAMPLE history.
- Perform a focused exam.
- **Consider the H's and T's.**

ALS Level 1

- Establish IV or IO access; give normal saline KVO.
- Administer epinephrine (1:10,000) 0.01 mg/kg IV/IO (maximum dose = 1 mg). If unable to establish an IV or IO, administer epinephrine (1:1000) 0.1 mg/kg ETT (maximum ETT dose = 2 mg). Repeat every 3–5 minutes for the duration of pulselessness.
- Perform a glucose test with a finger stick. If glucose < 60 mg/dL, administer:
  - If < 8 years: D_{25} 2 mL/kg IV/IO.
  - If > 8 years: D_{50} 1 mL/kg IV/IO (see Medical Procedure 4.39) (b).
- Perform five cycles of CPR and then reevaluate the heart rhythm.
- If a pulse is present, begin post-resuscitative care.
- Consider sodium bicarbonate (8.4%) 1 mEq/kg IV/IO (c).

ALS Level 2

None.

Note

(a) Give 1 breath every 6 seconds or 1 breath every 10 compressions.
(b) To avoid infiltration and resultant tissue necrosis, dextrose 25% and 50% should be given via slow IV with intermittent aspiration of the IV line to confirm IV patency, followed by saline flush.
(c) Sodium bicarbonate (4.2%) 1 mEq/kg IV/IO should be administered to infants (dilute 8.4% 1:1 with normal saline to make 4.2%).

3.3.2 Bradycardia

Causes of symptomatic bradycardia include hypoxemia, hypothermia, head injury, heart block, heart transplant (special situation), and toxin/poison/drug overdose.

Supportive Care

- Medical Supportive Care Protocol 3.1.3.
- Assure adequate ventilation and oxygenation.
- If heart rate < 60/min in an infant or child associated with poor systemic perfusion, start chest compressions (see Medical Procedure 4.2, Cardiopulmonary Resuscitation).
- Obtain a SAMPLE history.
- Perform a focused exam.
- **Consider the H's and T's.**

ALS Level 1

- Administer epinephrine (1:10,000) 0.01 mg/kg IV or IO (maximum dose = 1 mg IV or IO). If unable to establish IV or IO access, administer epinephrine (1:1000) 0.1 mg/kg ETT, up to a maximum dose of 2 mg (a). Repeat every 3–5 minutes at the same dose (b).
- Administer atropine 0.02 mg/kg IV or IO (minimum single dose = 0.1 mg) (c). If unable to establish IV or IO access, administer atropine 0.03 mg/kg ETT (a) (same minimum dose as IV or IO). May repeat atropine once (b)(d)(e).

ALS Level 2

- If the patient is conscious and aware of the situation, consider sedation with one of the following benzodiazepines:
  - Diazepam (Valium®) 0.1 mg/kg IV.

  or

  - Midazolam (Versed®) 0.05 mg/kg IV.

  or

  - Lorazepam (Ativan®) 0.05 mg/kg IV.
- Use an external pacemaker (see Medical Procedure 4.30, External Pacemaker).

NOTE

(a) Flush with 5 mL of normal saline and follow with five ventilations.
(b) Administer atropine before epinephrine for bradycardia due to suspected increased vagal tone or primary AV block.
(c) Small doses of atropine (≤ 0.1 mg) may produce paradoxical bradycardia.
(d) Maximum single dose for a child is 0.5 mg.
(e) Maximum single dose for an adolescent is 1 mg.

3: pediatric protocols

3.3.3 Narrow Complex Tachycardia

Pediatric patients suffering from tachycardia may or may not exhibit symptoms. Narrow complex tachycardia (QRS ≤ 0.08 second) may be either sinus tachycardia or supraventricular tachycardia. The following rates should be considered:

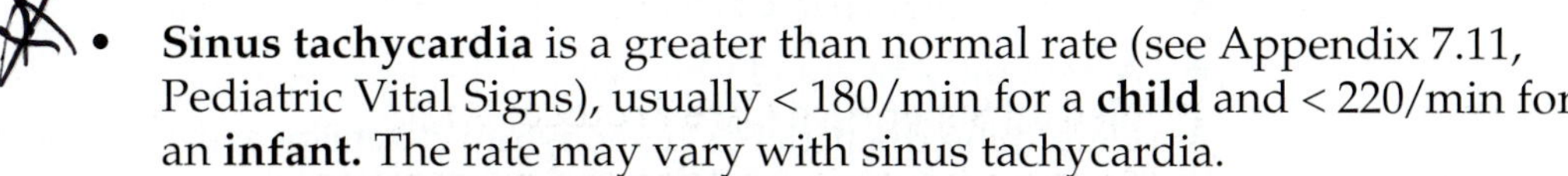

- **Sinus tachycardia** is a greater than normal rate (see Appendix 7.11, Pediatric Vital Signs), usually < 180/min for a **child** and < 220/min for an **infant.** The rate may vary with sinus tachycardia.
- **Supraventricular tachycardia** is usually a rate ≥ 220/min for infants. If the patient > 2 years of age, SVT may be slower (e.g., 180–220/min). The rate will not vary with SVT.

Wide complex SVTs are rare in children and, therefore, should initially be considered as ventricular in origin, unless proven otherwise (e.g., documented QRS morphology consistent with preexisting BBB or Wolff-Parkinson-White syndrome).

Unstable Sinus Tachycardia (Diminished Perfusion)

Supportive Care

- Medical Supportive Care Protocol 3.1.3.

ALS Level 1

- If suspected hypovolemia, administer a fluid challenge of normal saline 20 mL/kg IV.
- Consider other causes (e.g., **the H's and T's**).

ALS Level 2

None.

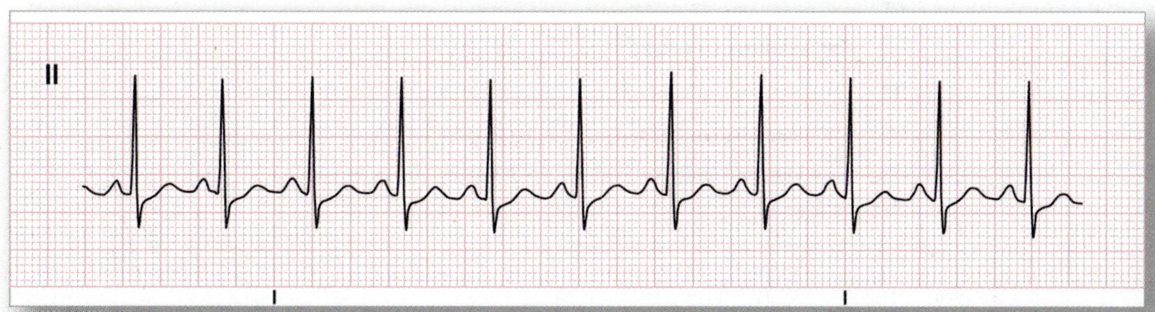

ECG of sinus tachycardia.

X all sync shocking in peds, pt is considered AL2 call for orders

3.3.3 Narrow Complex Tachycardia

Stable SVT (Normal Perfusion)

Supportive Care

- Medical Supportive Care Protocol 3.1.3.
- Assess the ABCs and vital signs.
- Determine the patient's hemodynamic stability and symptoms.
- Apply SpO_2 monitor and administer oxygen to maintain $SpO_2 \geq 92\%$.
- Obtain a SAMPLE history.
- Perform a focused exam.
- **Consider the H's and T's.**

ALS Level 1

- Apply an ECG; record a rhythm strip and obtain a 12-lead ECG.
- Establish IV access; give normal saline KVO.
- If the patient is asymptomatic, provide Medical Supportive Care Protocol 3.1.3 and transport.

ALS Level 2

- Attempt vagal maneuvers; begin with ice water (see Medical Procedure 4.35, Vagal Maneuvers) (a).
- Administer adenosine triphosphate (Adenocard®) 0.1 mg/kg (6 mg is the maximum first dose) via rapid IVP, followed by 6 mL normal saline flush (a).
- Repeat in 2 minutes: adenosine 0.2 mg/kg (12 mg is the maximum second dose) via rapid IVP, followed by 6 mL normal saline flush (a).

3.3.3 Narrow Complex Tachycardia

Unstable SVT (Diminished Perfusion)

Supportive Care

- Medical Supportive Care Protocol 3.1.3.
- Assess the ABCs and vital signs.
- Determine the patient's hemodynamic stability and symptoms.
- Apply SpO_2 monitor and administer oxygen to maintain $SpO_2 \geq 92\%$.
- Obtain a SAMPLE history.
- Perform a focused exam.
- **Consider the H's and T's.**

ALS Level 1

- Consider sinus tachycardia as the underlying rhythm, not SVT.
- Apply an ECG; record a rhythm strip and obtain a 12-lead ECG.
- Establish IV/IO access; give normal saline KVO.
- If the patient is responsive, administer adenosine triphosphate (Adenocard®) 0.1 mg/kg (maximum dose = 6 mg) via rapid IVP, followed by 6 mL normal saline flush (a).
- If the patient is responsive, repeat in 2 minutes: adenosine 0.2 mg/kg (maximum dose = 12 mg) via rapid IVP, followed by 6 mL normal saline flush. May repeat once in 2 minutes as needed (a).

ALS Level 2

- If the patient is conscious and aware of the situation, consider sedation with one of the following benzodiazepines:
  - Diazepam (Valium®) 0.1 mg/kg IV.

  or

  - Midazolam (Versed®) 0.05 mg/kg IV.

  or

  - Lorazepam (Ativan®) 0.05 mg/kg IV.
- If the patient is poorly responsive, apply synchronized cardioversion at 0.5 joule/kg to 1 joule/kg (b).
- If the patient is poorly responsive, apply synchronized cardioversion at 2 joule/kg (b).

Note

(a) Record the patient's heart rhythm while attempting to convert the rhythm so as to capture conversion data.
(b) Do not delay synchronized cardioversion to establish an IV for sedation purposes.

3: pediatric protocols

3.3.4 Pulseless Electrical Activity (PEA)

This protocol is used for electromechanical dissociation (EMD), pseudo-EMD, idioventricular rhythms, bradyasystolic rhythms, and post-defibrillation idioventricular rhythms.

Supportive Care

- Medical Supportive Care Protocol 3.1.3.
- Determine the patient's (un)responsiveness and check the ABCs.
- Oxygenate with 15–25 L/min via bag-valve mask with an appropriate airway adjunct device at 8–10 BPM (see Airway Protocol 3.1.2) (a).
- Begin immediate chest compressions at a rate of 100/min for 2 minutes while the monitor is being attached.
- **Do not interrupt CPR to check the heart rhythm. Continuous uninterrupted compressions are paramount to patient survival.**
- Check the heart rhythm.
- Resume 2 minutes of continuous compressions at 100/min; check the heart rhythm.
- If available, attach an impedance threshold device (ITD).
- Obtain a SAMPLE history.
- Perform a focused exam.
- **Consider the H's and T's.**

ALS Level 1

- Establish IV/IO access; give normal saline KVO.
- Administer epinephrine (1:10,000) 0.01 mg/kg IV or IO (maximum dose = 1 mg IV or IO). If unable to establish IV or IO access, administer epinephrine (1:1000) 0.1 mg/kg ETT (maximum ETT dose = 2 mg) (c). Repeat every 3–5 minutes for the duration of pulselessness (b).
- Administer five cycles of CPR.
- Evaluate the heart rhythm.
- If a pulse is present or there is a change in rhythm, treat the patient according to the applicable protocol or begin post-resuscitative care.
- Consider the cause (e.g., **the H's and T's**) and possible treatment options (e.g., glucose) (see specific protocols).
- Administer a fluid challenge of normal saline 20 mL/kg IV or IO.
- Consider sodium bicarbonate (8.4%) 1 mEq/kg IV or IO (c).

ALS Level 2

None.

NOTE

(a) Give 1 breath every 6 seconds or 1 breath every 10 compressions.
(b) Do not interrupt CPR for the administration of medications.
(c) Sodium bicarbonate (4.2%) 1 mEq/kg IV/IO should be administered to infants (dilute 8.4% 1:1 with normal saline to make 4.2%).

3.3.5 Wide Complex Tachycardia with a Pulse (Ventricular Tachycardia)

This protocol is used in wide complex tachycardia (QRS > 0.08 second) with a heart rate > 150/min.

Stable (Normal Perfusion)

Supportive Care

- Medical Supportive Care Protocol 3.1.3.
- Determine the patient's (un)responsiveness and check the ABCs.
- Obtain a SAMPLE history.
- Perform a focused exam.
- **Consider the H's and T's.**

ALS Level 1

None.

ALS Level 2

- Administer amiodarone 5 mg/kg IV over 20–60 minutes.

Unstable (Diminished Perfusion)

Supportive Care

- Medical Supportive Care Protocol 3.1.3.
- Determine the patient's (un)responsiveness and check the ABCs.
- Obtain a SAMPLE history.
- Perform a focused exam.
- **Consider the H's and T's.**

ALS Level 1

None.

3.3.5 Wide Complex Tachycardia with a Pulse (Ventricular Tachycardia)

ALS Level 2

- If the patient is conscious and aware of the situation, consider sedation with one of the following benzodiazepines (a):
  - Diazepam (Valium®) 0.1 mg/kg IV.

  or
  - Midazolam (Versed®) 0.05 mg/kg IV.

  or
  - Lorazepam (Ativan®) 0.05 mg/kg IV.
- Apply synchronized cardioversion at 0.5 joule/kg to 1 joule/kg.
- Apply synchronized cardioversion at 2 joule/kg.
- Administer amiodarone 5 mg/kg IV over 20 minutes.

Note

(a) Do not delay synchronized cardioversion to establish an IV for sedation purposes.

3.3.6 Wide Complex Tachycardia Without a Pulse and Ventricular Fibrillation

Supportive Care

- Medical Supportive Care Protocol 3.1.3.
- Determine the patient's (un)responsiveness and check the ABCs.
- Oxygenate with 15–25 L/min via bag-valve mask with an appropriate airway adjunct device at 8–10 BPM (see Airway Protocol 3.1.2) (a).
- Begin immediate chest compressions at a rate of 100/min for 2 minutes while the monitor is being attached.
- **Do not interrupt CPR to check the heart rhythm. Continuous uninterrupted compressions are paramount to patient survival.**
- Check the heart rhythm.
- Resume 2 minutes of continuous compressions at 100/min; check the heart rhythm.
- If available, attach an impedance threshold device (ITD).
- Obtain a SAMPLE history.
- Perform a focused exam.
- **Consider the H's and T's.**

ALS Level I

- Defibrillate at 2 joule/kg. The EMT should apply the AED (see Medical Procedure 4.1, Automated External Defibrillator).
- Resume CPR immediately. Administer five cycles of CPR.
- Check the heart rhythm. Treat according to the applicable protocol.
- Defibrillate at 4 joule/kg; continue CPR while the defibrillator is charging.
- Resume CPR immediately.
- Administer epinephrine (1:10,000) 0.01 mg/kg IV or IO (maximum dose = 1 mg). If unable to establish IV/IO, as a last resort administer epinephrine (1:1000) 0.1 mg/kg ETT (maximum dose = 2 mg) (a). Repeat every 3–5 minutes for the duration of pulselessness.
- Reevaluate the heart rhythm after five cycles of CPR.
- Defibrillate at 4 joule/kg; continue CPR while the defibrillator is charging.
- Resume CPR immediately.

3.3.6 Wide Complex Tachycardia Without a Pulse and Ventricular Fibrillation

- Administer one of the following antiarrhythmics:
  - Amiodarone 5 mg/kg IV or IO.

  or

  - If the patient has torsades de pointes, magnesium sulfate 25–50 mg/kg IV/IO, up to a maximum dose of 2 g.
- Administer sodium bicarbonate 1 mEq/kg IV (b).

ALS Level 2

None.

NOTE

(a) Give 1 breath every 6 seconds or 1 breath every 10 compressions.
(b) Sodium bicarbonate (4.2%) 1 mEq/kg IV or IO should be administered to **infants** (dilute 8.4% 1:1 with normal saline to make 4.2%).

Skill Drill 3-1: Performing Chest Compressions on a Child

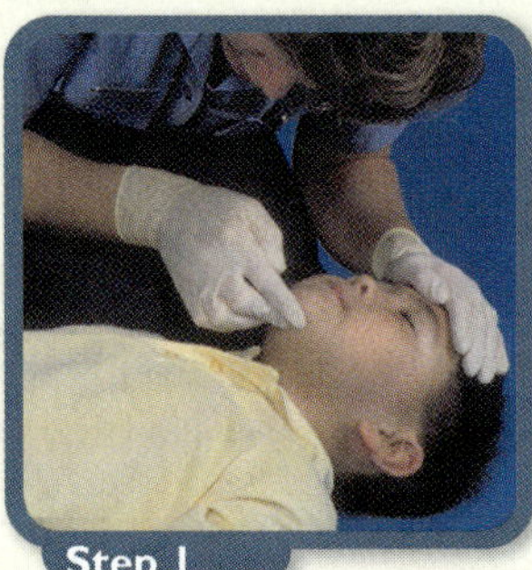

Step 1

Place the child on a firm survace, and use one hand to maintain the head tilt–chin lift.

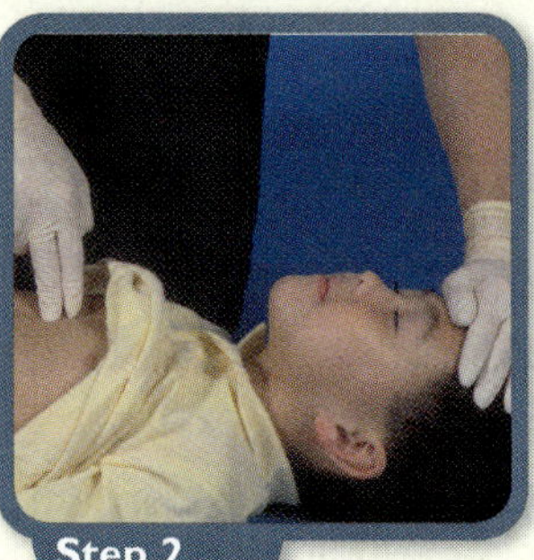

Step 2

Place the heel of your hand over the middle of the sternum (between the nipples); avoid compression of the xiphoid process.

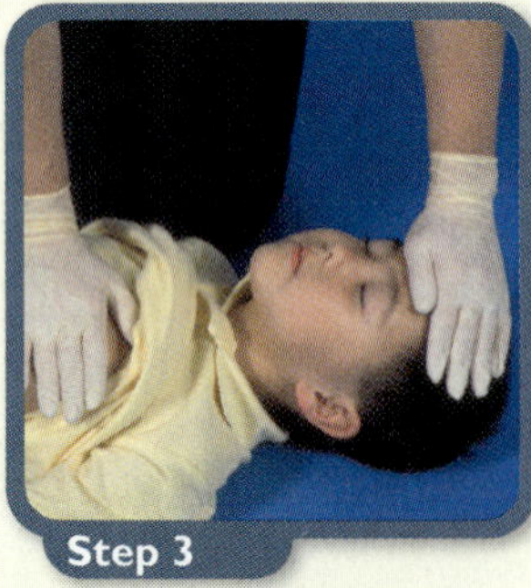

Step 3

Coordinate compression with ventilation in a 30:2 ration, pausing for ventilation.

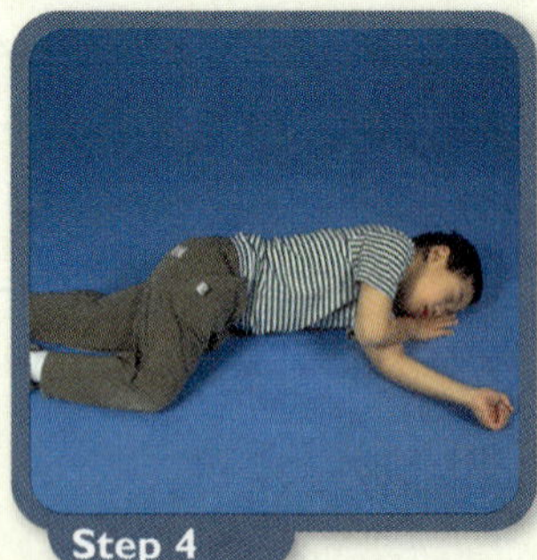

Step 4

Reassess breathing and pulse after 2 minutes and at 2-minute intervals thereafter. If the child resumes effective breathing, place him or her in the recovery posistion.

3.4 Newborn/Infant Cardiopulmonary Arrest

Infant and newborn cardiopulmonary arrest is usually a result of prolonged poor oxygenation and\or severe circulatory collapse. **Newborns** should be resuscitated using Pediatric Protocol 3.4.1. Unless there are obvious signs of death (see General Protocol 1.4, Death in the Field), the **infant** in cardiopulmonary arrest should be resuscitated using the protocols in Pediatric Protocol 3.3. While some infants may not be salvageable, the paramedic may determine a resuscitation attempt is warranted for psychological reasons (e.g., the parent's peace of mind). Consideration should also be given to SIDS (see Pediatric Protocol 3.4.2).

Skill Drill 3-2: Performing Infant Chest Compressions

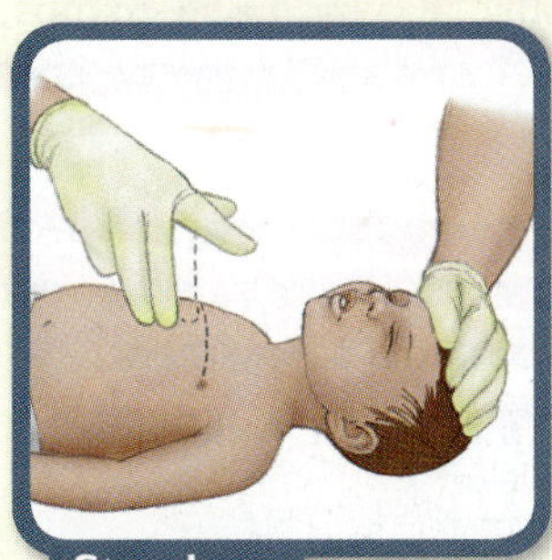

Step 1

Position the infant on a firm surface while maintaining the airway. Place two fingers in the middle of the sternum, one fingerbreadth below the imaginary intermammary line.

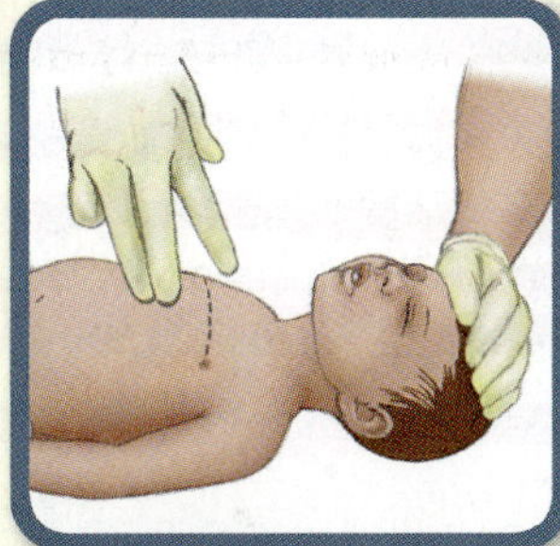

Step 2

Using two fingers, compress the sternum about one-third to one-half the depth of the chest. Push hard and fast, at a rate of 100 compressions/min. Allow the sternum to return briefly to its normal position between compressions.

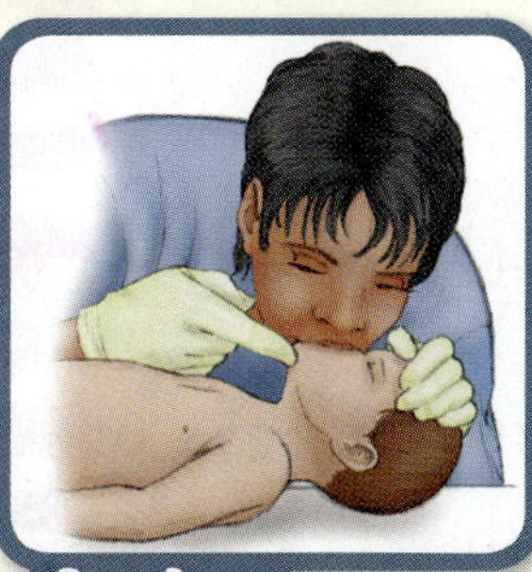

Step 3

Coordinate rapid compression and ventilation in a 30:2 ration. Check for the return of breathing and pulse after 2-minute intervals.

3.4.1 Newborn Resuscitation

This protocol is to be used for newborns who are in need of resuscitation immediately following delivery.

Supportive Care

- Dry and keep the baby warm (cover with a thermal blanket or dry towel, and cover the scalp with a stocking cap).
- Position the patient so as to open the airway (a).
- Clear the airway; suction the mouth and nose with a bulb syringe as needed.
- **Paramedic Only:** If the newborn has signs of thick meconium after suctioning with a bulb syringe **and if the child is not vigorous and crying,** intubate and suction the trachea (see Medical Procedure 4.9, Flexible Suctioning, Medical Procedure 4.10, Rigid Suctioning) (b).
- Stimulate the baby (rub the baby's back).
- Clamp and cut the cord, if not already done. Apply two umbilical clamps, 2 inches apart and at least 8 inches from the navel, and cut between clamps.
- Assess skin color, respirations, and heart rate.
- Administer 100% oxygen via blow-by method to newborns who are breathing but have central cyanosis or have no improvement in respiratory, circulatory, or neurological status within 90 seconds of initial assessment.
- Ventilate at 40–60 breath/min with 100% oxygen under the following conditions:
  - Apnea.
  - Heart rate < 100 beat/min.
  - Persistent central cyanosis after high-flow oxygen.
- **Paramedic Only:** Intubate under the following conditions (see Medical Procedure 4.18, Intubation):
  - Bag-valve mask ventilation is ineffective (> 2 minutes).
  - Tracheal suctioning is required, especially for thick meconium, **and the child is not vigorous and crying** (b).
  - Prolonged positive-pressure ventilation is needed.
- Perform chest compressions at 120/min (3:1 ratio; one-third of the anterior–posterior diameter of chest in depth), using two thumbs placed side by side (or superimposed one on top of the other) over the midsternum, just below the nipple line, with the fingers encircling the chest and supporting the back, under the following conditions:
  - Heart rate < 60 beat/min and not rapidly increasing despite adequate ventilation with 100% oxygen for approximately 30 seconds.

ALS Level 1

- Administer epinephrine (1:10,000) 0.01–0.03 mg/kg IV/IO (or ETT as a last resort) under the following conditions:
  - Asystole.
  - Heart rate < 60 beat/min despite adequate ventilation with 100% oxygen and 30 seconds of chest compressions.

3.4.1 Newborn Resuscitation

- Repeat every 3–5 minutes as needed.
- Administer a fluid challenge of normal saline 10 mL/kg IV under the following conditions:
  - Pallor that persists after adequate oxygenation.
  - Faint pulses with a good heart rate.
  - Poor response to resuscitation with adequate ventilations.
- Check the blood glucose level for all resuscitated newborns who do not respond to initial therapy. Use a heel stick (see Medical Procedure 4.39, Glucometer).
  - If blood glucose < 40 mg/dL, administer D_{10} 5 mL/kg IV/IO (dilute D_{50} 1:4 with normal saline to make D_{10}).
- Perform Pediatric Assessment Triangle: Rapid Cardiopulmonary Assessment (see Pediatric Protocol 3.1.1, Initial Assessment) frequently.

ALS Level 2

- If the neonate is unresponsive with depressed respirations, consider naloxone (Narcan®) 0.1 mg/kg (1 mg/mL concentration) IV/IO/IM (or ETT as a last resort) (c).

NOTE

(a) The neonate should be placed on his/her back or side with the neck in a neutral position. To help maintain correct position, a rolled blanket or towel may be placed under the back and shoulders of the supine neonate to elevate the torso 0.75 or 1 inch off the mattress to extend the neck slightly. If copious secretions are present, the neonate should be placed on his/her side with the neck slightly extended to allow secretions to collect in the mouth rather than in the posterior pharynx.

(b) Tracheal suctioning for thick meconium should be done via an endotracheal tube using a meconium aspirator attached to the 15-mm adaptor of the ETT. The suction unit is then attached and placed on low pressure (no more than 100 mm Hg). Suctioning should be performed until the ETT is clear (maximum 5 seconds). It may be necessary to repeat the intubation and continue suctioning until clear (maximum three times).

(c) Avoid the use of naloxone if the mother has a history of drug use/abuse, as naloxone may precipitate seizures in the newborn due to acute withdrawal.

3.4.2 Sudden Infant Death Syndrome (SIDS)

Sudden infant death syndrome (SIDS), also known as "crib death," is the sudden and unexpected death of an apparently healthy infant, usually younger than 1 year of age, which remains unexplained after a complete medical history, death scene investigation, and postmortem examination. SIDS almost always occurs when the infant is asleep or thought to be asleep.

Although there may be obvious signs of death (see Appendix 7.17, Sudden Infant Death Syndrome), the paramedic may attempt resuscitation of the infant for psychological reasons (e.g., the parent's peace of mind). There may also be some infants in whom the Paramedic determines that a resuscitation attempt is not warranted (see General Protocol 1.4, Death in the Field). In either event, **the paramedic should be prepared for a myriad of grief reactions from the parents and/or caregiver.**

Some SIDS deaths are mistaken for child abuse. If there are possible signs of abuse (see Appendix 7.16, Signs of Child Abuse), the paramedic should continue as if it were a SIDS death, to avoid any unnecessary grief on the part of the parents and/or caregiver. The paramedic should not attempt to determine whether child abuse has taken place. The scene should be treated as any other death scene, with attention to preservation of potential evidence.

Supportive Care

- In most instances, resuscitation should be attempted (see the appropriate Pediatric Protocols).
- Assign a crew member to assist the parents and/or caregiver and to explain the procedures.
- If time permits, elicit a brief history and perform an environmental check. Document all findings on the EMS Run Report.
- Once resuscitation is started, do not stop until directed to do so in the hospital by a physician.

ALS Level 1

None.

ALS Level 2

None.

3.5 Pediatric Neurologic Emergencies

This section covers the most common pediatric neurologic emergencies, altered mental status, and seizures. It is important for the paramedic to understand appropriate behavior for the child/infant's age to properly assess level of consciousness (see Appendix 7.7, Glasgow Coma Scale Score, for pediatric patients). Attention should be given to how the child interacts with parents and the environment and whether the patient can make good eye contact. Parents may be invaluable for a baseline comparison of level of consciousness. The parents may simply state that the patient is not acting right. Causes of pediatric altered mental status may include hypoxia, head trauma, ingestion/poisoning, infection, and hypoglycemia.

Approximately 4–6% of all children will have at least one seizure. Seizures may be due to an underlying disease (e.g., epilepsy) or may simply be a result of fever. Other potential causes of pediatric seizures include trauma, hypoxia, infection of brain and spinal cord (e.g., meningitis), hypoglycemia, and ingestion/poisoning.

3.5.1 Altered Level of Consciousness (Altered Mental Status)

Common signs of altered mental status in pediatric patients include combative behavior, decreased responsiveness, lethargy, weak cry, moaning, hypotonia, ataxia, and changes in personality. The initial management approach should be based on the assumption that the patient is suffering from infection, hypoxia, ischemia, hypoglycemia, or dehydration. Secondary considerations should include medications, illicit drugs/alcohol, plants, trauma, and other factors.

Supportive Care

- Medical Supportive Care Protocol 3.1.3; consider the need for spinal immobilization (see Medical Procedure 4.52, Spinal Immobilization).
- Consider the need for ventilatory assistance.

ALS Level 1

- If the child remains unresponsive and prolonged ventilatory assistance is needed, consider use of an appropriate airway adjunct device (a).
- Perform a glucose test with a finger stick. If glucose < 60 mg/dL, administer:
  - If < 8 years: D_{25} 2 mL/kg IV/IO.
  - If > 8 years: D_{50} 1 mL/kg IV/IO (see Medical Procedure 4.39, Glucometer) (b).
- If the patient's mental status is depressed and signs of dehydration exist, administer a fluid challenge of normal saline 20 mL/kg IV.
- If the patient's mental status and respiratory effort are depressed, administer naloxone (Narcan®) 0.1 mg/kg (maximum dose = 2 mg) IV/IO/IM (c). May repeat every 5 minutes as needed.
- **If toxicology (poisoning) is suspected, contact the Poison Information Center (1-800-222-1222).**

ALS Level 2

None.

Note

(a) Use appropriate discretion regarding the immediate use of airway adjuncts in pediatric patients, as they may quickly regain consciousness.

(b) To avoid infiltration and resultant tissue necrosis, dextrose 25% should be given via slow IV, with intermittent aspiration of the IV/IO line to confirm IV/IO patency, followed by saline flush.

(c) Intranasal administration of naloxone requires the use of a mucosal atomization device.

3.5.2 Seizure Disorders

This protocol should be used when the patient has shown continuous convulsions or repeating episodes without regaining consciousness or sufficient respiratory compensation. Consider an underlying etiology such as fever, hypoxia, head trauma, infection (e.g., meningitis), hypoglycemia, electrolyte imbalance, and ingestion/poisoning.

Supportive Care

- Medical Supportive Care Protocol 3.1.3. Apply gentle support to the patient's head to avoid trauma, and loosen tight-fitting clothing.

ALS Level 1

- Perform a glucose test with a finger stick. If glucose < 60 mg/dL, administer:
  - If < 8 years: D_{25} 2 mL/kg IV/IO.
  - If > 8 years: D_{50} 1 mL/kg IV/IO (see Medical Procedure 4.39, Glucometer) (a)(b).
  - If unable to establish IV/IO access and patient > 8 years: Glucagon 1 mg IM.
- If the seizure continues, administer one of the following benzodiazepines:
  - Diazepam (Valium®) 0.5 mg/kg (maximum 10 mg) rectally or 0.2 mg/kg intranasally. If IV/IO access is available prior to seizure, administer diazepam 0.2 mg/kg IV (c)(d).

  or

  - Lorazepam (Ativan®) 0.1 mg/kg (maximum dose = 2 mg) IM. If IV access is available prior to seizure, administer lorazepam 0.1 mg/kg (maximum dose = 2 mg) IV (c).

  or

  - Midazolam (Versed®) 0.1 mg/kg (maximum dose = 2 mg) IV or intranasal (c).

ALS Level 2

- If seizure continues for 5 minutes, administer one of the following benzodiazepines:
  - Diazepam (Valium®) 0.5 mg/kg (maximum dose =10 mg) rectally. If IV/IO access is available prior to seizure, administer diazepam 0.2 mg/kg IV (c)(d).

  or

  - Lorazepam (Ativan®) 0.1 mg/kg (maximum total dose = 4 mg) IM. If IV access is available prior to seizure, administer lorazepam 0.1 mg/kg (maximum total dose = 4 mg) IV (c).

  or

  - Midazolam (Versed®) 0.1 mg/kg (maximum dose = 2 mg) IV (c).

3.5.2 Seizure Disorders

NOTE

(a) For newborns and infants, perform a heel stick. In newborns and infants < 12 months of age with blood glucose < 40 mg/dL, administer D_{10} 5 mL/kg IV/IO (dilute D_{50} 1:4 with normal saline to make D_{10}).

(b) To avoid infiltration and resultant tissue necrosis, dextrose 10%, 25%, and 50% should be given via slow IV with intermittent aspiration of the IV/IO line to confirm IV/IO patency, followed by saline flush.

(c) Intranasal administration of benzodiazepines requires the use of a mucosal atomization device (same as IV dose).

(d) Use a lubricated tuberculin or 3–5 mL syringe **without the needle.** Position the patient in a decubitus knee position or supine the with legs held apart, and insert the lubricated syringe approximately 5 cm into the rectum. Inject the Valium, remove the syringe, and tape the buttocks closed.

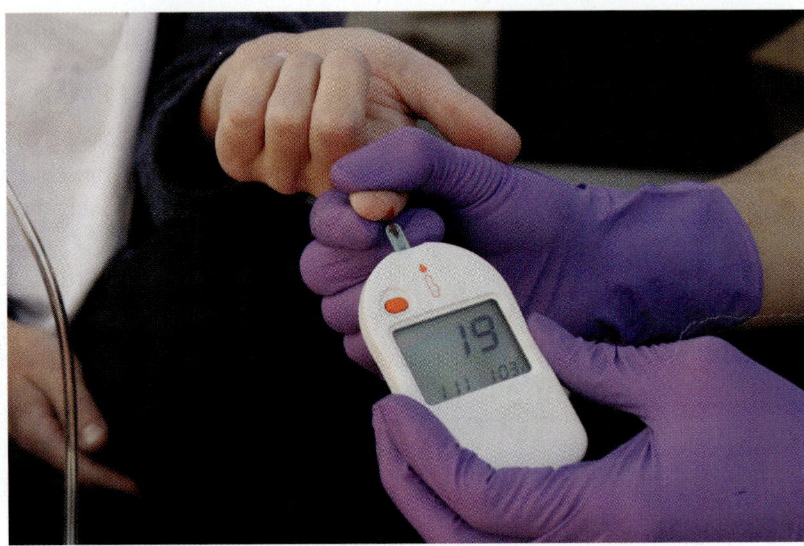

Perform a bedside blood glucose test.

3.6 Pediatric Toxicologic Emergencies

This protocol is to be used for those patients suspected of exposure to toxic substances via any route of exposure (e.g., drug overdose, snake bite). Each of the subprotocols gives specific considerations for each type of exposure as well as general treatment guidelines. Additional assistance may be necessary in certain cases (e.g., hazardous materials team for toxic exposure; police for scene control, including the presence of violent and/or impaired patient—see Pediatric Protocol 3.7.5). Also refer to the Pediatric Chemical Treatment Guidelines (found in Chapter 8) as needed.

A history of the events leading to the illness or injury should be obtained from the patient and bystanders, to include the following information:

1. To which drugs, poisons, or other substances was the patient exposed? Consider multiple substances, especially on overdoses. Also consider plants and herbal remedies.
2. When did the exposure occur, and how much exposure was there?
3. What is the duration of symptoms?
4. Is the patient depressed or suicidal? Does he/she have a history of previous overdose? (if applicable)
5. Was the exposure accidental? What was the nature of the accident?
6. What was the duration of exposure? (if applicable)

Collect all pill bottles—empty or full—and check for a "suicide note" (if applicable). Transport any/all information or items that may assist in the treatment of the patient to the emergency department.

Contact the Poison Information Center (1-800-222-1222) for consultation regarding specific therapy.

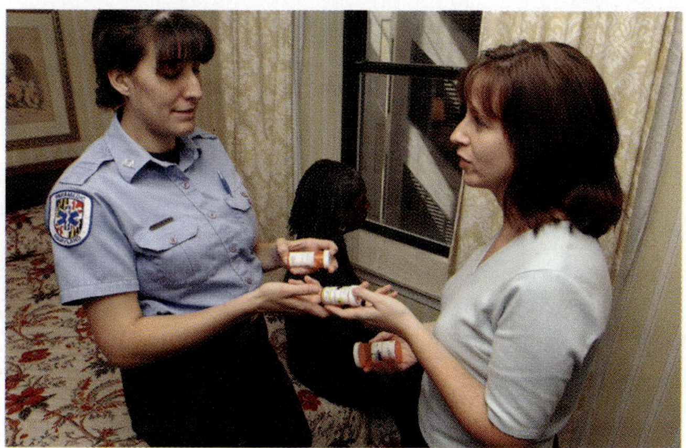

Bring any bottles or plant samples to the Emergency Department.

3.6.1 Pediatric Ingestion (Overdose)

This protocol should be used on most types of ingestion/poisoning (e.g., acetaminophen, benzodiazepines, narcotics, tricyclic antidepressants, vitamins with iron). See Adult Protocol 2.6 for lists of different types of medications. Symptoms vary with the substance involved. Also refer to the Pediatric Chemical Treatment Guidelines (found in Chapter 8) as needed.

Supportive Care

- Medical Supportive Care Protocol 3.1.3.
- Consider the need for ventilatory support (see Medical Procedure 4.4).
- **Contact the Poison Information Center (1-800-222-1222).**

ALS Level 1

- Consider the need for use of an airway adjunct device. If an endotracheal tube is used, attempt to utilize a "cuffed tube" to prevent aspiration.
- Perform a glucose test with a finger stick. If glucose < 60 mg/dL, administer:
  - If < 8 years: D_{25} 2 mL/kg IV/IO.
  - If > 8 years: D_{50} 1 mL/kg IV/IO (see Medical Procedure 4.39) (a)(b).
  - If unable to establish IV/IO access: Glucagon 1 mg IM.
- If narcotic overdose is suspected in a non-neonate, administer naloxone (Narcan®) 0.1 mg/kg (maximum dose = 2 mg) IV/IO/IM/intranasal. May repeat every 5 minutes as needed (c).
- If tricyclic antidepressant overdose is suspected, administer sodium bicarbonate 1 mEq/kg IV/IO (d).

ALS Level 2

None.

NOTE

(a) For newborns and infants, perform a heel stick. In newborns and infants < 12 months of age and with blood glucose < 40 mg/dL, administer D_{10} 5 mL/kg IV/IO (dilute D_{50} 1:4 with normal saline to make D_{10}).

(b) To avoid infiltration and resultant tissue necrosis, dextrose 10%, 25%, and 50% should be given via slow IV with intermittent aspiration of the IV/IO line to confirm IV/IO patency, followed by saline flush.

(c) Intranasal administration of naloxone requires the use of a mucosal atomization device (same as IV dose).

(d) If the patient is seizing, also see Pediatric Protocol 3.5.2.

3.6.2 Bites and Stings

This protocol includes the treatment for snake and spider bites, dog and cat bites, insect stings, and marine animal envenomations and stings. All bite patients should be transported to the hospital.

Snake Bites

Supportive Care

- Trauma Supportive Care Protocol 3.1.4.
- Consider the need for Pediatric Protocol 3.7.1, Allergic Reactions/Anaphylaxis.
- **Contact the Poison Information Center (1-800-222-1222).**
- Splint the affected area. Place the patient in a supine position with the extremities at a neutral level. Keep the patient quiet. Remove and secure all jewelry.
- Wash the area of the bite with copious amounts of water.
- Attempt to identify the snake, if it is safe to do so.
- Check the temperature and pulse distal to a bite on an extremity, and mark level of swelling and time with pen every 15 minutes.

ALS Level 1

- Refer to Pediatric Protocol 3.1.5 for pain management guidelines.

ALS Level 2

None.

Dog, Cat, and Wild Animal Bites

Supportive Care

- Trauma Supportive Care Protocol 3.1.4.
- Wound care: BLS. Do not use hydrogen peroxide on deep puncture wounds or wounds exposing fat.
- Advise dispatch to contact animal control and the police department for identification and quarantine of the animal.
- **Contact the Poison Information Center (1-800-222-1222).**

ALS Level 1

- Refer to Pediatric Protocol 3.1.5 for pain management guidelines.

ALS Level 2

None.

3.6.2 Bites and Stings

Insect Stings (Including Centipedes, Scorpions, and Spiders)

Supportive Care

- Trauma Supportive Care Protocol 3.1.4.
- Consider the need for Pediatric Protocol 3.7.1, Allergic Reactions/ Anaphylaxis.
- Remove the stinger by scraping the skin with the edge of a flat surface (e.g., a credit card). Do not attempt to pull the stinger out, as this may release more venom.
- Clean the wound area with soap and water.
- **Contact the Poison Information Center (1-800-222-1222).**

ALS Level 1

- Refer to Pediatric Protocol 3.1.5 for pain management guidelines.

ALS Level 2

None.

Marine Animal Envenomations: Stingray, Scorpionfish (Lionfish, Zebrafish, Stonefish), Catfish, Weeverfish, Starfish, and Sea Urchin

Supportive Care

- Trauma Supportive Care Protocol 3.1.4.
- Consider the need for Pediatric Protocol 3.7.1, Allergic Reactions/ Anaphylaxis.
- Immerse the punctures in nonscalding hot water to tolerance (110–113°F) to achieve pain relief (30–90 minutes). Transport should not be delayed for this purpose; immersion in nonscalding hot water may be continued during transport.
- Remove any visible pieces of the spine(s) or sheath. Gently wash the wound with soap and water, and then irrigate it vigorously with fresh water (avoid scrubbing).
- **Contact the Poison Information Center (1-800-222-1222).**

ALS Level 1

- Refer to Pediatric Protocol 3.1.5 for pain management guidelines.

ALS Level 2

None.

3.6.2 Bites and Stings

Marine Animal Stings: Jellyfish, Man-of-War, Sea Nettle, Irukandji, Anemone, Hydroid, and Fire Coral

Supportive Care

- Trauma Supportive Care Protocol 3.1.4.
- Consider the need for Pediatric Protocol 3.7.1, Allergic Reactions/ Anaphylaxis.
- Rinse the skin with sea water. Do not use fresh water, do not apply ice, and do not rub the skin.
- Apply soaks of acetic acid 5% (vinegar) until pain is relieved. If vinegar is not available, use a paste of baking soda or unseasoned meat tenderizer.
- Remove any large tentacle fragments using forceps. Use gloves to avoid contact with your bare hands.
- Apply a lather of shaving cream or a paste of baking soda and shave the affected area with the edge of a flat surface (e.g., a credit card).
- **Contact the Poison Information Center (1-800-222-1222).**

ALS Level 1

- Refer to Pediatric Protocol 3.1.5 for pain management guidelines.

ALS Level 2

None.

Human Bites

Supportive Care

- Trauma Supportive Care Protocol 3.1.4 (see General Protocol 1.12, Personal Exposure to Infectious Diseases).
- Wound care: BLS. Do not use hydrogen peroxide on deep puncture wounds or wounds exposing fat. Clean the wound area with soap and water.
- Advise dispatch to contact the police department for possible domestic disturbance.

ALS Level 1

- Refer to Pediatric Protocol 3.1.5 for pain management guidelines.

ALS Level 2

None.

3.7 Other Pediatric Medical Emergencies

The paramedic should use these protocols to guide him/her through the treatment of patients with other medical emergencies who are exhibiting signs and symptoms. In addition to these protocols, the paramedic may need to refer to other protocols for continued treatment.

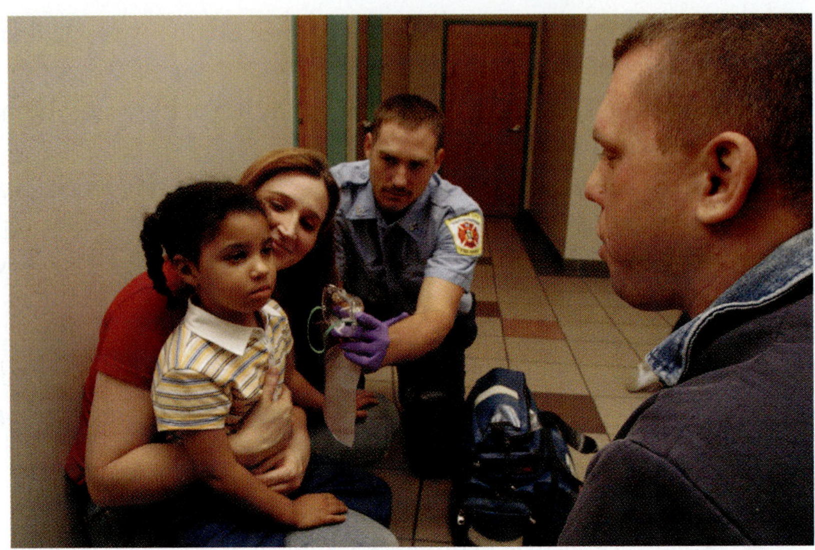

3.7.1 Allergic Reactions/Anaphylaxis

This protocol should be used for patients who are exhibiting signs and symptoms consistent with allergic reaction:

- **Skin:** flushing, itching, hives, swelling, cyanosis.
- **Respiratory:** dyspnea, sneezing, coughing, wheezing, stridor, laryngeal edema, laryngospasm, bronchospasm.
- **Cardiovascular:** vasodilatation, increased heart rate, decreased blood pressure.
- **Gastrointestinal:** nausea/vomiting, abdominal cramping, diarrhea.
- **CNS:** dizziness, headache, convulsions, tearing.

Treatment is outlined according to the severity of the allergic reaction (mild, moderate, and severe or anaphylaxis).

Mild Reactions

Mild reactions consist of redness and/or itching, but normal perfusion without dyspnea.

Supportive Care

- Trauma Supportive Care Protocol 3.1.4.

ALS Level 1

- For severe itching, administer diphenhydramine (Benadryl®) 1 mg/kg IM or IV (maximum dose = 50 mg IM or 25 mg IV).

ALS Level 2

- Epinephrine (1:1000) 0.01 mg/kg SQ (maximum dose = 0.3 mg).

Moderate Reactions

Moderate reactions are characterized by edema, hives, dyspnea, wheezing, and normal perfusion.

Supportive Care

- Trauma Supportive Care Protocol 3.1.4.

3.7.1 Allergic Reactions/Anaphylaxis

ALS Level 1

- Diphenhydramine (Benadryl®) 1 mg/kg IM/IV (maximum dose = 50 mg IM or 25 mg IV).
- Epinephrine (1:1000) 0.01 mg/kg SQ (maximum dose of 0.3 mg) (a).
- If the patient remains in respiratory distress, administer albuterol (Ventolin®): one nebulizer treatment (see Medical Procedure 4.27, Nebulizer).
    - If < 1 year or < 10 kg: mix 1.25 mg in 1.5 mL of normal saline (0.083%).
    - If > 1 year or > 10 kg: mix 2.5 mg in 3 mL of normal saline (0.083%).
- If respiratory distress is severe, administer one of the following steroids:
    - Methylprednisolone sodium succinate (Solu-Medrol®) 2 mg/kg IV/IM (maximum dose = 125 mg), if available.

  or

    - Dexamethasone (Decadron®) 0.6 mg/kg IM/IV (maximum dose = 10 mg).

ALS Level 2

None.

Severe Reactions

Severe reactions are characterized by edema, hives, severe dyspnea and wheezing, poor perfusion, and possible cyanosis and laryngeal edema.

Supportive Care

- Trauma Supportive Care Protocol 3.1.4.

ALS Level 1

- Diphenhydramine (Benadryl®) 1 mg/kg IM/IV (maximum dose = 50 mg IM or 25 mg IV).
- Epinephrine (1:1000) 0.01 mg/kg SQ (maximum dose = 0.3 mg) (a).
- If patient remains in respiratory distress, administer albuterol (Ventolin®): 1 nebulizer treatment (see Medical Procedure 4.27, Nebulizer).
    - If < 1 year or < 10 kg: mix 1.25 mg in 1.5 mL of normal saline (0.083%).
    - If > 1 year or > 10 kg: mix 2.5 mg in 3 mL of normal saline (0.083%).
- If bronchodilators are administered, may add ipratropium bromide (Atrovent®) 0.5 mg (0.5 mL) to either albuterol nebulizer treatment **for the first nebulizer treatment only.**

3.7.1 Allergic Reactions/Anaphylaxis

- If respiratory distress is severe, administer one of the following steroids:
    - Methylprednisolone sodium succinate (Solu-Medrol®) 2 mg/kg IV/IO/IM (maximum dose = 125 mg), if available.

  or

    - Dexamethasone (Decadron®) 0.6 mg/kg IV/IO/IM (maximum dose = 10 mg).
- May repeat epinephrine (1:1000) 0.01 mg/kg SQ (maximum dose = 0.15 mg) (a).

ALS Level 2

- If the patient's distress continues, repeat epinephrine (1:1000) 0.01 mg/kg SQ (maximum dose = 0.3 mg). May repeat every 15 minutes for two additional doses.

NOTE

(a) The EpiPen® or EpiPen Jr.® may be used if other means of epinephrine administration are not available.

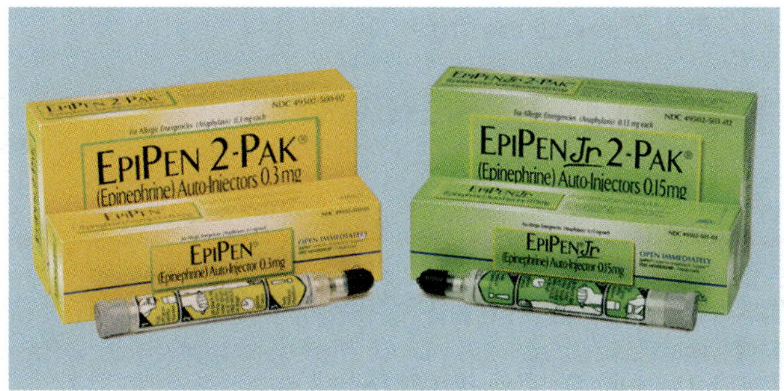

EpiPen® and EpiPen Jr.®

3.7.2 Hypoglycemia/Hyperglycemia

This protocol is to be used for those patients whose blood glucose < 60 mg/dL (see Pediatric Protocol 3.4.1 for newborn guidelines). Consider medication errors, overdoses, accidental ingestions, and other factors related to etiology. Look for pill bottles.

Supportive Care

- Medical Supportive Care Protocol 3.1.3.

ALS Level 1

- If the patient is conscious with an intact gag reflex, assist with self-administration of oral glucose, if possible.
- Perform a glucose test with a finger stick. If glucose < 60 mg/dL, administer:
  - If < 8 years: D_{25} 2 mL/kg IV/IO.
  - If > 8 years: D_{50} 1 mL/kg IV/IO (see Medical Procedure 4.39, Glucometer) (a)(b).
  - If unable to obtain IV/IO access and the patient is > 8 years: Glucagon 1 mg IM.
- Repeat a glucose test with a finger stick. If glucose < 60 mg/dL, administer:
  - If < 8 years: D_{25} 2 mL/kg IV/IO.
  - If > 8 years: D_{50} 0.5 mL/kg IV/IO (see Medical Procedure 4.39, Glucometer) (a)(b).

ALS Level 2

None.

NOTE

(a) For newborns and infants, perform a heel stick. In newborns and infants < 12 months of age with blood glucose < 40 mg/dL, administer D_{10} 5 mL/kg IV/IO (dilute D+ 1:4 with normal saline to make D_{10}).

(b) To avoid infiltration and resultant tissue necrosis, dextrose 25% and 50% should be given via slow IV with intermittent aspiration of the IV line to confirm IV patency, followed by saline flush.

3.7.3 Nontraumatic Abdominal Pain

This protocol should be used for patients who complain of abdominal pain without a history of trauma (refer to Appendix 7.16, Signs of Child Abuse).

Assessment should include specific questions pertaining to the GI/GU systems.

Abdominal physical assessment:

- Ask patient to point to the area of pain (palpate this area last).
- Gently palpate for tenderness, rebound tenderness, distention, rigidity, guarding, and pulsatile masses. Also palpate the flank for CVAT (costovertebral angle tenderness).

Abdominal history:

- History of pain (OPQRST).
- History of nausea/vomiting (color, bloody, coffee grounds, dark bilious).
- History of bowel movement (last BM, diarrhea, bloody, tarry).
- History of urine output (painful, dark, bloody).
- History of abdominal surgery.
- History of medication ingestions.
- SAMPLE history (pay attention to last meal).

Additional questions should be asked of the female adolescent patient regarding OB/GYN history (see Adult Protocol 2.7, Adult OB/GYN Emergencies).

An acute abdomen can be caused by appendicitis, diabetic ketoacidosis, incarcerated hernia, intussuception, cholecystitis, cystitis–UTI (bladder inflammation), duodenal ulcer, diverticulitis, abdominal aortic aneurysm, kidney infection, urinary tract infection (UTI), kidney stone, pelvic inflammatory disease (PID; female), or pancreatitis (see Appendix 7.1, Abdominal Pain Differential).

Supportive Care

- Medical Supportive Care Protocol 3.1.3.

ALS Level 1

- In case of decreased perfusion (see Appendix 7.11, Pediatric Vital Signs), administer a fluid challenge of normal saline 20 mL/kg IV.

ALS Level 2

- Consider pain control management (see Pediatric Protocol 3.1.5 for pain scale and medication dosage—same as isolated extremity fracture pain protocol).

3.7.4 Nontraumatic Chest Pain—Undifferentiated

Most chest pains in children are non-cardiac related. Causes of nontraumatic chest pain in the pediatric patient include wheezing-associated illness, spontaneous pneumothorax, pleurisy, costochondritis, pulmonary embolism, pneumonia, peptic ulcer, drug usage (e.g., stimulants—cocaine), dissecting aortic aneurysm, pericarditis, hiatal hernia, esophageal spasm, cholecystitis, pancreatitis, cervical disk problem, and, rarely, cardiac problems (see Appendix 7.5, Chest Pain Differential). Also refer to Appendix 7.16, Signs of Child Abuse.

Supportive Care

- Medical Supportive Care Protocol 3.1.3.
- Consider the need for other protocols (e.g., Pediatric Protocol 3.2, Pediatric Respiratory Emergencies).

ALS Level 1

None.

ALS Level 2

- Consider pain control management (see Pediatric Protocol 3.1.5 for pain scale and medication dosage—same as isolated extremity fracture pain control).

3.7.5 Violent and/or Impaired Patient

This treatment protocol is used in conjunction with General Protocol 1.2, Behavioral Emergencies. If the patient is violent and poses an immediate threat to self, EMS crew, or bystander safety, restraints should be used to prevent the patient from harming self or others. If the patient is not violent, be observant for the possibility of violence and avoid provoking the patient. **Particular caution should be exercised when any "nonlethal" law enforcement device (e.g., pepper spray, Taser) has been employed.**

Supportive Care

- Have the patient placed under the Baker Act provisions when appropriate and refer to the Impaired/Incapacitated Persons Act (see General Protocol 2.1).
- Medical Supportive Care 3.1.3.
- Rule out causes other than psychiatric (e.g., drug overdose, ETOH, head trauma, hypoxia, hypoglycemia).
- Physically restrain the patient **only** when appropriate (see Medical Procedure 4.41, Physical Restraints).

ALS Level 1

- Administer one of the following benzodiazepines.
  - Diazepam (Valium®) 0.2 mg/kg (maximum dose = 5 mg) IV or intranasal; may repeat once as needed (up to a maximum dose of 10 mg) (a).

  or

  - Midazolam (Versed®) 0.1 mg/kg (maximum dose = 2 mg) IV or intranasal; may repeat once as needed (up to a maximum dose of 4 mg) (a).

  or

  - Lorazepam (Ativan®) 0.1 mg/kg (maximum dose = 2 mg) IV/IM; may repeat once as needed (up to a maximum dose of 4 mg) (a)(b).
- Diphenhydramine HCl (Benadryl®) 1 mg/kg (maximum dose = 50 mg IM or 25 mg IV) IM or IV (b).

ALS Level 2

None.

Note

(a) Intranasal administration of benzodiazepines requires the use of a mucosal atomization device (same as IV dose).

(b) In some instances, IV administration may present a safety concern. As a consequence, IM or intranasal administration of sedatives may be the more desirable route.

3.7.6 Suspected Child Abuse

This protocol should be used when the paramedic suspects that child abuse may have occurred. See Appendix 7.16, Signs of Child Abuse, and Appendix 7.14, Report of Abuse. **Child abuse** is when a person intentionally inflicts, or allows to be inflicted, physical or psychological injury to a child, which causes or results in risk of death, disfigurement, or distress. **Child neglect** is when a child's physical, mental, or emotional condition is impaired or endangered because of failure of the legal guardian to supply basic necessities, including adequate food, clothing, shelter, education, or medical care.

Supportive Care

- Trauma Supportive Care Protocol 3.1.4.
- Advise police that child abuse is suspected.
- Protect the child from further abuse.
- Obtain information in a nonjudgmental manner.
- Do not confront the caregiver and/or parent.
- Transport the patient to the hospital for evaluation and possible treatment (a).
- Report suspected child abuse—Florida Child Abuse Hotline: 1-800-342-9152 (b).

ALS Level 1

None.

ALS Level 2

None.

NOTE

(a) If the parent refuses to have the pediatric patient transported to a hospital, request police assistance.
(b) Reporting of suspected child abuse is required by law.

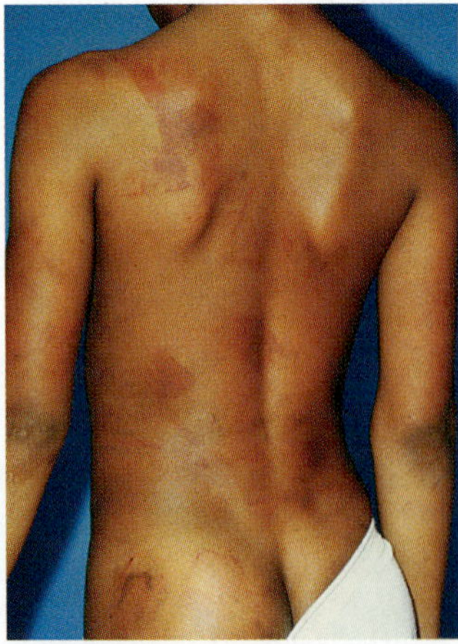

Multiple bruises or injuries that are in different stages of healing are concerns for abuse.

3.7.7 Sickle Cell Anemia

Sickle cell anemia is a chronic hemolytic anemia occurring frequently in African Americans and Hispanics; it is characterized by sickle-shaped red blood cells. Sickle cell crisis results from the occlusion of a blood vessel by masses of sickle-shaped red blood cells. Pain is the principal manifestation—it represents the most common type of crisis. This pain typically occurs in the patient's joints and back. Hepatic pulmonary or central nervous system involvement can occur, with each manifestation having its own group of symptoms. Patients with sickle cell disorder have a high incidence of life-threatening disorders at a very young age.

Supportive Care

- Medical Supportive Care Protocol 3.1.3. Administer 100% oxygen.
- Administer a fluid challenge of normal saline 20 mL/kg IV.
- Provide emotional support.

ALS Level 1

- If pain persists and systolic BP is adequate (see Appendix 7.11, Pediatric Vital Signs), choose one of the following medications:
  - Ketorolac (Toradol®) 1 mg/kg IV (maximum dose = 30 mg) or 2 mg/kg IM (maximum dose = 60 mg).

  or

  - Morphine sulfate—may be given intravenously in increments every 3–5 minutes, titrated to pain, to a maximum dose of 10 mg. Administer at a rate not to exceed 1 mg/min. *Pediatric dose:* 0.1 mg/kg IV. *Infant dose:* 0.05 mg/kg IV (a).

ALS Level 2

None.

Note

(a) Extreme caution should be used with administering narcotic analgesics to a patient with an $SpO_2 < 95\%$.

3.8 Pediatric Environmental Emergencies

The following protocols cover a range of problems related to the environment, including trauma due to changes in atmospheric pressure, exposure to heat and cold extremes, water submersion, and exposure to electricity. Initial management efforts should focus on removing the patient from the harmful environment.

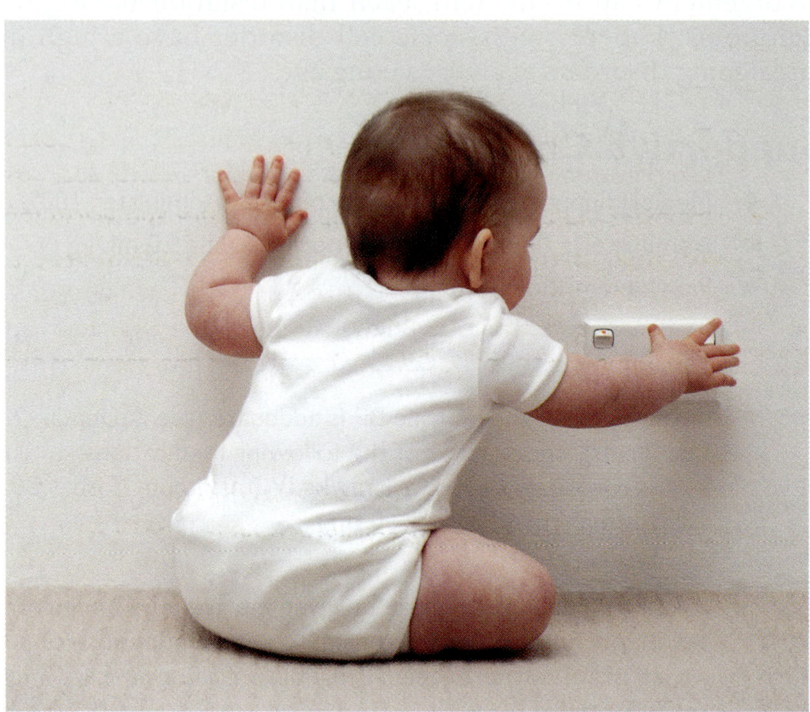

3.8.1 Near Drowning

Near-drowning patients are those persons who have been submerged in fresh or salt water and may or may not be conscious. If the patient is still in open water upon arrival of EMS crew members, a Dive Rescue Team should be used to remove the patient from the water whenever possible. Additional protocols may be needed for treatment decisions (e.g., Pediatric Protocol 3.8.4, Barotrauma/Decompression Illness: Dive Injuries).

Supportive Care

- Trauma Supportive Care Protocol 3.1.4: protect the c-spine (a).
- Determine any pertinent history (duration of submersion, depth, water temperature, possible seizure, drug and/or alcohol use, possible trauma).
- Maintain the patient's body temperature; dry and warm the patient.
- **All near-drowning patients should be transported to the hospital,** regardless of how well they may seem to have recovered. Delayed death or complications due to pulmonary edema or aspiration pneumonia are not uncommon. The most devastating injury is the result of asphyxia.

ALS Level 1

- Treat dysrhythmias per specific protocol (see Pediatric Protocol 3.3).
- Consider insertion of a nasogastric tube (see Medical Procedure 4.19, Nasogastric Tube Insertion) (b).

ALS Level 2

None.

Note

(a) The routine use of abdominal thrusts for near-drowning victims is not recommended. This maneuver should be used only in cases of FBAO (see Medical Procedure 4.3, Suspected Foreign Body Airway Obstruction).

(b) Any near-drowning patient with a decreased ability to protect his/her airway, who has gross abdominal distention, or who requires ventilatory assistance needs an NG tube.

3.8.2 Heat-Related Emergencies

Hyperthermia occurs when the patient is exposed to increased environmental temperature. It can manifest as heat cramps, heat exhaustion, or heat stroke. Certain drugs may also cause an increase in body temperature (e.g., cocaine, ecstasy).

Some tympanic thermometers (e.g., Braun Thermoscan™ Pro-1 and Pro 3000) will register temperatures in the range of 68–108°F. Tympanic thermometers should not be used in infants < 1 year.

- **Heat cramps:** Signs and symptoms include muscle cramps of the fingers, arms, legs, or abdomen; hot, sweaty skin; weakness; dizziness; tachycardia; normal BP; and normal temperature.
- **Heat exhaustion:** Signs and symptoms include cold and clammy skin, profuse sweating, nausea/vomiting, diarrhea, tachycardia, weakness, dizziness, transient syncope, muscle cramps, headache, positive orthostatic vital signs, and normal or slightly elevated temperature.
- **Heat stroke:** Signs and symptoms include hot dry skin (sweating may be present), confusion and disorientation, rapid bounding pulse followed by slow weak pulse, hypotension with low or absent diastolic reading, rapid and shallow respirations (which may later slow), seizures, coma, and elevated temperature (> 105°F).

Heat Cramps and Heat Exhaustion

Supportive Care

- Medical Supportive Care Protocol 3.1.3.
- Remove the patient from the warm environment; cool the patient.
- Monitor the patient's temperature.
- For mild to moderate heat cramps and heat exhaustion, if the patient is conscious, encourage the patient to drink salt-containing fluids (e.g., half-strength Gatorade®).

ALS Level 1

- If heat cramps are severe or if the patient's level of consciousness is diminished, administer a fluid challenge of normal saline 20 mL/kg IV.

ALS Level 2

None.

3.8.2 Heat-Related Emergencies

Heat Stroke

Supportive Care

- Medical Supportive Care Protocol 3.1.3.
- Remove the patient from the warm environment; aggressively cool the patient. Remove the patient's clothing, and cover the patient with sheets soaked in ice water. Also, turn air-conditioning units and fans on high, and apply ice packs to the patient's head, neck, chest, and groin.
- Monitor the patient's temperature. Cool the patient to 102°F, then remove wet sheets and ice packs, and turn off fans (avoid lowering the patient's temperature too much).

ALS Level 1

- Treat hypotension with IV fluids. Avoid using vasopressors and anticholinergic drugs, as they may potentiate heat stroke by inhibiting sweating. Administer a fluid challenge of normal saline 20 mL/kg IV.

ALS Level 2

None.

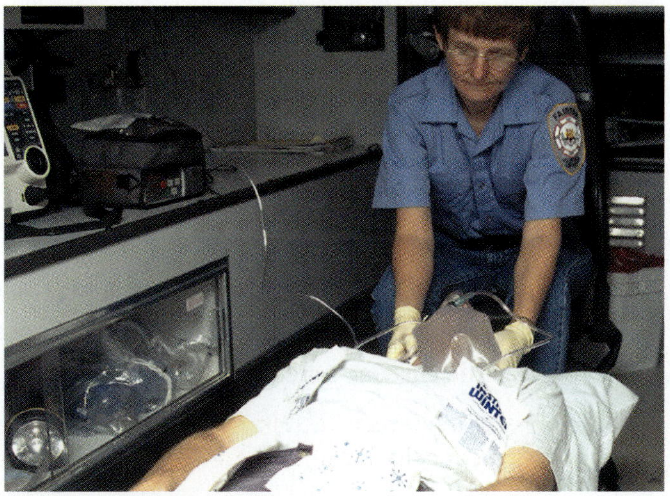

Apply cool packs to the patient's neck, groin, and armpits.

3.8.3 Cold-Related Emergencies

Factors that predispose and/or cause a patient to develop hypothermia include geriatric and pediatric age, poor nutrition, diabetes, hypothyroidism, brain tumors or head trauma, sepsis, use of alcohol and certain drugs, and prolonged exposure to water or low atmospheric temperature. Hypothermia patients can be classified into three categories:

- **Mild hypothermia:** temperature 94–97°F.
- **Moderate hypothermia:** temperature 86–94°F.
- **Severe hypothermia:** temperature < 86°F.

Most oral thermometers will not register temperatures of less than 96°F. However, some tympanic thermometers (e.g., Braun Thermoscan™ Pro-1 and Pro 3000) will register temperatures in the range of 68–108°F. Tympanic thermometers should not be used in infants < 1 year.

Patients with **mild to moderate hypothermia** will generally present with shivering, lethargy, and stiff, uncoordinated muscles. Patients with **severe hypothermia** may have altered mental status, ranging from confusion to lethargy or coma. Shivering will usually stop and physical activity will be uncoordinated. In addition, severe hypothermia will frequently produce an Osborn wave or J wave on the ECG, as well as dysrhythmias (bradycardia, ventricular fibrillation).

Supportive Care

- Medical Supportive Care Protocol 3.1.3 (a).
- Remove all wet clothes; dry the patient.
- Protect the patient from heat loss and wind chill.
- Maintain the patient in a horizontal position.
- Avoid rough movement and excess activity.
- Monitor the patient's temperature.
- Add heat to the patient's head, neck, chest, and groin.
- In cases of severe hypothermia, warm IV fluids, if possible.

For severe hypothermic cardiac arrest:

- Start CPR.

3.8.3 Cold-Related Emergencies

ALS Level 1

- For VF or pulseless VT, see Pediatric Cardiac Dysrhythmia Protocol 3.3.6.
- Intubate and hyperventilate the patient with warm humidified oxygen, if possible.
- Establish IV access; give warm normal saline.

If temperature > 86°F:

- Follow the appropriate dysrhythmia treatment (see Pediatric Protocol 3.3).

If temperature < 86°F:

- Continue CPR and transport the patient immediately. Do not treat dysrhythmias in patients with severe hypothermia; warm the patient prior to treatment.

ALS Level 2

None.

Note

(a) Areas of frostbite should be bandaged with dry sterile dressings. Patients with frostbite should be transported without attempting rewarming in the prehospital setting.

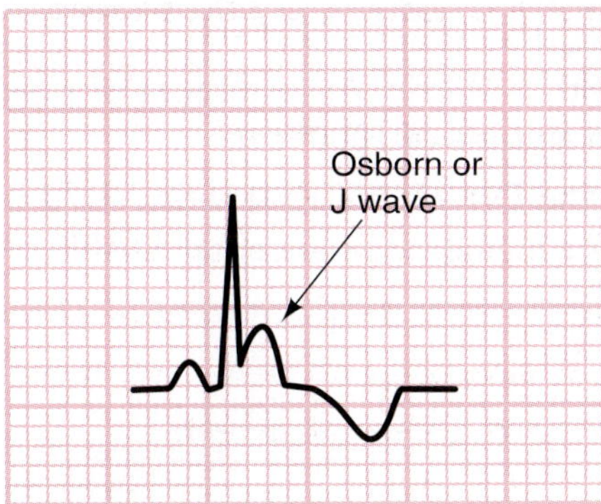

Osborn or J wave.

3.8.4 Barotrauma/Decompression Illness: Dive Injuries

Barotrauma and decompression illness are caused by changes in the surrounding atmospheric pressure beyond the body's capacity to compensate for the excess gas load. These injuries are most commonly associated with the use of SCUBA (Self-Contained Underwater Breathing Apparatus). SCUBA diving emergencies can occur at any depth, with the most serious injuries manifesting symptoms after a dive. If a patient took a breath underwater from any source of compressed gas (e.g., submerged vehicle, SCUBA), while at a depth greater than 3 feet, the patient may be a victim of barotrauma. Barotrauma may cause several injuries to occur, including arterial gas embolism (AGE), pneumothorax, pneumomediastinum, subcutaneous emphysema, and the "squeeze." Decompression illnesses may also include decompression sickness ("bends").

Supportive Care

- Trauma Supportive Care Protocol 3.1.4: Give high-flow O_2.
- Place the patient in a supine position.
- Complete the Dive Accident Signs and Symptoms checklist (see Appendix 7.6).
- Start a Dive History Profile, if possible (the patient's dive buddy may be helpful in answering many of these questions).
- Whenever possible, have the legal authority in charge (e.g., police, Florida Marine Patrol, U.S. Coast Guard) secure all of the victim's dive gear, following the proper chain of custody for testing, analysis, and other purposes.
- Manage the patient according to the appropriate protocol(s).
- Transport the patient to the closest emergency department or trauma center with a helipad. Air transport of a diving accident victim must remain below an altitude of 1000 feet.
- Contact the Diver's Alert Network (DAN) at Duke University Medical Center for further assistance; call DAN collect at 919-684-4326 (a).

ALS Level 1

None.

ALS Level 2

None.

Note

(a) DAN may be contacted while on scene or after arrival at the hospital. If the contact is made at the hospital, provide the name of the ED physician and ED phone number.

3.8.5 Electrical Emergencies

A wide range of injuries can be caused by a lightning strike or contact with electricity. Electrical injury can occur from direct contact, an arc, or a flash of electricity, and by a direct hit or a splash from lightning. The movement of electrical current through the body can cause violent muscle contractions that can lead to fractures; for this reason, the c-spine of a patient who has experienced an electrical emergency should be protected. The thermal energy can cause external burns, but in many cases the majority of thermal damage is internal, with few external signs of injury. Dysrhythmias are also common (e.g., ventricular fibrillation). The rescuer should be sure that the patient is no longer in contact with the electrical current before initiating treatment.

Supportive Care

- Trauma Supportive Care Protocol 3.1.4: Protect the c-spine.
- Treat burns per Pediatric Protocol 3.9.7.
- Consider the need to transport the patient to a trauma center (see General Protocol 1.10).

ALS Level 1

- Treat dysrhythmias per specific protocol (see Pediatric Protocol 3.3).

ALS Level 2

None.

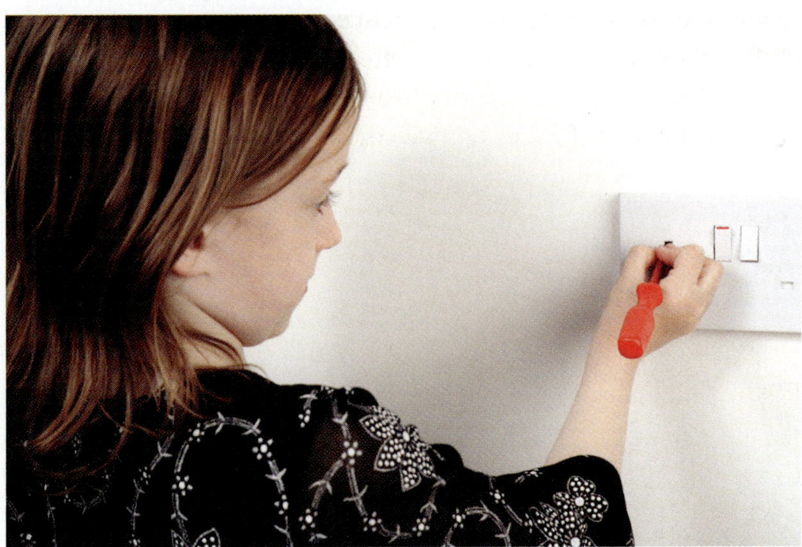

The human body is a good conductor of electricity.

3.9 Pediatric Trauma Emergencies

These protocols cover specific types of injuries and their treatment. The initial assessment of the trauma patient should include determination of Trauma Alert criteria (see General Protocol 1.10, Trauma Transport). When the situation demands it (e.g., when Trauma Alert criteria are met), scene time should be limited as much as possible (e.g., 10 minutes), and the patient should be expeditiously transported to a trauma center. Do not delay transport to establish vascular access or to bandage and splint every injury. Priority should be given to airway management, rapid preparation for transport (e.g., full immobilization on a backboard), and control of gross hemorrhage.

If a vascular access is obtained and hypovolemia is suspected (e.g., the patient shows signs and symptoms of shock), a fluid challenge of 20 mL/kg should be administered. If the patient is still in shock, repeat the fluid challenge at 20 mL/kg until a maximum of 60 mL/kg of fluid is administered. Be aware that administration of large volumes of IV fluids has been found to be deleterious to the survival of patients with uncontrolled hemorrhage, internally or externally. Studies (*NEJM,* 1994) have shown that maximal fluid resuscitation may increase bleeding, thereby preventing the formation of a protective thrombus or dislodging it once the intraluminal pressure exceeds the tamponading pressure of the thrombus. **Therefore, consultation with the physician should be made prior to the administration of large volumes of IV fluids when the transport time is relatively short (e.g., less than 20 minutes).**

Avoid the use of vasopressor agents (e.g., dopamine) in trauma patients who are hypotensive (see Appendix 7.11, Pediatric Vital Signs).

The adolescent female in her third trimester of pregnancy should be placed on her left side for transport. If the injuries require the use of a backboard, following full immobilization to the backboard, the backboard should be tilted to the left. Failure to follow this practice may cause hypotension due to decreased venous return.

3.9.1 Head and Spine Injuries

If history, symptoms, or signs of head or spinal injuries are present, manually immobilize the patient's head and neck while maintaining a patent airway using a modified jaw-thrust method. Immobilization of the entire spine is indicated following initial stabilization.

Supportive Care

- Trauma Supportive Care Protocol 3.1.4.
- If the patient is not hypotensive (see Appendix 7.11, Pediatric Vital Signs), elevate the head of the backboard 30 degrees (12–18 inches).

ALS Level 1

- If signs of brain stem herniation exist (e.g., pupillary dilation, asymmetric pupillary reactivity, or motor posturing), consider intubation and ventilate at 20 breaths/min for a child and 30 breaths/min for an infant (see Medical Procedure 4.18, Intubation, and Medical Procedure 4.4, Rescue Breathing).

ALS Level 2

- If the patient is seizing, see Pediatric Protocol 3.5.2. Avoid administration of glucose-containing solutions and medications.

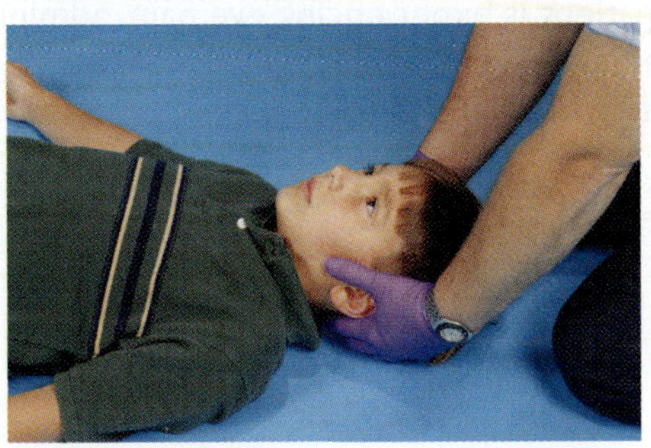

Manually immobilize the patient's head and neck.

3.9.2 Eye Injuries

This protocol covers a variety of injuries to the eye. If other injuries to the body exist, priority of care should be determined as appropriate.

Supportive Care

- Trauma Supportive Care Protocol 3.1.4: Establish IV access as needed.
- Remove, or ask the patient to remove, contact lenses, if still in the affected eye(s).
- For a penetrating object, stabilize the object and cover the affected eye with an ocular shield or similar rigid device. Cover both eyes to minimize eye movement. Avoid placing direct pressure on the eye or penetrating object.
- If the eyeball has been forced out of the socket, cover the entire eye area with a rigid container, such as a disposable drinking cup. Avoid contact with the exposed globe. If bleeding is present, control it by applying direct pressure with a sterile dry dressing.
- If there are signs and symptoms or suspicion of ocular exposure to chemicals or foreign body, without obvious or suspected penetrating injury or laceration of the cornea or globe, irrigate with a normal saline IV solution (see Medical Procedure 4.45, Morgan Lens).

ALS Level 1

- If the patient is experiencing eye pain, administer tetracaine 1 drop in each affected eye. Tetracaine is contraindicated in penetrating eye injuries or patients with allergies to lidocaine.

ALS Level 2

None.

3.9.3 Chest Injuries

This protocol covers both blunt and penetrating chest trauma and should be part of the initial resuscitation effort if the patient's breathing is compromised.

Supportive Care

- Trauma Supportive Care Protocol 3.1.4.
- Penetrating injuries to the chest or upper back should be covered immediately with an occlusive dressing (e.g., Vaseline gauze).
- Do not attempt to remove an impaled object; instead, stabilize it with bulky dressing or other means. If the impaled object is very large or unwieldy, attempt to cut the object to no less than 6 inches from chest.

ALS Level 1

- For tension pneumothorax, with evidence of respiratory and circulatory compromise, decompress the chest **on the affected side** (see Medical Procedure 4.14, Chest Decompression).
- For massive flail chest with severe respiratory compromise, intubate and ventilate at 20 breaths/min for a child and 30 breaths/min for an infant. If the flail chest does not cause severe respiratory compromise, stabilize the chest externally by placing the ipsilateral arm in a sling and swathe.
- For crush injury, establish two large-bore IVs. If the crushing object is still on the patient, infuse a minimum of 20 mL/kg of fluid before attempting to lift the object off the patient.
- For traumatic asphyxia, administer sodium bicarbonate (8.4%) 1 mEq/kg IV (a).

ALS Level 2

None.

Note

(a) Sodium bicarbonate (4.2%) 1 mEq/kg IV/IO should be administered to **infants** (dilute 8.4% 1:1 with normal saline to make 4.2%).

3.9.4 Abdomino-Pelvic Injuries

This protocol covers blunt and penetrating abdomino-pelvic trauma. Penetrating injuries may also affect the chest (see Pediatric Protocol 3.9.3, Chest Injuries). Also refer to Appendix 7.16, Signs of Child Abuse.

Supportive Care

- Trauma Supportive Care Protocol 3.1.4.
- For penetrating injuries, cover the wound with an occlusive dressing (e.g., Vaseline gauze).
- For evisceration, cover the organs with a saline-soaked sterile dressing, and then cover it with an occlusive dressing (e.g., foil). Do not attempt to put the organs back into the abdomen.
- Do not log-roll any patient with suspected pelvic fracture; you may use a scoop stretcher if it is appropriate given the patient's size.

ALS Level 1

None.

ALS Level 2

None.

3.9.5 Extremity Injuries

This protocol covers open and closed injuries to the extremities, including amputation.

Supportive Care

- Trauma Supportive Care Protocol 3.1.4.
- Any fracture or suspected fracture should be splinted appropriately, with ice being applied to the affected area. Remove and secure all jewelry. Check the pulse, sensation, and movement in the extremity before and after splinting.
- Angulated fractures should be aligned using proximal and distal traction during splinting, except in fractures that involve a joint, which should be splinted in the position in which they are found.
- Traction splints should be used in cases of femur fractures, unless a pelvic fracture is suspected. PASG may be used for splinting lower extremities where a traction splint is not applicable, if available.
- Amputations should be dressed with bulky dressings. The amputated part should be wrapped in moistened sterile gauze and placed in a plastic bag; this bag should then be placed on ice for transportation to the hospital.

ALS Level 1

- See Pediatric Protocol 3.1.5, Pain Management.

ALS Level 2

None.

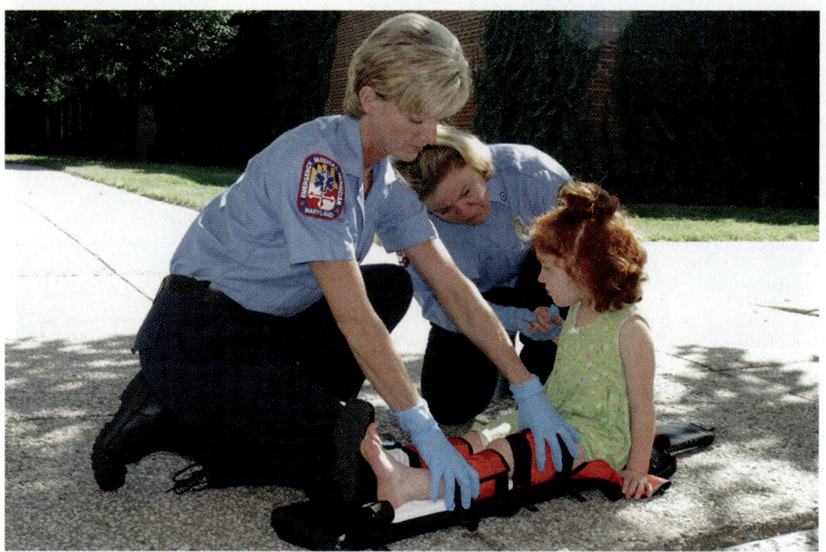

Splinting.

3.9.6 Traumatic Arrest

The decision to attempt resuscitation of a patient in traumatic arrest should be based on the paramedic's judgment as to the possibility of survival and/or the possibility of organ harvest. In some instances, attempted resuscitation of a traumatic arrest is not warranted (see General Protocol 1.4, Death in the Field).

Supportive Care

- Trauma Supportive Care Protocol 3.1.4.
- Rapidly prepare the patient for transport and then expeditiously transport the patient to the trauma center.

ALS Level 1

- If IV access can be established, infuse normal saline 20 mL/kg, up to a maximum of 60 mL/kg IV.
- Avoid use of vasopressors in cases of suspected hypovolemia.

ALS Level 2

None.

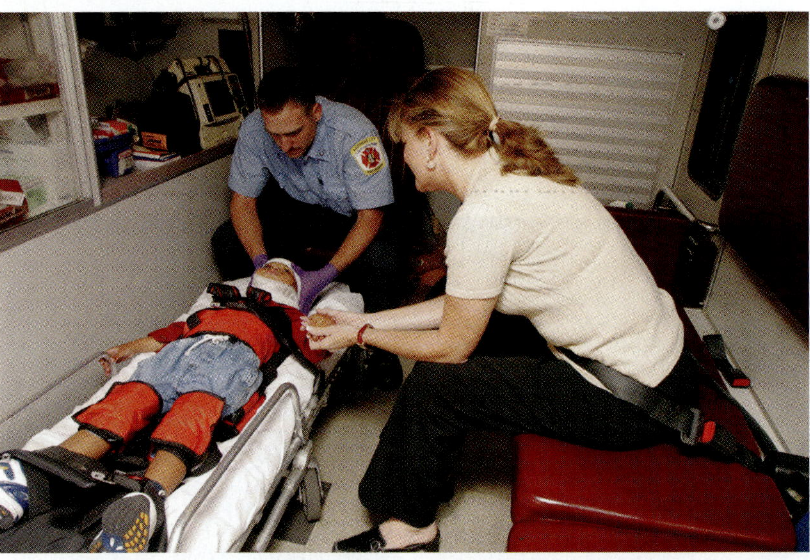

Transport as quickly as possible.

3.9.7 Burn Injuries

Burns can be caused by thermal, chemical, and electrical sources. If an electrical burn is suspected, also see Pediatric Protocol 3.8.5, Electrical Emergencies. Remember that burn patients are volume depleted. Burns do not bleed, however, so look for other sources if bleeding is present. Assume that any patient with compromised perfusion has other injuries and treat him/her accordingly.

Many burn injuries are associated with inhalation injury. Signs and symptoms of inhalation injury include nasal and oropharyngeal burns, charring of the tongue or teeth, sooty (blackened) sputum, singed nasal and facial hair, abnormal breath sounds (e.g., stridor, rhonchi, wheezing), and respiratory distress. In cases of inhalation injury, attention should be given to the patency of the airway. Acute swelling can cause an airway obstruction. The paramedic should consider the need for early intubation to avoid a complete airway obstruction that requires a cricothyroidotomy.

Supportive Care

- Trauma Supportive Care Protocol 3.1.4.
- Stop the burning process, if necessary, but do not cause hypothermia.
  - **Thermal burns:** Lavage the burned area with tepid water (sterile, if possible) to cool skin. Do not attempt to wipe off semisolids (e.g., grease, tar, wax).
  - **Dry chemical burns:** Brush off dry powder, then lavage with copious amounts of tepid water (sterile, if possible) for 15 minutes.
  - **Liquid chemical burns:** Lavage the burned area with copious amounts of tepid water (sterile, if possible) for 15 minutes. (When *phenol* has caused the burn, flush with copious amounts of tepid water and then apply vegetable oil to the burned area, if available. Isopropyl alcohol may be used for *very* small areas.)
- Remove clothing from around the burned area, but do not remove or peel off any skin or tissue.
- Remove and secure all jewelry and tight-fitting clothing.
- Assess the extent of the burn using the modified Rule of Nines and the degree of burn severity (see Appendix 7.4, Burn Severity Categorization, and Appendix 7.15, Rule of Nines). An alternative method is to use the palmar surface of the patient as an estimate of 1% BSA.

3.9.7 Burn Injuries

- Apply a dressing to the burned area:
  - If there is greater than or equal to 20% second-degree or 5% third-degree burns, cover the burned areas with dry sterile dressings or Water Gel™ wraps.
  - If there is less than 20% second-degree or 5% third-degree burns, apply wet sterile dressings to the burned areas for 15 minutes to aid in pain control. Alternatively, Burn Free™ gel pads or Water Gel™ wraps may be applied continuously to aid in pain control.
- Prevent hypothermia, keep the patient warm, and ensure that all outer layers of dressings are dry.

ALS Level 1

- Pain Management Protocol 3.1.5.

ALS Level 2

None.

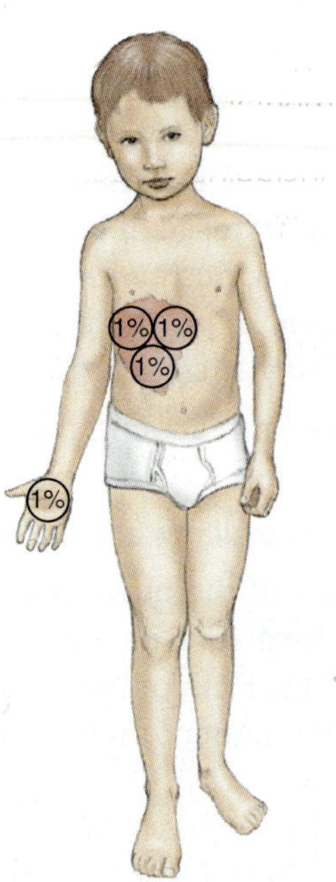

The palm plus fingers is approximately 1% of the body surface area.

3.10 Children with Special Healthcare Needs

These protocols cover specific types of special healthcare needs in pediatric patients. "Children with special health care needs are those who have or are at risk for chronic physical, developmental, behavioral, and emotional conditions that necessitate use of health and related services of a type or amount not usually required by typically developing young children."[2]

The general approach to children with special healthcare needs includes the following measures:

1. Priority is given to the ABCs.
2. Do not be overwhelmed by the machines.
3. Listen to the caregiver.
4. If a nurse is present, rely on his/her judgment.
5. Remember that the child's cognitive level of function may be altered.
6. Assume that the child can understand exactly what you say.
7. Bring all medications and equipment to the hospital.

Obtaining a history includes asking the patient/caregiver about the following issues:

1. The child's normal vital signs.
2. The child's actual weight.
3. The child's developmental level.
4. The child's allergies, including to latex.
5. Pertinent medications/therapies.

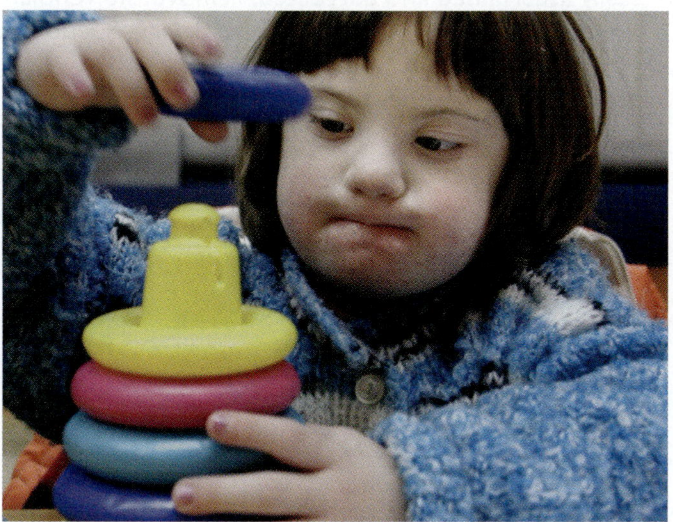

A child with Down Syndrome.

[2]American Heart Association, *PALS Provider Manual, 2002,* p. 287.

3.10.1 Home Mechanical Ventilator

Home mechanical ventilators may be indicated for chronically ill children with abnormal respiratory drive, severe chronic lung disease, or severe neuromuscular weakness. Some children require continuous mechanical ventilation, whereas others require only intermittent support during sleep or acute illness. Home ventilators may either be limited or pressure limited. All are equipped with alarms.

Types of Ventilator Alarms

- **Low pressure or apnea:** may be caused by a loose or disconnected circuit or an air leak in the circuit or at the tracheostomy, resulting in inadequate ventilation.
- **Low power:** caused by a depleted battery.
- **High pressure:** may be caused by a plugged or obstructed airway or circuit tubing, by coughing, or by bronchospasm.
- **Setting error:** caused by ventilator settings that exceed the capacity of the equipment.
- **Power switchover:** occurs when the unit switches from alternating-current power to the internal battery.

Supportive Care

- ◆ Medical Supportive Care Protocol 3.1.3.
- ◆ If a ventilator-dependent child is in respiratory distress and the cause is not easily ascertained and corrected, remove the ventilator and provide assisted manual ventilations with a bag-valve device. Suction as needed.
- ◆ Consider the need for other protocols (e.g., Pediatric Protocol 3.2, Pediatric Respiratory Emergencies).

ALS Level 1

None.

ALS Level 2

None.

3.10.2 Tracheostomy

Tracheostomies are indicated for long-term ventilatory support, to bypass an upper airway obstruction, and to aid in the removal of secretions. Tracheostomies come in neonatal, pediatric, and adult sizes and can include either a single lumen or a double lumen. Special attachments include a tracheostomy nose (filtration device), tracheostomy collar (for oxygen or humidification), and Passy-Muir valve (speaker valve).

Signs of Tracheostomy Tube Obstruction

- Excess secretions.
- No chest wall movement.
- Cyanosis.
- Accessory muscle use.
- No chest wall rise with bag-valve ventilations.

Supportive Care

- Medical Supportive Care Protocol 3.1.3.
- If an obstruction is present, inject 1–3 mL of normal saline into the tracheostomy tube and suction as needed (set the suction pressure at 100 mm Hg or less).
- If unable to clear the obstruction by suctioning, remove the tracheostomy tube and insert a new tube (the same size or one size smaller). **Do not force the tube.**
- If unable to insert a new tracheostomy tube or if one is unavailable, insert an endotracheal tube of similar size into the stoma and ventilate with a bag-valve mask as needed.
- If unable to insert an endotracheal tube, ventilate with a bag-valve mask over the stoma or over the patient's mouth while covering the stoma as needed.
- Consider the need for other protocols (e.g., Pediatric Protocol 3.2, Pediatric Respiratory Emergencies).

ALS Level 1

None.

ALS Level 2

None.

3.10.3 Central Venous Lines

Central venous lines are indicated for administration of medications, delivery of chemotherapy, nutritional support, infusion of blood products, and blood draws. Types of central venous lines include Broviac/Hickman, Port-a-Cath/Med-a-Port, and percutaneous intravenous catheters (PIC). Central venous line emergencies include the catheter coming completely out, bleeding at the site, the catheter broken in half, blood embolus, thrombus, air embolus, and internal bleeding. **Use of SQ ports requires special training; these ports should not be used for IV access.**

Signs of Blood Embolus, Thrombus, Air Embolus, and Internal Bleeding

- Chest pain.
- Cyanosis.
- Dyspnea.
- Shock.

Supportive Care

- Medical Supportive Care Protocol 3.1.3. CVP and PUC lines may be used for emergency IV access under sterile conditions.
- If the catheter has come completely out, apply direct pressure to the site.
- If there is bleeding at the site, apply direct pressure.
- If the catheter is broken in half, clamp the end of the remaining tube.
- If a blood embolus, thrombus, or internal bleeding is suspected, clamp the line.
- If an air embolism is suspected, clamp the line and place the patient on his/her left side.
- Consider the need for other protocols (e.g., Pediatric Protocol 3.2, Pediatric Respiratory Emergencies).

ALS Level 1

None.

ALS Level 2

None.

3.10.4 Feeding Tubes

Feeding tubes are indicated for administration of nutritional supplements and in patients who have an inability to swallow. Types of feeding tubes include nasogastric tubes (temporary) and gastrostomy tubes (G tube). Types of G tubes include those that are surgically placed, percutaneous endoscopic gastrostomy tubes (PEG tubes), and jejunal tubes (J tubes). Potential complications include leaks, bleeding around the site, and the displacement of the tube.

Supportive Care

- Medical Supportive Care Protocol 3.1.3.
- If the catheter has come completely out, cover the site with Vaseline gauze and apply direct pressure to the site.
- If there is bleeding at the site, apply direct pressure.

ALS Level 1

None.

ALS Level 2

None.

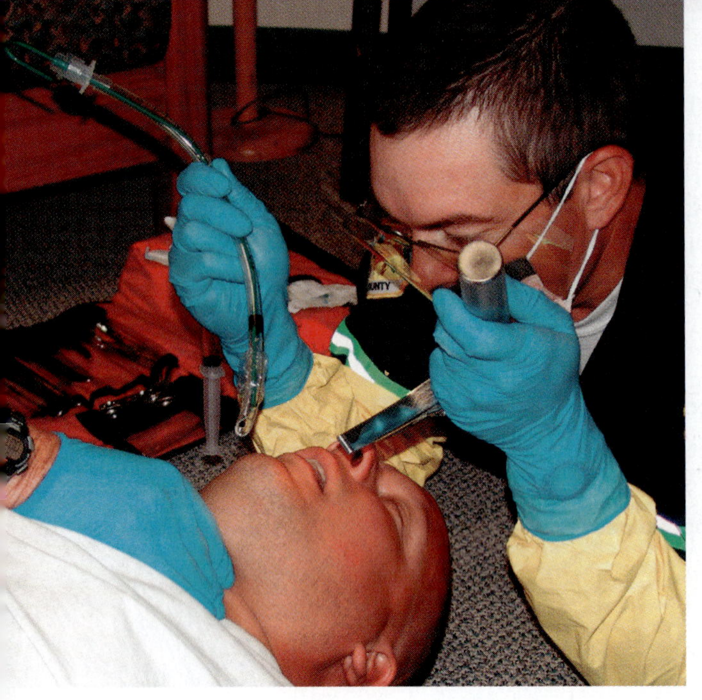

chapter 4

Medical Procedures

4.1 Automated External Defibrillator (AED)

Automated external defibrillators are to be used by the first responder and EMT, when Advanced Life Support providers (e.g., paramedics with monitors/defibrillators) are not available, for treatment of the patient in nontraumatic cardiac arrest. Two types of AEDs are distinguished: fully automatic and semiautomatic.

1. Perform continuous CPR until the AED is applied.
2. Apply the AED pads to the patient according to the manufacturer's recommendation.
3. Activate the unit and follow the AED prompts.
4. If the AED advises to "shock," clear everyone from touching the patient.
5. Push the "shock" button to defibrillate the patient.
6. Immediately resume chest compressions.
7. Analyze per AED prompt after 2 minutes of uninterrupted compressions.

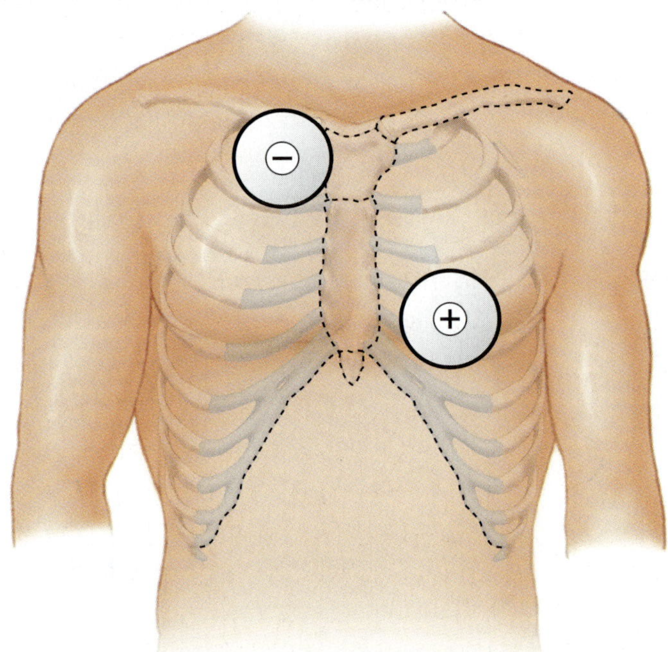

Position the paddles for defibrillation.

4.2 Cardiopulmonary Resuscitation (CPR)

Adult

1. Establish unresponsiveness (call for backup as needed).
2. A: Open the ***airway*** using an appropriate method.
3. B: Assess ***breathing*** by looking, listening, and feeling (5–10 seconds).
4. If breathing is absent, give two breaths.
5. C: Assess ***circulation*** via carotid pulse (5–10 seconds).
6. If a pulse is absent, start chest compressions (push hard, push fast).
7. Administer compressions at a rate of 100 per minute (place the heel of hand on the sternum between the nipples and compress to a depth of 1½ to 2 inches).

8a. Administer 30 compressions and then 2 ventilations.

or

8b. If an ETT/supraglottic airway is in place and there are two rescuers, administer continuous compressions and unsynchronized ventilations at a rate of 1 breath every 6 seconds or 1 breath every 10 compressions.

9. Continue compressions and ventilations until the return of a pulse is noted. Intermittently check for the return of a spontaneous pulse.

Child

1. Establish unresponsiveness (call for backup as needed).
2. A: Open the ***airway*** using an appropriate method.
3. B: Assess ***breathing*** by looking, listening, and feeling (5–10 seconds).
4. If breathing is absent, give two breaths to make the chest rise.
5. C: Assess ***circulation*** via carotid pulse (5–10 seconds).
6. If a pulse is absent, start chest compressions.
7. Administer compressions at a rate of 100 per minute (place the heel of one hand or two hands on the lower half of the sternum and compress to one-third to one-half the depth of the chest).

8a. For one rescuer, administer 30 compressions and then 2 ventilations.

or

8b. For two rescuers, administer 15 compressions and then 2 ventilations.

or

8c. If an ETT/supraglottic airway is in place and there are two rescuers, administer continuous compressions and unsynchronized ventilations at a rate of 1 breath every 6 seconds or 1 breath every 10 compressions.

9. Continue compressions and ventilations until the return of a pulse is noted. Intermittently check for the return of a spontaneous pulse.

4.2 Cardiopulmonary Resuscitation (CPR)

Infant

1. Establish unresponsiveness (call for backup as needed).
2. A: Open the ***airway*** using an appropriate method.
3. B: Assess ***breathing*** by looking, listening, and feeling (5–10 seconds).
4. If breathing is absent, give two breaths to make the chest rise.
5. C: Assess ***circulation*** via brachial pulse (5–10 seconds).

6a. For one rescuer, use two fingers on the sternum, one finger width below the nipple line; administer 100 compressions per minute, at one-third to one-half the depth of the chest.

or

6b. For two rescuers, use two thumbs side by side at the center of breast bone just below the nipple line. Squeeze the infant's posterior chest with the encircled fingers, and administer 100 compressions per minute at one-third to one-half the depth of the chest.

7a. For one rescuer, administer 30 compressions and then 2 ventilations.

or

7b. For two rescuers, administer 15 compressions and then 2 ventilations.

or

7c. If an ETT/supraglottic airway is in place and there are two rescuers, administer continuous compressions and unsynchronized ventilations at a rate of 1 breath every 6 seconds or 1 breath every 10 compressions.

8. Continue compressions and ventilations until the return of a pulse is noted. Intermittently check for the return of a spontaneous pulse.

Skill Drill 4-1: Performing Infant Chest Compressions

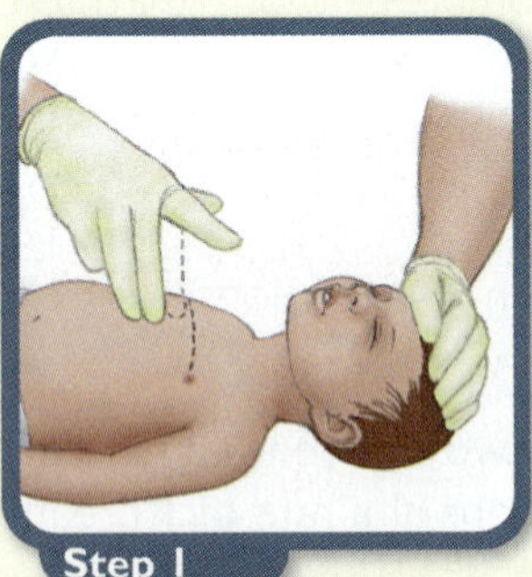

Step 1

Position the infant on a firm surface while maintaining the airway. Place two fingers in the middle of the sternum, one fingerbreadth below the imaginary intermammary line.

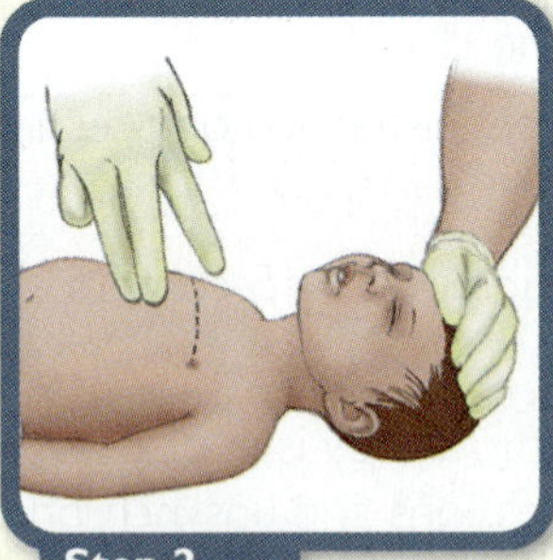

Step 2

Using two fingers, compress the sternum about one-third to one-half the depth of the chest. Push hard and fast, at a rate of 100 compressions/min. Allow the sternum to return briefly to its normal position between compressions.

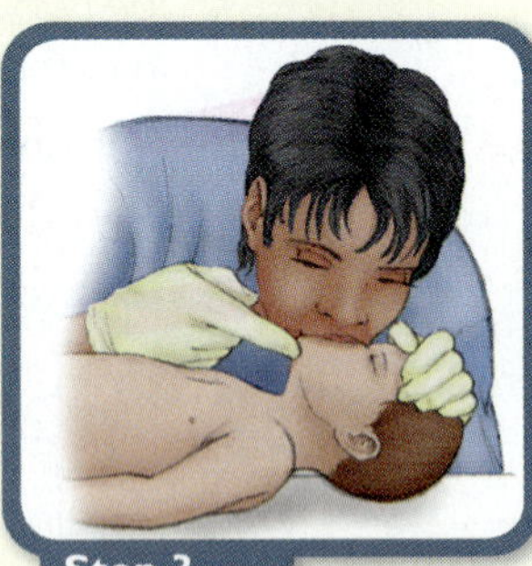

Step 3

Coordinate rapid compression and ventilation in a 30:2 ration. Check for the return of breathing and pulse after 2-minute intervals.

4.3 Suspected Foreign Body Airway Obstruction (FBAO)

Adult

1. If the patient is conscious, ask, "Are you choking?"
2. If the patient is unable to speak and/or nods his/her head "yes," give abdominal thrusts, or chest thrusts if the patient is pregnant or obese.
3. Repeat the abdominal thrusts until they are effective or the patient becomes unconscious.

If the patient becomes unconscious, continue with the following steps:

4. Open the airway. If able to visualize the obstruction, perform a finger sweep to remove the object.
5. Attempt to ventilate; if the airway is still obstructed, reposition the airway and try to ventilate again.
6. Give 30 chest compressions.
7. Repeat Steps 4 through 6 until the FBAO is relieved.

Child

1. If the patient is conscious, ask, "Are you choking?"
2. If the patient is unable to speak and/or nods his/her head "yes," give abdominal thrusts.
3. Repeat the abdominal thrusts until they are effective or the patient becomes unconscious.

If the patient becomes unconscious, continue with the following steps:

4. Open the airway. If able to visualize the obstruction, perform a finger sweep to remove the object.
5. Attempt to ventilate; if the airway is still obstructed, reposition the airway and try to ventilate again.
6. Give 30 chest compressions.
7. Repeat Steps 4 through 6 until the FBAO is relieved.

Skill Drill 4-2: Managing Severe Airway Obstruction in a Conscious Adult or Child

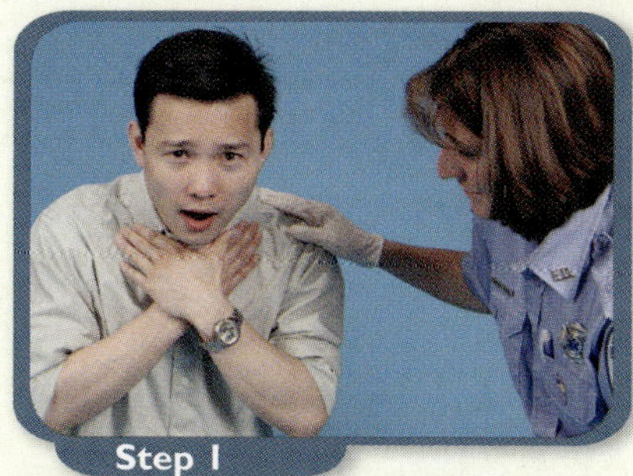

Step 1

Determine whether the patient is choking by asking, "Are you choking?" If the patient nods "yes," then help is needed.

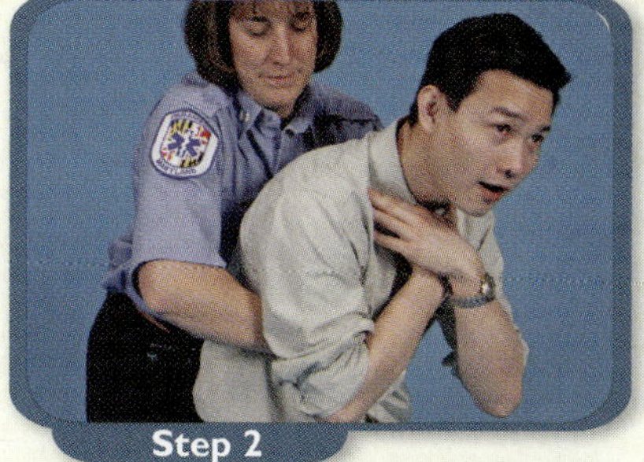

Step 2

Perform the Heimlich maneuver until the object is expelled or the patient becomes unresponsive.

4.3 Suspected Foreign Body Airway Obstruction (FBAO)

Infant

1. If the patient is conscious, determine airway patency.
2. If the patient is unable to move air or has poor air exchange, give 5 back slaps between the shoulder blades and then 5 chest thrusts with the patient in a head-dependent position.
3. Repeat the back slaps and chest thrusts until they are effective or the patient becomes unconscious.

If the patient becomes unconscious, continue with the following steps:

4. Open the airway. If able to visualize the obstruction, perform a finger sweep to remove the object.
5. Attempt to ventilate; if the airway is still obstructed, reposition the airway and try to ventilate again.
6. Give 30 chest compressions.
7. Repeat Steps 4 through 6 until the FBAO is relieved.

Skill Drill 4-3: Managing Severe Airway Obstruction in a Conscious Infant

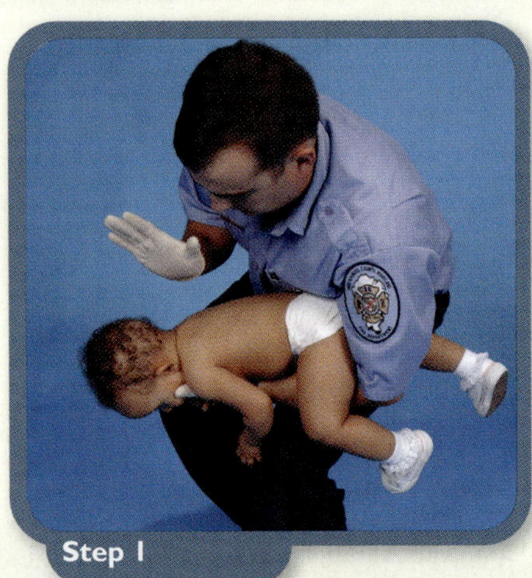

Step 1

Perform five back blows (slaps).

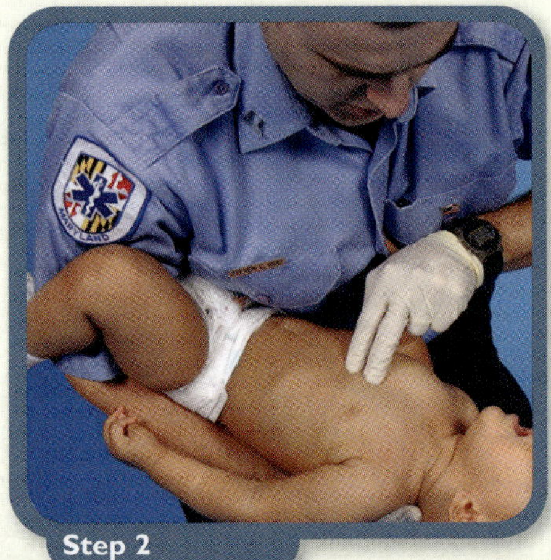

Step 2

Perform 5 chest thrusts. Repeat step 1 until the object is expelled or the infant becomes unresponsive.

4.4 Rescue Breathing

One Person

1. Position yourself directly above the patient's head.
2. Place the mask on the patient's face, using the bridge of the nose as a guide for correct positioning.
3. Use the E-C clamp technique to hold the mask in place while you lift the patient's jaw to hold the airway open.
    - Perform a head tilt.
    - Use the thumb and index finger of one hand to make a "C," pressing the edges of the mask to the face.
    - Use the remaining fingers to lift the angles of the jaw (three fingers form an "E") and open the airway.
4. Squeeze the bag to achieve chest rise. The delivery of breaths is the same whether you do or do not use supplementary oxygen.

    For perfusing rhythm:

    - Adult: 10–12 breaths/min.
    - Pediatric: 12–20 breaths/min.

    When CPR is being performed or if an advanced airway is in place:

    - Adult and pediatric: 8–10 breaths/min.
5. Insert an oral or nasal airway.

Two Persons

1. Rescuer one:
    - Take a position directly above the patient's head.
    - Place the mask on the patient's face, using the bridge of the nose as a guide for correct positioning.
    - Use the E-C clamp technique to hold the mask in place with both hands.
    - Use the thumb and index finger of one hand to make a "C," pressing the edges of the mask to the face.
    - Use the remaining three fingers to form an "E" to lift the angles of the jaw.

4.4 Rescue Breathing

2. Rescuer two:
   - Squeeze the bag for 1 second, while watching for chest rise.
   - Apply continuous cricoid pressure.
3. Squeeze the bag to achieve chest rise. The delivery of breaths is the same whether you do or do not use supplementary oxygen.

   For perfusing rhythm:
   - Adult: 10–12 breaths/min.
   - Pediatric: 12–20 breaths/min.

   When CPR is being performed or if an advanced airway is in place:
   - Adult and pediatric: 8–10 breaths/min.
4. Insert an oral or nasal airway.

4.5 Head Tilt–Chin Lift

1. Place one hand on the patient's forehead and push with your palm to tilt the head back.
2. Place the fingers of the other hand under the bony part of the patient's lower jaw near the chin. Do not press deeply into the soft tissue under the chin because it might obstruct the airway.
3. Lift the jaw to bring the chin forward.

Skill Drill 4-4: Head Tilt–Chin Lift Maneuver

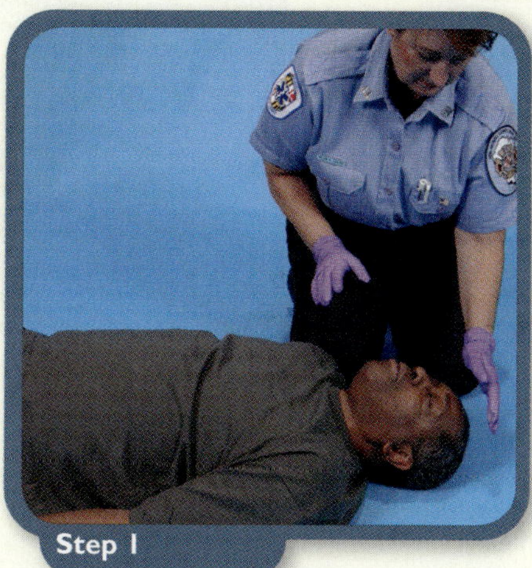

Step 1

Position yourself at the side of the supine patient.

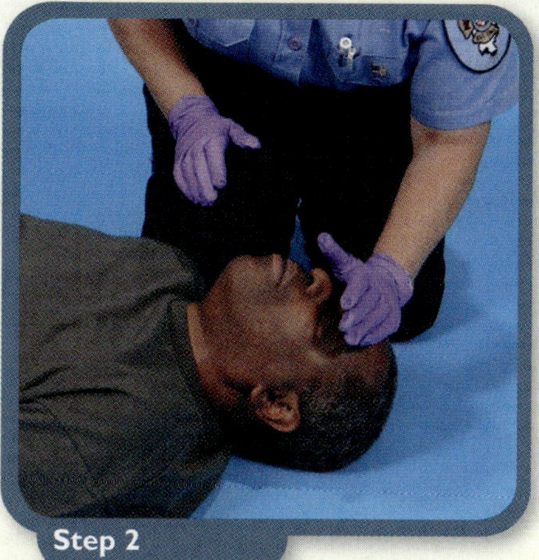

Step 2

Place your hand closest to the patient's head on the forehead.

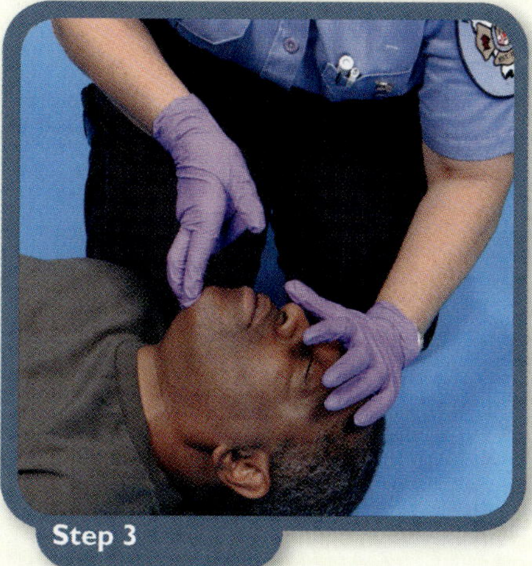

Step 3

With your other hand, place two fingers on the underside of the patient's chin.

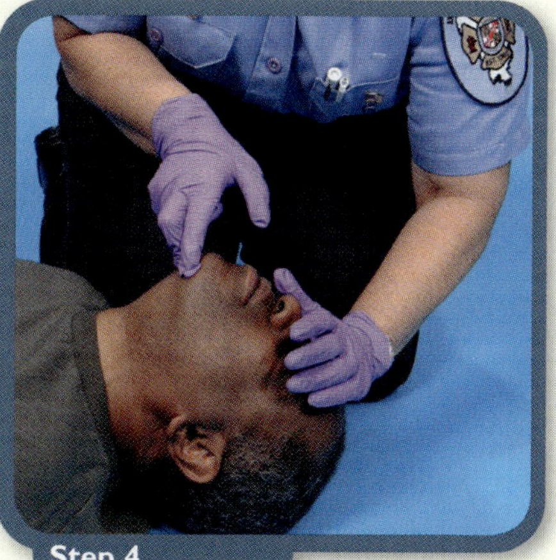

Step 4

Simultaneously apply backward and downward pressure to the patient's forehead and lift the jaw straight up. Do not depress the soft tissue below the chin.

4.6 Jaw Thrust

1. Place a hand on each side of the patient's face.
2. Grasp the angles of the patient's mandible and lift upward.
3. If there are not enough responders to maintain the jaw thrust or if the jaw thrust is not successful in opening the airway, proceed to the head tilt–chin lift maneuver (Medical Procedure 4.5).

Skill Drill 4-5: Jaw-Thrust Maneuver

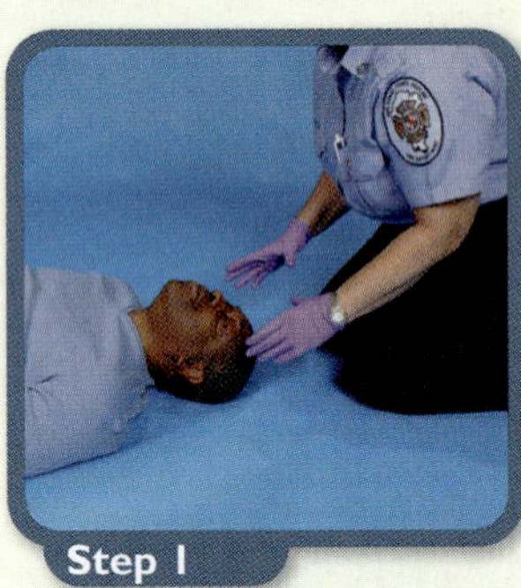

Step 1

Position yourself at the top of the patient's head.

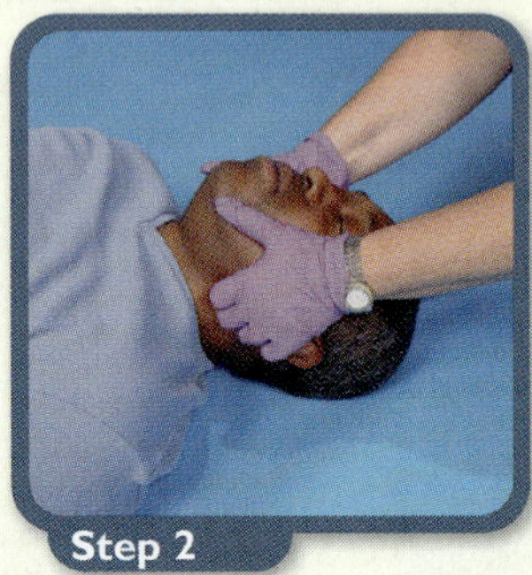

Step 2

Place the meaty portion of the base of your thumbs on the zygomatic arches, and hook the tips of your index fingers under the angle of the mandible, in the indent below each ear.

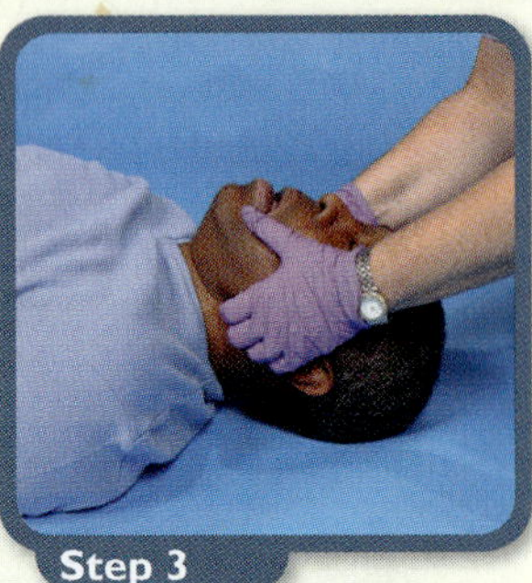

Step 3

While holding the patient's head still, displace the jaw upward and open the patient's mouth with your thumb tips.

4.7 Nasopharyngeal Insertion (NPA)

This procedure should not be performed in the presence of frontal head or midfacial trauma where the cribriform plate may be fractured.

1. Determine the proper size of tube (measure from the nostril to the earlobe).
2. Lubricate with a water-soluble lubricant (***optional: lidocaine gel***).
3. Position the patient's head in a neutral position, inspect the nose, and select the larger nostril. (***Optional: Spray Neo-Synephrine into nasopharynx.***)
4. Insert the nasopharyngeal tube with the bevel facing the nasal septum.
5. Gently insert the tube until the flange rests against the nostril.
   - If resistance is met, insert with a twisting motion.
   - If there continues to be resistance, attempt insertion in the other nostril.
6. Ventilation with a bag-valve device.

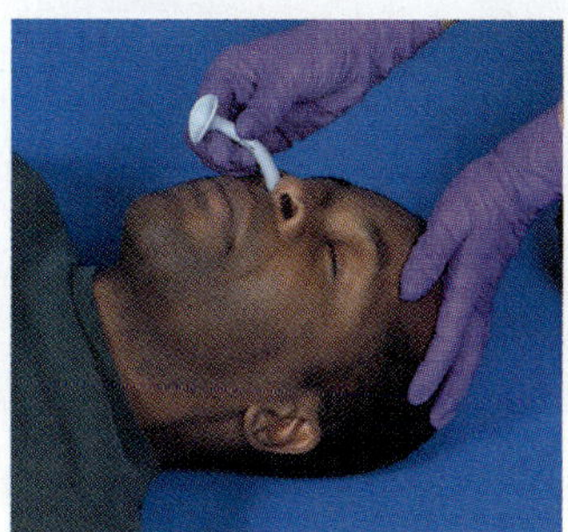

Gently insert the tube.

4.8 Oropharyngeal Insertion (OPA)

1. Determine the proper size of tube (measure from the corner of the mouth to the earlobe).
2. Open the patient's mouth by tongue/jaw-lift maneuver.
3. Insert the oropharyngeal tube with the tip toward the side of the mouth.
   - Prior to complete insertion, start to rotate the tube 90 degrees so that the flange rests on the lips.
   - If the patient has an intact gag reflex, perform a nasopharyngeal insertion.
4. Ventilate with a bag-valve device.

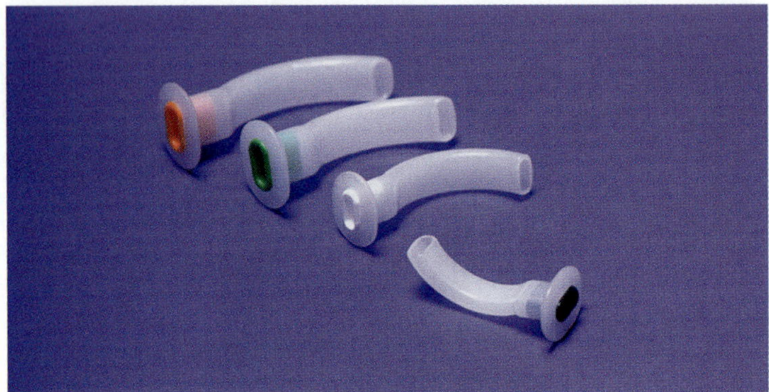

An oral airway is used for unconscious patients who have no gag reflex. It helps to keep the tongue from blocking the airway.

4.9 Flexible Suctioning

1. Wear protective eyewear, gloves, and face mask.
2. Preoxygenate the patient.
3. Turn on the suction unit.
4. Insert the catheter to an appropriate depth, place your thumb over the suction control orifice, and rotate the catheter between your fingertips while withdrawing catheter. (**Caution:** Do not suction for more than 10 seconds.)
5. Monitor the patient's heart rate, pulse, oxygen saturation, and clinical appearance during suctioning. If bradycardia occurs or the clinical appearance deteriorates, administer high-flow oxygen until the rate and clinical appearance return to normal.
6. Maintain ventilatory support with 100% oxygen.

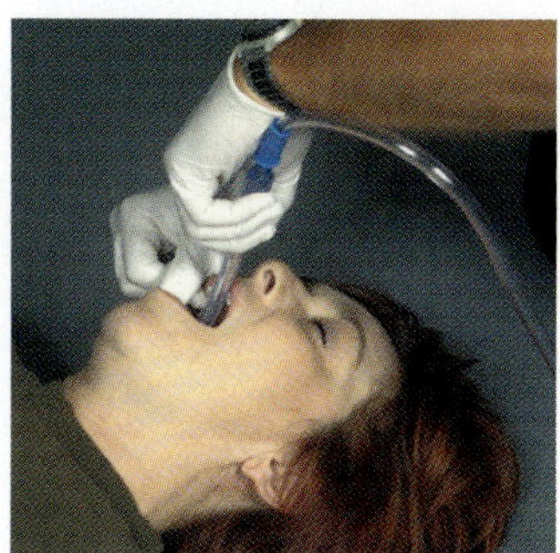

Do not suction for more than 10 seconds.

4.10 Rigid Suctioning

1. Wear protective eyewear, gloves, and face mask.
2. Preoxygenate the patient.
3. Turn on the suction unit.
4. Measure the depth of catheter insertion from the patient's earlobe to the corner of the mouth.
5. Insert the catheter to an appropriate depth, place your thumb over the suction control orifice, and suction the oropharynx. (**Caution:** Do not suction for more than 10 seconds.)
6. Monitor the patient's heart rate, pulse, oxygen saturation, and clinical appearance during suctioning. If bradycardia occurs or the clinical appearance deteriorates, administer high-flow oxygen until the rate and clinical appearance return to normal.
7. Maintain ventilatory support with 100% oxygen.

4.11 Combitube®

1. Assure a patent airway and ventilate with 100% O_2 before attempting placement of the Combitube. **Do not hyperventilate the patient.**
2. Assess for contraindications:
   - Patients younger than 16 years of age and/or less than 5 feet tall.
   - Patients who are conscious or who have an intact gag reflex.
   - Patients with known esophageal disease (e.g., esophageal varices, alcoholism).
   - Patients who have ingested caustic substances.
3. Prepare the Combitube for insertion by lubricating its distal end with a water-soluble gel.
4. Maintain the patient's neck in a neutral, semi-flexed position (only if there is no chance of cervical injury).
5. Lift the tongue and mandible anteriorly with one hand. (**Caution:** When facial trauma has resulted in sharp, broken teeth or dentures, remove the teeth/dentures and exercise extreme caution when passing the Combitube into the mouth to prevent the cuff from tearing.)
6. With your other hand, hold the Combitube so that it curves in the same direction as the natural curvature of the pharynx. Insert the tip into the patient's mouth and advance it gently until the printed ring is aligned with the teeth. (**Caution: Do not force the Combitube.** If the tube does not advance easily, redirect it or withdraw and reinsert it.)
7. Inflate line 1, the blue pilot balloon leading to the pharyngeal balloon, with the recommended volume of air for the tube size. (This may cause the Combitube to move slightly from the patient's mouth.)
8. Inflate line 2, the white pilot balloon leading to the distal cuff, with the recommended volume of air for the tube size.
9. Begin ventilation through the longer blue connecting tube. If auscultation of breath sounds is positive and auscultation of gastric insufflation is negative, continue ventilation.
10. If auscultation of breath sounds is negative and gastric insufflation is positive, immediately begin ventilation through the shorter, clear connecting tube. Reconfirm tracheal ventilation by auscultation of breath sounds and absence of gastric insufflation.
11. Confirm Combitube placement with an end-tidal CO_2 monitoring device.
12. Secure the Combitube with a commercially available device.
13. Monitor SpO_2 with a pulse oximeter.
14. Provide 100% O_2 with positive-pressure oxygen or a bag-valve device.

4.12 Laryngeal Mask Airway

1. Assure a patent airway and ventilate with 100% O_2 before attempting placement of the laryngeal mask airway (LMA). **Do not hyperventilate the patient.**
2. Tightly deflate the cuff so that it forms a smooth "spoon shape." Lubricate the posterior surface of the mask with a water-soluble lubricant.
3. Hyperextend the patient's neck (unless cervical spine injury is suspected).
4. Carefully flatten the laryngeal mask tip against the hard palate.
5. Advance the mask until definite resistance is felt at the base of the hypopharynx.
6. Without holding the tube, inflate the cuff to the recommended volume of air for the tube size.
7. Confirm LMA placement with an end-tidal CO_2 monitoring device.
8. Additional confirmation methods:
   - Negative epigastric sounds.
   - Positive bilateral breath sounds.
9. Secure the LMA with a commercially available device.
10. Monitor SpO_2 with a pulse oximeter.
11. Provide 100% O_2 with positive-pressure oxygen or a bag-valve device.

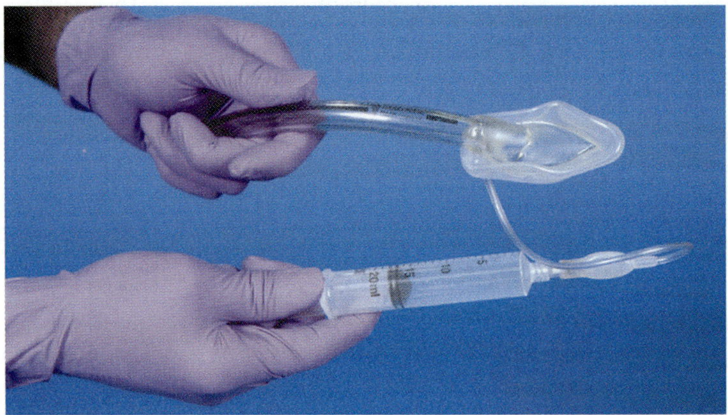

The laryngeal mask airway.

4.13 King Supraglottic Airway

1. Assure a patent airway and ventilate with 100% O_2 before attempting placement of the King airway device. **Do not hyperventilate the patient.**
2. Assemble and check the necessary equipment.
3. Lubricate the tip of the tube with a water-soluble gel.
4. Place the patient's head in a neutral position.
5. Apply the tongue/jaw-lift maneuver with one hand while passing the tube with the other hand. Insert the device at a 45- to 90-degree angle, and rotate it to midline as it passes the tongue.
6. Without exerting excessive force, advance the tube until the base of the connector gastric access lumen is aligned with the patient's teeth or gums.
7. Inflate the pharyngeal cuff with the recommended volume of air for the tube size.
8. Confirm placement of the King tube with an end-tidal CO_2 monitoring device.
9. Additional confirmation methods:
   - Negative epigastric sounds.
   - Positive bilateral breath sounds.
10. Secure the King tube with tape applied to the maxillary region of the patient's face or a commercially available device.
11. Monitor SpO_2 with a pulse oximeter.
12. Provide 100% O_2 with positive-pressure oxygen or a bag-valve device.

4.14 Chest Decompression

1. Assess the patient to make sure that his/her condition is due to a tension pneumothorax:
   - Absent or decreased breath sounds on the affected side.
   - Poor ventilation despite an open airway.
   - Tracheal deviation away from the side of the injury (may not always be present).
   - Neck vein distention (may not be present if there is associated severe hemorrhage).
   - Tympany (hyperresonance) to percussion on the affected side.
   - Shock.
   - Decreased SpO_2/end-tidal CO_2.
2. Provide the patient with high-flow oxygen and ventilatory assistance.

3a. Identify the second or third intercostal space (i.e., the space between the second and third ribs or between the third and fourth ribs) in the midclavicular line on the same side as the tension pneumothorax.

or

3b. (Alternate site) Identify the fourth or fifth intercostal space in the midaxillary line on the same side as the tension pneumothorax.

4. Quickly prepare the area with povidone-iodine.

5a. Make a one-way valve on a 14-gauge, 3- to 3½-inch IV catheter by inserting the IV catheter through the finger of a sterile glove that has been moistened with sterile water.

or

5b. Use a commercial decompression device.

6. (Optional) Attach the IV catheter to a syringe half-filled with saline to aid in visualizing air release.
7. Insert the catheter into the intercostal space.
8. Insert the catheter through the parietal pleura until air escapes. It should exit under pressure.
9. Remove the needle and/or syringe. Leave the plastic catheter in place until it is replaced by a chest tube at the hospital.
10. Monitor the patient, as the initial catheter may clog or kink, requiring reinsertion of another needle.

4.15 Needle Cricothyroidotomy for Pediatrics

1. Hyperextend the patient's neck (unless cervical spine injury is suspected).
2. Locate the cricothyroid membrane between the cricoid and thyroid cartilages by palpating the depression caudal (toward the feet) to the midline Adam's apple.
3. Clean the area well with a Betadine solution or povidone-iodine swabstick.
4. Prepare the necessary equipment:
    - 14-gauge, over-the-catheter needle
    - 10-cc syringe
    - 15-mm adaptor from 3.0 or 3.5 intubation tube
5. Insert the IV catheter through the skin and cricothyroid membrane into the trachea. Direct the needle at a 45-degree angle caudally (toward the feet). When the needle penetrates the trachea, a "pop" will be felt.
6. Aspirate with the syringe. If air is returned easily, the needle is in the trachea.
7. Withdraw the stylet while gently advancing the catheter downward into the position.
8. Attach the 15-mm adaptor to the needle hub.
9. Ventilate the patient with a bag-valve device using the 15-mm adaptor; provide high-flow oxygen.
10. Confirm placement:
    - Negative epigastric sounds.
    - Positive bilateral breath sounds.
11. Attach an end-tidal CO_2 monitoring device.
12. Monitor SpO_2 with a pulse oximeter.
13. Provide 100% O_2 with positive-pressure oxygen or a bag-valve device.
14. Monitor for changes in breathing or airway status.

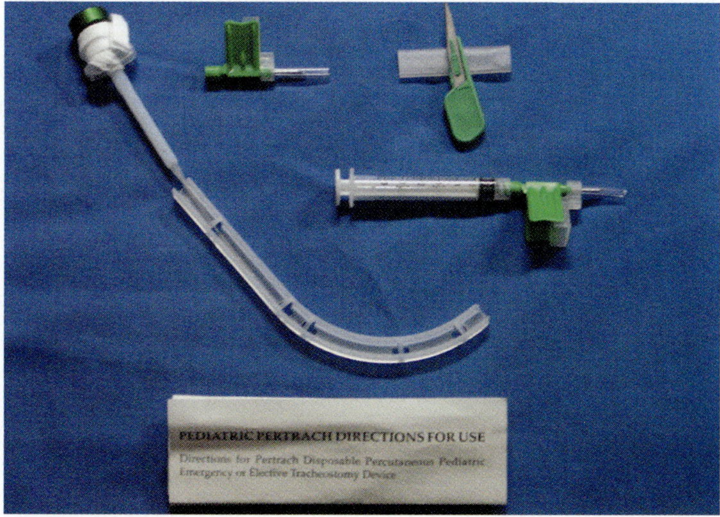

Cricothyrotomy kit.

4.16 Surgical Airway (Cricothyroidotomy)

1. If the patient <12 years of age, refer to the needle cricothyroidotomy protocol (Medical Procedure 4.15).
2. Hyperextend the patient's neck (unless cervical spine injury is suspected).
3. Locate the cricothyroid membrane between the cricoid and thyroid cartilages by palpating the depression caudal (toward the feet) to the midline Adam's apple.
4. Clean the area well with a Betadine solution or povidone-iodine swabstick.
5. Using a scalpel, make a vertical incision through the skin and then a horizontal incision through the cricothyroid membrane.
6. Once the scalpel has passed into the membrane, insert the handle into the opening and twist the handle to open a space between the cricoid and thyroid cartilages. **Do not aim the knife cephalad (toward the head), because injury to the vocal cords may occur.**

   - It is recommended to use a safety scalpel.

   or

   - A trach hook may also be used.

7. Insert a size 6.0 endotracheal tube or tracheostomy tube through the incision.
8. Inflate the cuff with the recommended amount of air.
9. Ventilate the patient with a bag-valve device using the 15-mm adaptor; provide high-flow oxygen.
10. Confirm placement:

    - Negative epigastric sounds.
    - Positive bilateral breath sounds.

11. Attach an end-tidal CO_2 monitoring device.
12. Monitor SpO_2 with a pulse oximeter.
13. Provide 100% O_2 with positive-pressure oxygen or a bag-valve device.
14. Monitor for changes in breathing or airway status.
15. If necessary, cut several 4 × 4 gauze pads down the middle to the center of the pads. Wrap the pads at the base of the tube and secure them to assist in bleeding control and/or to reduce air escape.

4.17 Nasotracheal Intubation

1. Assure the patient has a patent airway and ventilate with 100% O_2 before attempting placement of the airway device. **Do not hyperventilate the patient.**
2. Assemble and check the necessary equipment.
3. Lubricate the tip of tube with a water-soluble gel (*optional: lidocaine gel*).
4. Place the patient's head and neck in a relaxed position.
5. Inspect the patient's nose and select the larger nostril. (*Optional: Spray Neo-Synephrine into the nasopharynx.*)
6. Insert the tube (without a stylet) into the patient's nostril, with the flanged end of the tube facing the nasal septum.
7. Gently guide the tube. If you feel resistance, withdraw slightly and rotate the ETT to avoid the turbinates of the nose. Reinsert the ETT gently; **do not force it.**
8. Apply cricoid pressure and displace the mandible anteriorly.
9. Advance the ETT into the trachea during inhalation of the patient, as evidenced by the whistling Ballistic Airway Adjunct Mechanism (BAAM).
10. Hold the tube in place to prevent its dislodgement.
11. Inflate the distal cuff with 10 cc of air and remove the syringe.
12. Verify proper placement by monitoring for chest rise and breath sounds:
    - Absence of epigastric sounds.
    - CO_2 detector.
13. Secure the endotracheal tube.

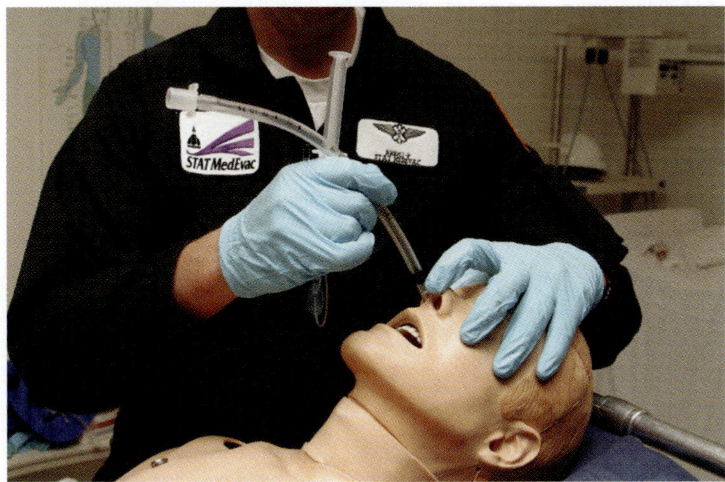

Insert the tube into the most compliant nostril.

4.18 Orotracheal Intubation by Direct Laryngoscopic Visualization

Adult

1. Assure a patent airway and ventilate with 100% O_2 before attempting placement of the airway device. **Do not hyperventilate the patient.**
2. Assemble and check the necessary equipment.
3. Hyperextend the patient's neck (unless cervical spine injury is suspected).
4.  Perform laryngoscopy in less than 30 seconds:
   - Hold the handle in your left hand.
   - Insert the blade from the right side of the patient's mouth.
   - Displace the tongue to the left.
   - Lift the laryngoscope forward to view the glottic opening.
   - Do not use the patient's teeth or lips as a fulcrum.
5. Advance the tube through the glottic opening until the proximal end of the cuff disappears past the vocal cords.
6. If the patient is having difficulty tolerating the intubation attempt, sedate with Versed 0.02 mg/kg IV.
7. Remove the stylet, inflate the cuff with 10 cc of air, and remove the syringe.
8. Hold the tube firmly in place, attach a bag-valve device, and confirm its placement.
9. Auscultate:
   - Negative epigastric sounds.
   - Positive bilateral breath sounds.
10. Attach an end-tidal CO_2 monitoring device.
11. Monitor SpO_2 with a pulse oximeter.
12. After positive confirmation of tube placement, secure it with a commercial device or tape applied to the maxillary region of the face.

Child

1. Assure a patent airway and ventilate with 100% O_2 before attempting placement of the airway device. **Do not hyperventilate the patient.**
2. Assemble and check the necessary equipment.
   - The endotracheal tube can be sized by several methods, including a weight-based tape or size of the nares or pinky finger.
3. Hyperextend the patient's neck (unless cervical spine injury is suspected).

4.18 Orotracheal Intubation by Direct Laryngoscopic Visualization

4. Perform laryngoscopy in less than 30 seconds:
   - Hold the handle in your left hand.
   - Insert the blade from the right side of the patient's mouth.
   - Displace the tongue to the left.
   - Lift the laryngoscope forward to view the glottic opening.
   - Do not use the patient's teeth or lips as a fulcrum.
5. Advance the tube through the glottic opening until the proximal end of the tube disappears past the vocal cords.
6. If the patient is having difficulty tolerating the intubation attempt, sedate with Versed 0.02 mg/kg IV.
7. Remove the stylet.
8. Hold the tube firmly in place, attach a bag-valve device, and confirm its placement.
9. Auscultate:
   - Negative epigastric sounds.
   - Positive bilateral breath sounds.
10. Attach an end-tidal CO_2 monitoring device.
11. Monitor SpO_2 with a pulse oximeter.
12. After positive confirmation of tube placement, secure it with a commercial device or tape applied to the maxillary region of the face.
13. Whenever a pediatric patient is intubated, or prolonged bag-valve mask ventilation (> 3 minutes) occurs, a nasogastric tube will be inserted. This procedure will ensure that gastric distention is relieved and maximum ventilatory support is achieved.

4.19 Nasogastric Tube Insertion

This procedure should not be performed in the presence of frontal head or midfacial trauma where the cribriform plate may be fractured.

1. Position the patient:
   - Conscious patient: upright or high Fowler's position.
   - Unconscious patient: horizontal.
2. Prepare the necessary equipment:
   - Adult: 18 French.
   - Pediatric: per the pediatric length/weight-based measurement device.
   - 60-cc syringe.
   - Water-soluble lubricant.
   - Tape.
   - Stethoscope.
3. Measure the tube by placing it over the patient's stomach region and extending it around the ear and then to the nose.
   - Mark the tube with tape.
   - Wrap the tube around two fingers and hold it for a second to remove packaging folds and form a slight curve in the tip of the tube.
4. Lubricate the end of the tube with lidocaine gel and insert into the largest nare, advancing until the tube mark from Step 3 is at the nare opening.
   - The conscious patient can assist while swallowing during insertion.
   - *Optional: Spray Neo-Synephrine into the nasopharynx.*
   - Instruct the conscious patient to flex his/her chin to the chest once the tube is past the nasal cavity. Unconscious patients require manual flexing by the inserter.
5. **Do not force the NG tube.** If resistance is felt, withdraw the tube slightly and gently reinsert it using a twisting motion.
6. Verify tube placement by auscultating epigastric sounds while inserting 20–30 cc of air.
7. Tape the tube in place and note the depth of tube on the Run Report.

4.20 Rapid Sequence Intubation

1. Evaluate the patient for the need to use paralytics.
2. Contraindications:
   - Penetrating eye injuries.
   - Renal failure (dialysis patients).
   - Patients with distorted midface/neck anatomy.
   - History of malignant hyperthermia.
   - Inability to ventilate with a bag-valve mask (BVM).
3. Prepare the necessary equipment:
   - BVM connected to a functioning O_2 delivery system.
   - Working suction with Yankauer suction tip attached.
   - Endotracheal tube(s) with stylet in place; tube shaped and lubricated, and cuff intact.
   - Laryngoscope handle with straight and curved blades.
   - Cricothyroidotomy kit.
4. Verify the patient has a functioning, secure IV line in place.
5. Ensure ECG monitoring and observe for dysrhythmia during induction.
6. Palpate the cricothyroid space and mark it with an ink pen.
7. Premedicate the patient as appropriate:
   - Versed 0.02 mg/kg via IV push, for sedation.

   or

   - Amidate (Etomidate) 20 mg (0.2 mg/kg) or 0.2–0.6 mg/kg via IV push, for sedation.
   - Atropine 0.02 mg/kg (minimum dose = 0.1 mg; maximum dose = 0.5 mg) via IV push, for pediatric patients.
   - Lidocaine 2% 1.5 mg/kg via IV push (wait 45 seconds before intubating).
8. Administer succinylcholine chloride (Anectine) 1 mg/kg via IV push.
9. Apply cricoid pressure to occlude the esophagus until intubation is successfully completed and the endotracheal tube cuff is inflated. Elevate the patient's head 15 degrees when possible.
   - After fasciculations stop (if they occur), demonstrate adequate relaxation by ventilating the patient four to five times with the BVM (hyperventilate to blow off CO_2).
   - Jaw relaxation and decreased resistance to BVM ventilation indicate that the cords are paralyzed and that it is time to proceed with intubation (approximately 45 seconds to 1 minute).

4.20 Rapid Sequence Intubation

10. Perform endotracheal intubation.
    - If unable to intubate during the first 20-second attempt, stop and ventilate with the BVM for 30–60 seconds.
    - If inadequate relaxation is present, give a second dose of succinylcholine chloride (1.0–1.5 times the initial dose). Observe for severe bronchospasm in pediatric patients.
    - If repeated intubation attempts fail, ventilate the patient via BVM until spontaneous ventilations return (usually 3–5 minutes).
11. If unable to intubate after the administration of succinylcholine chloride, ventilate the patient with a BVM. If unable to appropriately ventilate the patient with a BVM, consider performing surgical cricothyroidotomy.
12. Treat bradycardia occurring during intubation by temporarily halting intubation attempts and continue ventilation of the patient via BVM with 100% O_2. If bradycardia does not resolve with oxygenation and ventilation, administer atropine 0.5–1.0 mg via IV push.
13. Auscultate:
    - Negative epigastric sounds.
    - Positive bilateral breath sounds.
14. Attach an end-tidal CO_2 monitoring device.
15. Monitor SpO_2 with a pulse oximeter.
16. After positive confirmation of tube placement, secure the tube with a commercial device or tape applied to the maxillary region of the face.
17. Release the cricoid pressure.
18. Administer vecuronium bromide 0.1 mg/kg via IV push, for continued paralysis.
    - Repeat doses may be required generally within 25–40 minutes of the initial dose (10–40 minutes in patients without anesthesia).
    - If the patient shows symptoms of regaining consciousness, sedate the patient with a repeat dose of Versed 0.02 mg/kg.

4.21 CO Monitoring (Rad-57) Carboxyhemoglobin

1. Press the green power button to activate the unit.
2. Place the sensor on the patient's finger (observe the top and bottom of the sensor). Do not place the sensor on the thumb or fifth digit (pinky). If available, utilized the pediatric sensor as instructed by the manufacturer.
3. Four green LED lights below the power button indicate the battery level.
4. The sensor is calibrated to penetrate the mid-nail area, not the cuticle area. Do not force the patient's finger in too far.
5. RAD-57 will calibrate on the patient in 5–8 seconds.
6. Displays will come up in pulse oximeter (SpO_2) mode.
7. The PI graph will display perfusion strength.
8. The display will show "SEN OFF" until the sensor is on the finger.
9. Press the orange "SpCO" button.
10. The display will show the SpCO level from 1% to 99%.
11. Record the level(s) on the patient report.
12. Press and hold the green power button to turn the unit off.

CO Level: Signs and Symptoms

Level	Signs and Symptoms
0–4	Minor headache
5–9	Headache
10–19	Dyspnea, headache
20–29	Headache, nausea, dizziness
30–39	Severe headache, vomiting, altered LOC
40–49	Confusion, syncope, tachycardia
50–59	Seizures, shock, apnea, coma
60–Up	Coma, death

4.22 Electronic Waveform CO_2 Detection

Intubated/Supraglottic Device

1. Follow the manufacturer's recommendation for inserting the airway device.
2. Verify placement of the airway device.
3. Attach the CO_2 detection tubing to the airway device.
4. Monitor the electronic readings.

Non-Intubated Device

1. Select the appropriate size of detection tubing.
2. Place the detection tubing on the patient.
3. Attach the detection tubing to the CO_2 detection device.
4. Monitor the electronic readings.

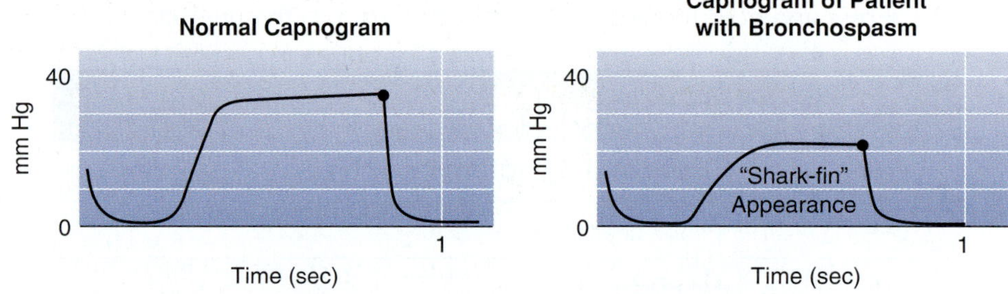

Capnography Waveform.

4.23 Color Metric End-Tidal CO_2 Detector

1. Remove the detector from the package and match the initial color of the indicator to the purple color labeled "CHECK" on the product dome.
   - The color should be the same or darker.
   - If the color is lighter, **do not use the unit.**
   - Use an appropriate CO_2 indicator based on the patient's weight.
2. After the tube is inserted, firmly attach the EASY CAP detector between the tube and the breathing device.
3. Ventilate the patient with **6 breaths** of moderate tidal volume. **Interpreting results with fewer than 6 breaths can yield false results.**
4. Compare the color of the indicator on full end-expiration to the color chart on the product dome. (The chemical indicator may become irreversibly yellow after contact with any liquid.)
   - If the color indicator is "yellow," the ETT is in the trachea.
   - If the color indicator is "tan," ventilate six more times and recheck.
   - If the color indicator is "purple," recheck ETT placement with direct laryngoscopy to confirm placement.
5. If the results are not conclusive, the tube should be immediately removed unless correct anatomic placement can be confirmed with certainty by other means.

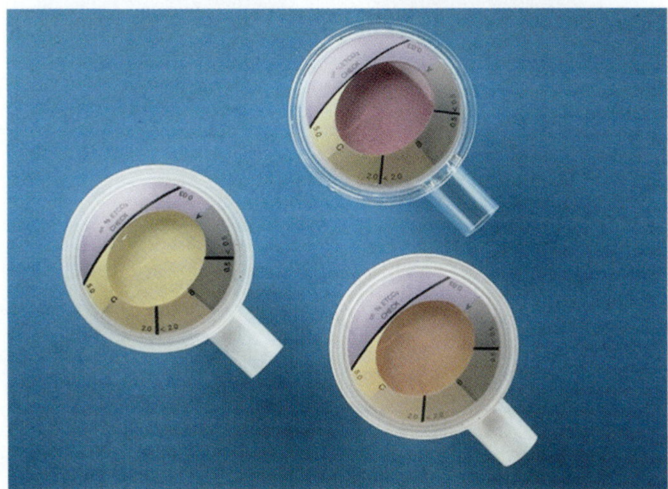

End-tidal carbon dioxide detectors.

4.24 CPAP (Whisper Flow Fixed-Flow O_2 Generator)

1. Place the patient in an upright or high Fowler's position.
2. Assess vital signs.
3. Attach a cardiac monitor, pulse oximeter, and capnography (if available).
4. Select a sealing face mask and ensure that the mask fits comfortably. The mask should form a seal with the bridge of the patient's nose and fully cover the nose and mouth.
5. Connect the generator to a 50-psi oxygen outlet.
6. Hold the mask or have the patient hold the mask to his/her face. If the patient seems anxious, it is acceptable to turn the generator "on" and have the gas flowing before placing the mask on the patient's face. When the patient is comfortable, use the head strap to hold the mask in place. Ensure it is not too tight. Some air leakage is acceptable, unless it is in the eye area.
7. Choose the appropriate PEEP valve 5–10 cm H_2O.
8. Treatment should be given continuously throughout transport.
9. Evaluate vital signs every 5 minutes.
10. In case of a life-threatening complication, stop treatment and consider the need for intubation.

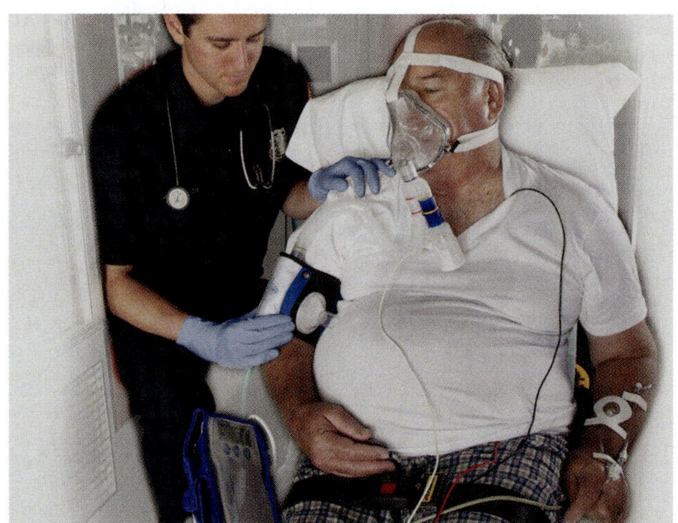

CPAP.

4.25 Esophageal Detection Device (TubeCheck)

1. Perform a leak test: Compress the bulb, apply a gloved thumb over the adapter, and release. Discard the TubeCheck device if an air leak is detected.
2. Warning:
   - Tube obstruction, morbid obesity, pulmonary edema, main stem bronchus intubation, severe bronchospastic disease, or obstructive lung disease may lead to equivocal results due to decreased air available for aspiration.
   - Use care if the unit's storage temperature is near the freezing point. The bulb will not function properly if it is frozen due to loss of self-inflating properties.
   - **Do not use** an esophageal detection device in children younger than 5 years old or weighing less than 20 kg (44 lb).
3. Insert the tube and check for proper depth.
4. Compress the bulb and attach it to the end of the tube.
5. Allow the bulb to self-inflate.
   - If air returns and fills the bulb rapidly (less than 5 seconds), the tube is likely in correct position.
   - If air slowly fills the bulb (5–30 seconds), the tube is likely positioned incorrectly.

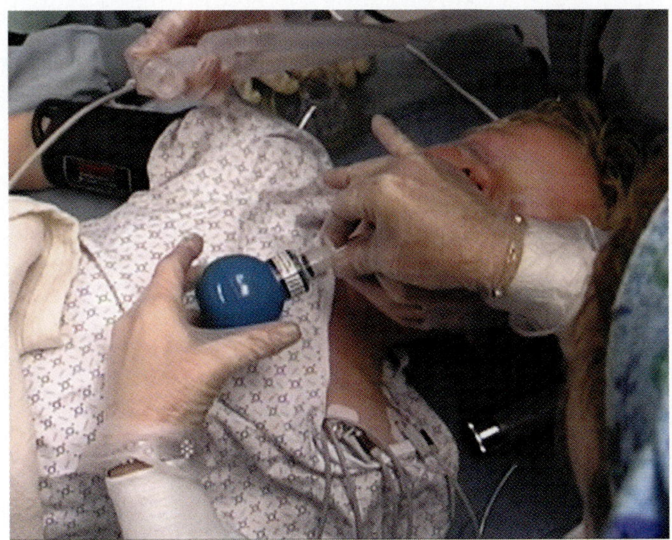

If the ET tube is in the trachea, air will freely inflate the bulb of the EDD.

4.26 Esophageal Detection Device (TubeCheck-B)

The TubeCheck-B device is used as an adjunct to assist in verifying placement of the endotracheal tube in the trachea. It does not eliminate the need for clinical judgment, however.

1. Apply a gloved finger over the adapter, compress the bulb, and release it to conduct a leak test.
   - If a leak is detected, discard the unit and obtain a new one.
2. Prior to ventilation, compress the TubeCheck-B.
3. Attach an adapter to the endotracheal tube and release.
4. Allow the bulb to self-inflate.
   - The endotracheal tube is probably in the trachea if the bulb fills with air in less than 5 seconds.
   - Intubation needs to be visually confirmed if tube fills slowly (5–30 seconds).
   - The endotracheal tube is probably in the esophagus if the bulb does not fill with air or if vomitus returns.
5. If proper endotracheal tube placement cannot be confirmed, reintubate the patient or continue ventilation with a bridge device.

4.27 Nebulizer

1. Prepare the equipment for appropriate application:
    - Mask application: mask, mist chamber, oxygen supply tubing, and cylinder.
    - Self-administration application: mouthpiece, mist chamber, oxygen supply tubing, and cylinder.
2. Add medication to the nebulizer mist chamber. Make sure the nebulizer mist chamber cap is tightly secured.
3. Gently swirl the nebulizer to mix the contents.
4. Attach the mouthpiece or mask.
5. Connect the nebulizer to the oxygen tubing and oxygen cylinder.
6. Set the flow:
    - Adult: 6–8 L/min
    - Pediatric: 3 L/min
7. The patient should breathe as calmly, deeply, and evenly as possible until no more mist is formed in the nebulizer chamber (5–15 minutes).

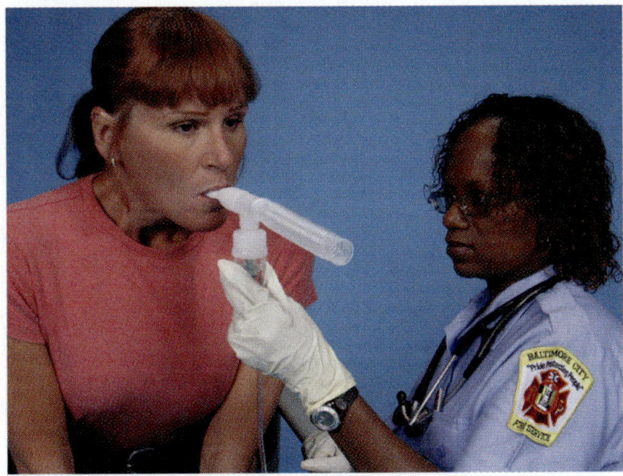

Nebulizer treatment.

4.28 Nitrous Oxide—Nitronox

1. Prepare the equipment. Nitronox units consist of a nitrous oxide cylinder, a blending regulator, an oxygen cylinder, and a mask.
2. Contraindications: altered state of consciousness, COPD, acute pulmonary edema, pneumothorax, decompression sickness, air embolus, pregnancy (except during delivery), abdominal pain with distention or suspicion of obstruction, and inability to self-administer the medication.
3. Turn the oxygen and nitrous oxide cylinder valves to the "on" position. Make sure the device shows appropriate blending of the gases.
4. Attach a mask to the Nitronox unit regulator and provide it to the patient for self-administration. **The patient must be able to self-administer the medication; if he/she cannot, Nitronox cannot be used.**
5. Monitor the patient's vital signs and pulse oximeter. If the patient's vital signs become unstable or the patient becomes symptomatic from the side effects, discontinue Nitronox.

4.29 Pulse Oximeter

Pulse oximeters are used for the detection of hypoxemia in arterial oxyhemoglobin. Peripheral oxygen is obtained by placing a sensor probe on the peripheral capillary bed.

1. Attach the appropriate sensor to the patient's finger or toe. Remove any nail polish.
2. Turn on the pulse oximeter unit.
3. Evaluate the results:
   - Normal range: oxygen saturation of 92–100%
   - Mild distress: oxygen saturation of 90–92%
   - Moderate distress: oxygen saturation of 80–89%
   - Severe distress: oxygen saturation of less than 80%
4. Oxygenate the patient with the appropriate delivery device based on the reading and the patient's condition.
5. Evaluate the patient for possibly false **high** readings:
   - **Carbon monoxide poisoning:** Elevated carboxyhemoglobin can falsely elevate saturation readings because carboxyhemoglobin modulates light similar to oxyhemoglobin as it passes through the tissue.
   - **Trauma:** Despite a normal saturation level, severe hemorrhage can cause the patient to not have enough blood to perfuse the organs, so that the patient is hypoxic.
6. Evaluate the patient for possibly false **low** readings:
   - **Deeply pigmented patients:** may diminish light transmission.
   - **Nail polish or fake nails:** may diminish light transmission.
   - **Patient movement:** may cause the pulse oximeter to not register.
   - **Low blood flow states:** may cause the pulse oximeter to not register.
7. Continuously monitor and document readings.

4.30 External Pacemaker

Several different external pacers are available. While their control panels may look different, all of them have several features in common.

1. Turn on the device.
2. Attach an ECG monitor and therapy electrodes and cables.
   - Place electrodes over the heart on the anterior and posterior locations.

   or

   - Place one electrode in the upper right torso (lateral to the sternum and below the clavicle). Place the other electrode in the left upper midaxillary area (lateral to patient's left nipple).
3. Evaluate the patient:
   - Medication patches: Remove the patches.
   - Patient located on wet surface: Relocate the patient to a dry area.
   - Patient with fluid on chest or back area: Dry with a towel.
4. **Record a strip of the patient's rhythm prior to initiating pacing.**
5. Consider sedation for conscious patients.
6. Set the unit to pacer mode.
7. Set the heart rate at 70 or 80 beats per minute.
8. Increase the energy setting until electrical capture is achieved (evidenced by a pacer spike followed by a wide QRS complex).

4.30 External Pacemaker

9. Evaluate pacing effectiveness and perform one of the following options:

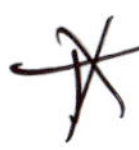

- Electrical capture is achieved: Check pulse and blood pressure (right carotid, right femoral, or either brachial pulse due to muscle twitching).

or

- Electrical capture is achieved but no pulse: Treat with the PEA protocol.

or

- No electrical capture: Increase pacer to maximum energy setting and recheck all settings, cables, battery charge, electrode placement, and patient's own rhythm.

10. ECG rhythm strips should be recorded and retained for documentation.
11. Continue all other supportive measures. (There is no risk of electrical shock from touching the patient or from performing other procedures during pacing.)

4.31 Auto-Pulse

A load-distributing band device is designed to deliver consistent uninterrupted chest compressions during cardiac arrest.

1. Initiate CPR.
2. Maintain high-quality compressions.
3. Power up the Auto-Pulse by pressing the ON/OFF button at the top of the device.
4. Remove the clothing on the patient's torso:

    - Sit the patient up and perform a single cut down the back of the patient's clothing. Then slide the Auto-Pulse platform into position behind the sitting patient, and have the patient lie down on the platform.

    or

    - Log-roll the patient to one side and perform a single cut down the back of the patient's clothing. Then log-roll the patient onto the Auto-Pulse platform.

5. Align the patient on the platform. The patient's armpit should be positioned on the "yellow" indicator line on the Auto-Pulse platform.
6. Close the LifeBand over the patient's chest.

    - Therapy electrodes or defibrillation pads should be in place before applying the LifeBand.
    - Make sure the LifeBand is not twisted.
    - The LifeBand is secure when the mating slot is placed over the alignment tab and the bands are pressed together to engage the Velcro.
    - Center the LifeBand on the patient's chest.

7. Begin compressions by pressing the green Start/Continue button once. The Auto-Pulse device will automatically adjust the bands on the chest.
8. The Auto-Pulse unit will pause for 3 seconds to allow for a check of proper alignment.

    - If patient is not aligned correctly, push the orange Stop/Cancel button.
    - Realign the LifeBand and press the green Start/Continue button.

9. Select the desired mode of compressions by pushing the gray Menu/Mode button.

    - 30:2 mode: 30 compressions and a pause for 2 ventilations.

    or

    - Continuous mode: uninterrupted compressions.

4.31 Auto-Pulse

10. Complete the process of securing the patient for transport.
    - Clip the straps for the shoulder restraint to the Auto-Pulse platform and tighten them.
    - Secure the patient's head to the Auto-Pulse platform with the manufacturer's head immobilizer or tape applied across the patient's forehead.
11. After successful resuscitation or termination of activities, press the orange Stop/Cancel button.

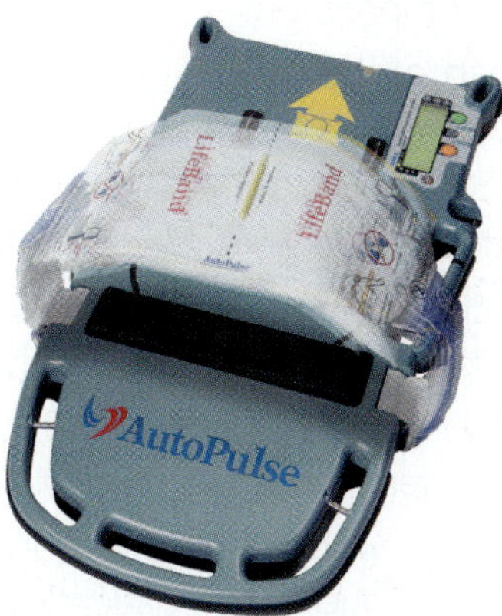

The AutoPulse non-invasive cardiac support pump.

4.32 Lucas Chest Compression System

1. Initiate CPR.
2. Maintain high-quality compressions.
3. Open the LUCAS carrying bag to expose the unit.
4. Make certain the On/Off knob is in the "adjust" position.
5. Connect the high-pressure air line to the regulator on the air source.
6. Take the back plate out of the bag. With one rescuer on each side of patient, grab the patient's arm to lift the upper body. One person should lift the patient and support the head, and the other person should lift the patient and slide the back plate below the armpits.
7. Continue manual compressions.
8. Take the upper part of the LUCAS unit out of the bag. Hold the LUCAS device by the handles on the support legs and make sure the support legs have reached their outer position.
9. Pull up once on the release rings to check that the claw locks are open.
10. Interrupt manual chest compressions and place the upper part of the LUCAS unit over the patient's chest. The claw locks at the end of each support leg should be aligned with the back plate to lock the components together.
11. Check by pulling upward that both support legs are locked into the back plate.
12. Lower the suction cup with the height adjustment handles until the pressure pad inside the suction cup touches the patient's chest without compressing the chest.
13. Turn the ON/OFF knob to activate the chest compressions.
14. Attach the neck pad by raising the patient's head slightly. Clip the pad into each buckle attached to the support arms. Pull the excess slack out of each strap by pulling gently and simultaneously until the pad positions itself into place.
15. Attach the wrist straps to each of the patient's wrists to assist with securing the arms during movement/transportation. Use caution to determine that the intravenous site is not compromised due to a slight bend that will occur in the patient's arm. If this does occur, release the arm and secure the unit by other means.
16. After successful resuscitation or termination of activities, turn the ON/OFF knob to the "Off" position.

4.33 12-Lead ECG Application

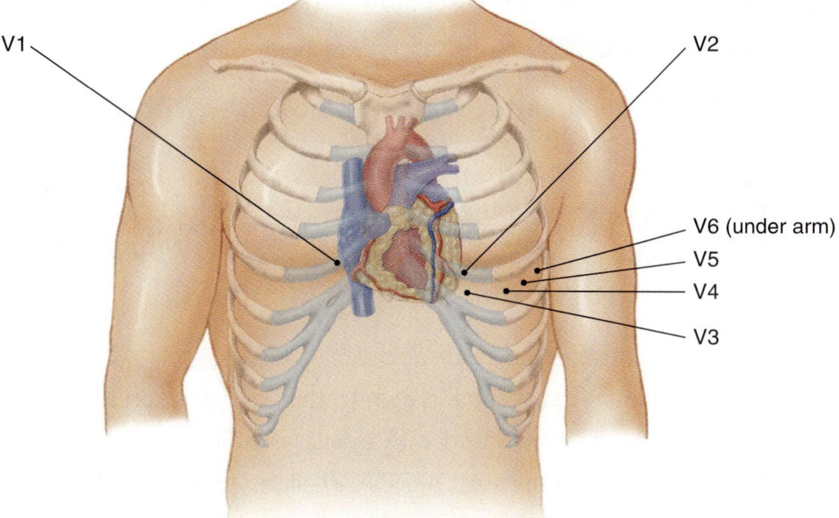

12-Lead ECG Electrode Placement.

1. RA: right arm, upper arm, or upper chest near the shoulder.
2. LA: left arm, upper arm, or upper chest near the shoulder.
3. RL: right leg or lower abdominal quadrant near the hip.
4. LL: upper leg or lower abdominal quadrant near the hip.
5. V1: fourth intercostal space, immediately to the right of the sternum.
6. V2: fourth intercostal space, immediately to the left of the sternum.
7. V4: fifth intercostal space in the midclavicular line. (***Note:*** V4 must be placed prior to V3.)
8. V3: placed between V2 and V4.
9. V5: fifth intercostal space in the anterior axillary line.
10. V6: fifth intercostal space in the midaxillary line.

4.34 ResQPOD® Circulatory Enhancer

The ResQPOD Circulatory Enhancer is a device for enhancing blood circulation in patients who require cardiopulmonary resuscitation.

1. Attach the ResQPOD Circulatory Enhancer:
   - Secure the unit directly to the face mask with a strap or with two-handed mask seal.

   or

   - Secure the unit directly to the airway tube. (If an electronic CO_2 monitoring device is used, place that device's tubing *after* the ResQPOD Circulatory Enhancer is placed.)
2. Attach a positive-pressure device with 100% oxygen.
3. Slide the "timing assist light" switch to the "on" position.
4. Administer ventilation timed with the flashing light.
5. Discontinue use of the ResQPOD Circulatory Enhancer when there is a return of spontaneous circulation.

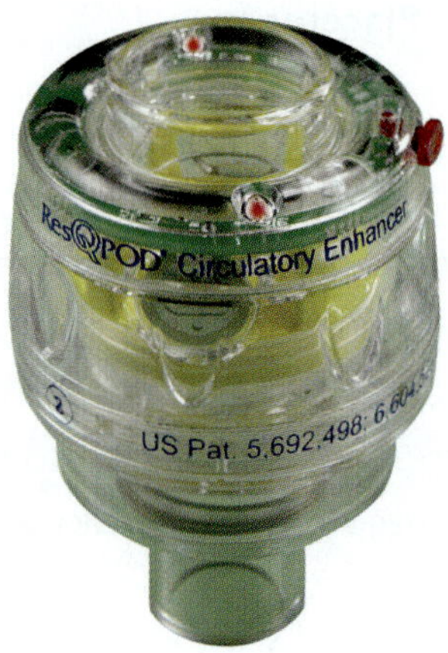

ResQPOD.

4.35 Vagal Maneuvers

The degree of stimulation of the vagus nerve affects the heart rate. The greater the degree of vagal stimulation, the more the vagus nerve will slow the heart rate, thereby inhibiting the SA node.

4.35.1 Ice Water Immersion of the Face (Vagal Maneuvers)

1. Attach the patient to an ECG for continuous monitoring.
2. Establish intravenous access.
3. Determine that patient is conscious and cooperative.
4. Note that this procedure is contraindicated for patients with history of acute coronary syndrome, hypertension, and heart transplant.
5. Document the ECG and any dysrhythmia.
6. Describe the procedure to the patient.
   - Fill a large basin or sink with ice water. It must be **very** cold.
   - Ask the patient to hold his/her breath and put the entire face into the water for several seconds.

   or

   - Fill a large latex exam glove with ice water.
   - Place the glove on the patient's face for several seconds.
7. Continue to monitor the heart rhythm during the procedure. Stop the procedure if:
   - The patient becomes confused.
   - The heart rate drops below 100 BPM.
   - Asystole occurs.

4.35.2 Valsalva Maneuver (Vagal Maneuvers)

1. Attach the patient to an ECG for continuous monitoring.
2. Establish intravenous access.
3. Determine that the patient is conscious and cooperative.
4. Document the ECG and any dysrhythmia.
5. Describe the procedure to the patient.

    - Have the patient inhale and hold his/her breath.
    - Bear down as if to have a bowel movement.
    - Hold for 20–30 seconds.
    - Try to turn the face red.

    or

    - Have the patient blow forcefully through a straw or IV catheter for as long as possible.

6. Continue to monitor the heart rhythm during the procedure. Stop the procedure if:

    - The patient becomes confused.
    - The heart rate drops below 100 BPM.
    - Asystole occurs.

4.36 Cyanokit (Hydroxycarbolomin for Injection)

This kit is for intravenous use. The hydroxycarbolomin is to be reconstituted with 100 mL per vial of 0.9% sodium chloride injection. The starting dose is 5 g (two vials).

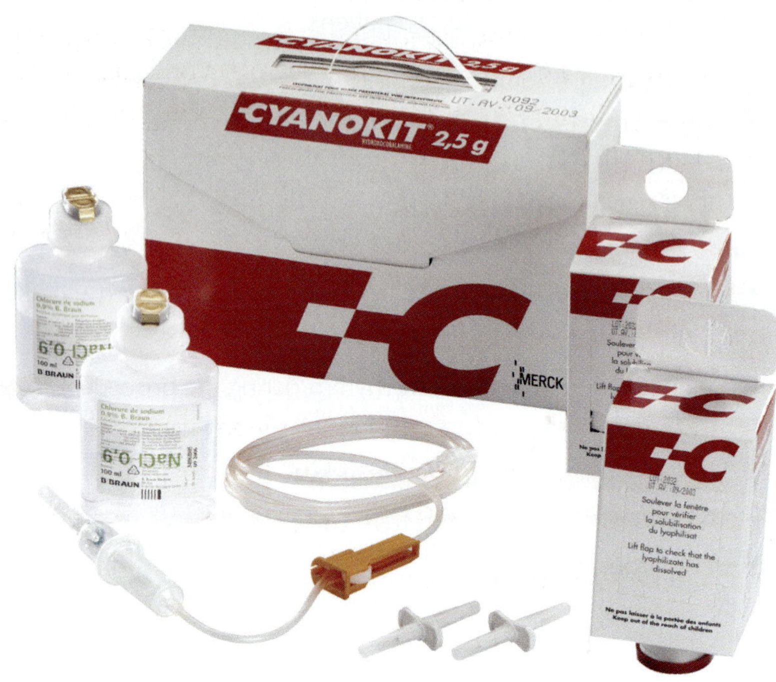

Cyanokit Administration Set-Up.

1. **Reconstitution:** Add 100 mL of 0.9% sodium chloride injection to the vial using a transfer spike. **Fill to the line (with the vial in an upright position).**
2. **Mix:** Rock or rotate the vial for 30 seconds to mix the solution. Do not shake.
3. **Infuse the first vial:** Use vented IV tubing to hang the bag and infuse over 7.5 minutes.
4. **Infuse the second vial:** Repeat Steps 1 and 2 before the second infusion. Use vented IV tubing to hang the bag and infuse over 7.5 minutes.

See Drug Summary 5.25, Hydroxycarbolomin.

4.37 Blood Alcohol Sampling

Drawing a blood alcohol sample **should not delay treatment or transport** of the critical patient.

1. The EMS Run Report should contain the following information:
   - A blood alcohol kit was used.
   - A Betadine (povidone-iodine) solution (or hydrogen peroxide/acetone if the patient is allergic to iodine) was used for the skin preparation.
   - Name of the law enforcement officer requesting blood sample.
   - Time of draw.
   - If the paramedic drawing sample is different from the one signing the report, that paramedic will sign under the above information.
2. All blood samples taken must be surrendered to the requesting law enforcement officer.
3. The paramedic:
   - May be required to obtain multiple samples.
   - **Must follow all blood sampling kit guidelines.**
   - Must obtain blood alcohol samples only at the request of a law enforcement officer, either in the field or upon arrival in the emergency department.

4.38 Fibrinolytic Screening

The intent of fibrinolytic screening is to determine whether the prehospital patient can or cannot receive fibrinolytics. The screening procedure includes assessing the criteria for both indications and contraindications to fibrinolytic therapy.

A fibrinolytic screening checklist should be completed on all patients who meet the criteria for fibrinolytic therapy. The checklist should include the indications and contraindications as specified above as a minimum data set. A copy of the fibrinolytic screening checklist should be attached to the EMS Run Report.

Indications for Fibrinolytic Therapy

1. Diagnosis of probable acute myocardial infarction.
   - There is a minimum of 2 mm of ST elevation in two or more related precordial leads or 1 mm of ST elevation in two or more limb leads on the 12-lead ECG, with a history suggestive of AMI.
2. Diagnosis of probable stroke or "brain attack."
   - Patients exhibit signs consistent with stroke/CVA/"brain attack" (e.g., altered mental status, slurred speech, loss of function of any body part, hemiplegia, loss of vision, weakness of facial muscles, loss of sensation, drooling). Other causes should be ruled out (e.g., hypoglycemia, drug overdose, hypoxia).
   - In "brain attack" patients, hemorrhagic causes of stroke (e.g., emergency CT scan) must be ruled out prior to administration of thrombolytics.

Contraindications to Fibrinolytic Therapy

1. Active or known bleeding problems.
   - Hemophilia.
   - Active ulcer (with or without signs of bleeding).
   - GI/GU bleeding. Signs and symptoms may include hematemesis, hemoptysis, melena, hematuria, bleeding from mouth/nose or rectum, and a rigid and/or tender abdomen.
   - Pregnancy or menses.
   - Other external signs of bleeding.
2. Recent trauma (within 2 weeks).
   - CPR.
   - Trauma.
   - Major surgery.
   - Organ biopsy.

4.38 Fibrinolytic Screening

3. CNS abnormalities.
    - Intracranial or intraspinal surgery or trauma within 2 months.
    - Brain tumor.
    - History of CVA or TIA. CT scan must confirm absence of hemorrhage.
4. Vascular deficiencies.
    - History of arteriovenous malformations.
    - History of aneurysm.
    - Suspected aortic aneurysm or dissection.
5. Severe uncontrolled hypertension (220/110 mm Hg).
6. Diabetic eye problems and/or other hemorrhagic ophthalmic condition.
7. Disoriented and/or uncooperative patient, which causes information to be unreliable.
    - May be eliminated if a relative can confirm the answers to the paramedic's questions.
8. Previous administration of or allergy to streptokinase.

4.39 Glucometer

The glucometer is designed to be used to test capillary blood for the level of glucose. Several types of glucometers are available. The paramedic should refer to the user's manual for his/her specific type for further information.

1. Select a sample site on the patient's finger and clean the area with an alcohol swab. Allow the alcohol to dry before sticking the finger for a sample.
2. Tear off a single test strip packet. Note the expiration date on the packet. Open the packet and fold back the foil ends to expose the **meter end** of the test strip.
3. Hold the test end of the test strip **between the foil.** Insert the test strip fully into the test slot located on the side of the meter; continue the insertion until a confirmation tone is heard.
4. Stick the patient's finger with a lancing device and press the finger to form a small drop of blood. If blood does not readily form on the surface of the patient's skin, have the patient lower his/her hand below the level of the heart to aid in this process.
5. Apply the drop of blood to the test strip.
6. Dispose of the sharp in a biohazard puncture-resistant container.
7. Following a brief delay, the blood glucose result appears in the display.
8. Remove and dispose of the test strip in biohazard garbage bag.

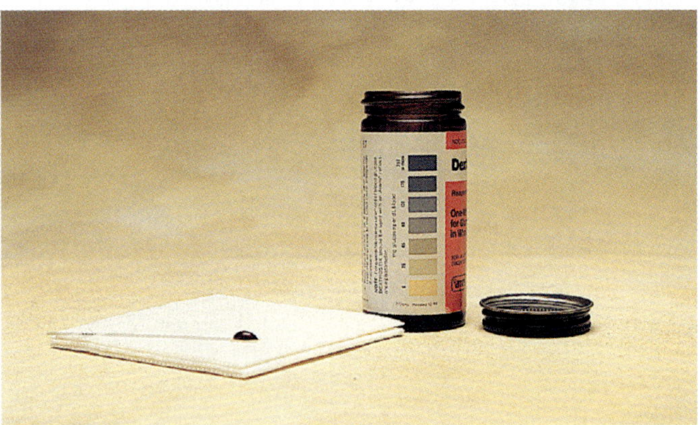

Glucose test strips for blood analysis.

4.40 Pediatric Weight-Based Emergency Tape: Broselow

The pediatric weight-based emergency tape is designed to be used as a quick reference for drug dosages and equipment sizing for pediatric patients. The tape is calibrated in different colors according to different lengths. The color that corresponds to the patient's length is used. If the pediatric weight-based emergency tape bag is also used, the color on the tape can be matched with the color on the pouch that contains the appropriately sized equipment and drugs.

1. Place the patient in a supine position.
2. Remove the tape from the package and unfold it.
3. Place the tape next to the patient, ensuring that the multicolored side faces up.
4. Place the red end of the tape even with the top of the patient's head.
5. Place the edge of one hand on the red end of the tape.
6. Starting from the patient's head, run the edge of your free hand down the tape.
7. Stop your hand even with the heel of the patient's foot. If the patient is larger than the tape, stop here and use the appropriate adult technique.
8. Verbalize the color block (on the edge of the tape) and weight range where your free hand has stopped. If the patient falls on the line, go to the next higher section.
9. Use the color block (on the edge of the tape) to identify the weight range of the patient.
10. Use the weight range to determine appropriate sizes of equipment and approximate dosages for medications.

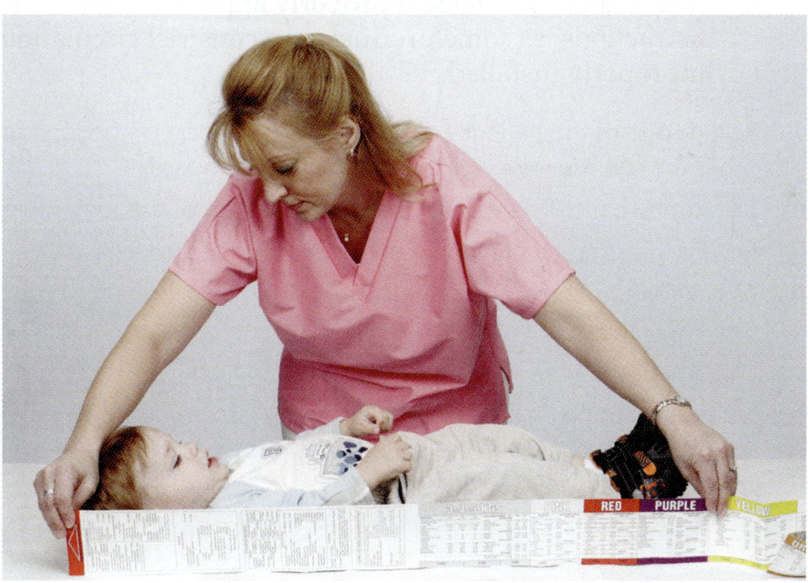

Pediatric weight-based tape.

4.41 Physical Restraints

A **restraint** is defined as any mechanism that physically restricts a person's freedom of movement, physical activity, or normal access to his/her body.

Restraints should be used only as a last resort because they have the potential to produce serious consequences, such as physical and psychological harm, loss of dignity, violation of the individual's rights, and even death. Justification for the restraints must be noted in the EMS Run Report.

Restraints should be used only when attempts at pharmacological, verbal, and family intervention have been deemed ineffective and when the patient is:

- Attempting to inflict intentional harm on self or others.
- Attempting to inflict bodily harm on EMS personnel.

Only a commercial soft restraint system should be used.

1. The patient should be placed supine on a long spine board (or backboard). **Never place a patient in the prone position.**
    - Use of a long spine board provides the flexibility to easily move the patient should he/she vomit.
    - It also provides a safe means of transfer from the stretcher to the bed.
2. Wrap the cuff pad around each limb.
    - Do not cinch the strap tight. You should be able to insert one finger between the limb and the device.
    - Ensure that the device is properly applied per the manufacturer's instructions, as some products can constrict circulation when improperly installed.
3. Secure one of the patient's arms on the upper part of the long spine board and the other arm on the lower part of the long spine board.
4. Secure the patient's ankles to the lower portion of the long spine board.
5. Secure the strap to the long spine board with a quick-release tie.
6. Check for and correct any circulatory, respiratory, or neurological compromise caused by the restraint.
7. Document the time when the restraint is applied.
8. Utilize the strapping mechanisms of the long spine board to provide additional security and support for the patient with moving.

4.41 Physical Restraints

9. Continuously monitor the patient for the following issues:
   - Tightening of the strap around the limb.
   - Changes in mental status.
   - Changes in vital signs.
   - Changes in pulse oximetry.
   - ECG changes.
   - Changes in respiratory effort (positional asphyxia).
   - Vomiting.
   - Signs of circulatory and/or neurological compromise at the site of the restraint.
10. Immediately address any changes in patient status.
11. Document the duration of the restraint.

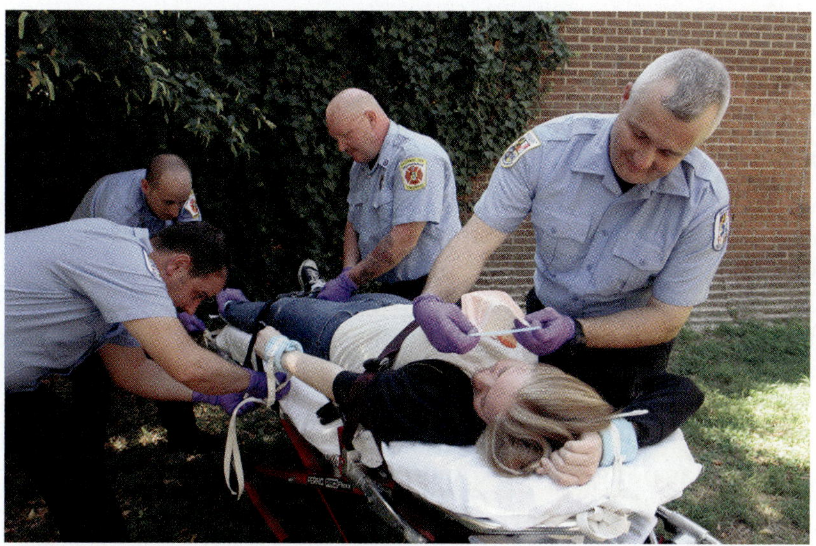

Continuously monitor the restrained patient.

4.42 The Autistic Patient

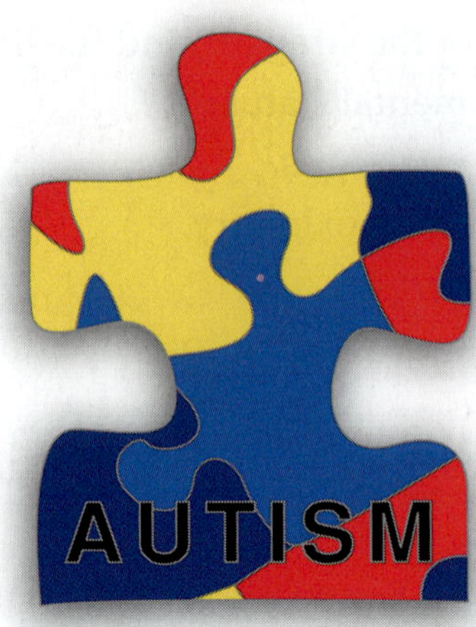

This protocol is intended to assist emergency personnel in dealing with the special challenges that they face when encountering an autistic patient.

Signs of Autism

Many parents are in denial or do not realize the possibility that their child is autistic. It is for this reason that careful consideration should be made before inquiring whether a child is autistic. Doing so may prompt the parent to "shut down" or become defensive, which could hamper the process of acquiring patient information. Signs of autism that the emergency care provider may recognize include these:

- Has not "babbled" or "cooed" by the age of 1 year.
- Has not gestured, pointed, or waved by 1 year.
- Has not spoken a single word by 16 months.
- Has not spoken a two-word phrase by 2 years.

4.42 The Autistic Patient

Special Considerations

When dealing with an autistic patient, special accommodations must be made during the encounter to achieve a positive outcome. Conditions that may affect the encounter include these:

- Autistic patients may respond aggressively to an unwanted touch.
- Autistic patients may appear to have a hearing impairment.
  - This may affect your assessment of the patient's level of consciousness and the Glasgow Coma Scale score.
  - It may also prevent the patient from coming to you if called, such as in motor vehicle accidents, fires, and evacuations (a).
- During stressful times, autistic persons may "bolt" or run away from the situation even if they are hurt. These patients will not respond to someone calling their name to stop! This behavior may result in the person running into traffic or other hazardous areas (b).
- Autistic patients cannot tell or describe what is hurt or what they want (c).
- Autistic patients will likely not follow any directions. This will present a great challenge during the patient assessment (c).
- Autistic children do not play with toys appropriately.
- Autistic patients have poor eye contact, which may affect the evaluation of pupils.
  - The autistic patient usually directs his/her eyes up, down, or away. This factor should be considered when head injuries are suspected.
- Autistic patients appear to be in their own world. This could pose a concern if a patient is in danger and is not aware of it (d).
- Autistic patients have odd movement patterns.
  - These movements may include hand flapping, hand washing motions, spinning motions, head slapping, and covering of the ears or eyes.
- Autistic patients exhibit an unusual attachment to toys or other objects.
  - To gain the trust of an autistic patient, provide him/her with a favorite object, which may not necessarily be a toy. Ask the parent/caregiver to assist you.
- Autistic patients often demonstrate repetitive behaviors.
  - Autistic persons feel compelled to complete certain tasks, such as lining up their toys.
  - Before allowing an intrusion, such as emergency workers examining them, autistic patients may feel compelled to complete a certain task such as lining up toys, opening a door, or going through a certain routine.

4.42 The Autistic Patient

- Autistic patients do not adjust well to a change in their surroundings or routines.
  - These patients are usually set in a certain routine and are extremely comfortable in their known surroundings. Any changes could result in an aggressive response.
- Autistic patients may walk on "tippy toes."
- Autistic patients may have an increased level of pain tolerance.
  - This may be a major consideration during the physical exam. A thorough physical exam is required, especially with suspected abdominal pain, fractures/sprains, and head/neck injuries.
- Autistic patients have an extreme sensitivity to touches and textures (i.e., smooth, rough, sticky, hot/cold, wet/dry).
  - Consideration should be given to this factor when applying dressings and bandages. The simplest of procedures, such as applying a Band-Aid or irrigating a wound, could result in a "meltdown."
- Autistic patients are extremely sensitive to having things on their heads or around their necks.
  - This factor should be considered when applying dressings to head injuries, as well as when utilizing a sling to secure an extremity.

"Meltdowns" and "Refocus" Periods

Children with autism can have frequent "meltdowns" (tantrums) due to any one of the factors mentioned in the "Special Considerations" section of this protocol. These meltdowns may also occur for no apparent reason and may result in aggressive behavior.

After a meltdown, autistic children will likely go through what is known as a "refocus" period. They will suddenly become quiet; they may crouch down and cover their ears or eyes. Typically they will look for a quiet, darkened, "sheltered" area. During this period, patients are trying to "refocus" their world; this is *their* time. The refocus period can last a few minutes to possibly 30 minutes or longer. If there is an attempt to rush this period, another meltdown may occur, to be followed by another refocus period; this process could become a vicious cycle.

4.42 The Autistic Patient

If you encounter a parent/caregiver who is aware of the autism, ask him/her for advice on how to handle the patient. Parents of autistic children are usually very actively involved with their children and understand their "quirks." Their help should enhance your treatment and be a major factor in lessening the stress level in an already stressful situation.

NOTE

(a) Clues that may indicate that you are dealing with an autistic patient may include car magnet "puzzle piece" ribbons on vehicles involved in motor vehicle accidents as well as window stickers on homes indicating the presence of a special needs person.

(b) Autistic patients are not aware of any present dangers. To safely secure the patient, reduce the risk of danger before encountering the patient.

(c) Ask the parent/caregiver to assist you during your interview.

(d) If possible, ask the parent/caregiver to assist with "refocusing" the patient. If such a person is not available, try clapping your hands to get the patient's attention if the situation is urgent. Be aware of a possibly aggressive response to an unwanted touch.

4.43 Eye Washing for Chemical and Small Foreign Body

1. Remove the patient from the contaminated area.
2. Attempt to identify the chemical and notify the receiving facility.
3. Remove the patient's clothing (if necessary) and decontaminate with copious amounts of water.
4. Remove contact lenses (if present) to ensure that chemicals are not trapped under the lenses.
5. To ensure adequate rinsing behind the eyelid, hold the lid with your thumb and index finger, as it is normal for the eye to close when splashed.
6. Flush the eye away from the nose to avoid contamination of the other eye for a minimum of 20 minutes. **Do not delay transport to complete the irrigation process.**
7. Use any of these methods:
    - Flush using a faucet spray from a sink or shower.
    - Flush using a bottle of normal saline or sterile water.
    - Flush using a basin filled with water.
    - Flush using nasal cannula tubing.

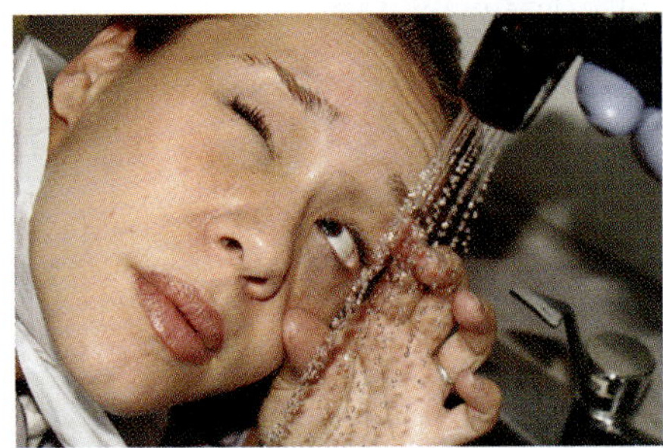

A. Sink or shower.

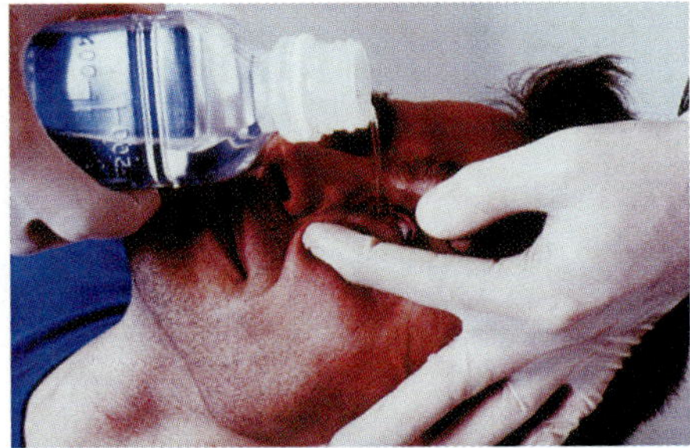

B. Bottle.

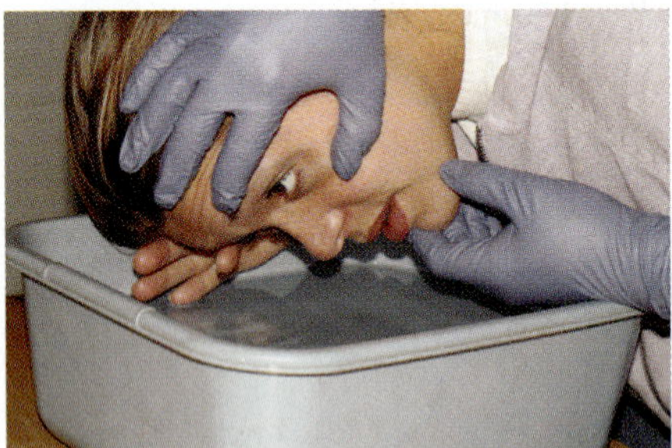

C. Basin.

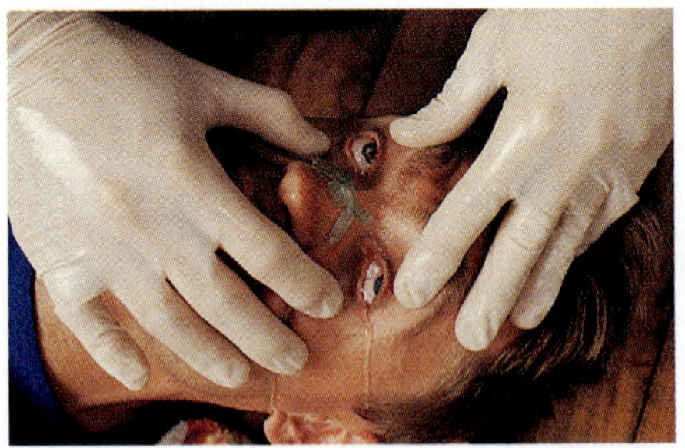

D. Nasal Cannula.

4.44 Football Helmet Face Mask Removal

1. Apply manual in-line stabilization.
2. Employ any of these face mask removal methods:

   - Use a cordless screwdriver to remove the screws attaching the face mask to the helmet.

   or

   - Use a face mask extractor or other cutting device to cut the face mask straps.

3. Secure the patient to a long spine board.
4. Perform cervical immobilization.

   - Apply towel rolls on each side of the helmet and tape the helmet to the long spine board.

   or

   - Use a commercial cervical immobilization device.

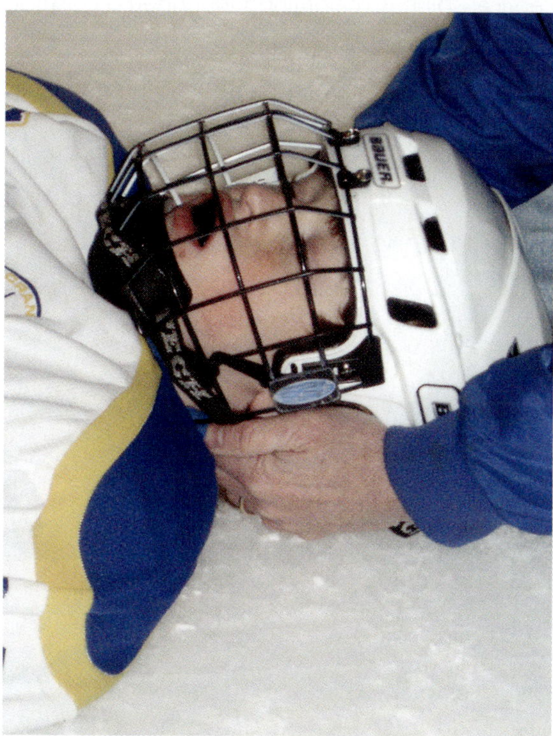

Apply manual in-line stabilization.

4.44.1 Football Helmet Removal

1. Apply manual in-line stabilization.
2. Consider completely removing the helmet in the following circumstances:
   - The face mask cannot be removed after a reasonable period of time to access the patient's airway.
   - The helmet chin strap does not hold the patient's head securely.
   - The helmet prevents immobilization during transport.
3. Cut or disconnect the chin straps.
4. Transfer manual in-line stabilization to the second rescuer by placing one hand on the patient's mandible (thumb on one side and fingers on the other side) and the other hand under the patient's head at the occipital area.
5. Laterally move the helmet to clear the patient's ears.
6. Tilt the helmet backward to raise it over the patient's nose and remove it.
7. Apply a cervical collar.
8. If the patient has a chest pad on, it is important to apply padding under the head so the cervical spine is maintained in a neutral position on the spinal board.
9. Secure the patient to a long spine board.
10. Perform cervical immobilization with a commercial cervical immobilization device.

4.44.2 Full Face Mask Helmet Removal

1. Apply manual in-line stabilization by placing your hands on each side of the helmet, with your fingers on the patient's mandible.
2. Cut or disconnect the chin straps.
3. Transfer manual in-line stabilization to the second rescuer by placing one hand on the patient's mandible (thumb on one side and fingers on the other side) and the other hand under the patient's head at the occipital area.
4. Inspect the patient for glasses; remove them, if present.
5. Laterally move the helmet to clear the patient's ears.
6. Tilt the helmet backward to raise over the patient's nose and remove it.
7. Apply a cervical collar.
8. Secure the patient to a long spine board.

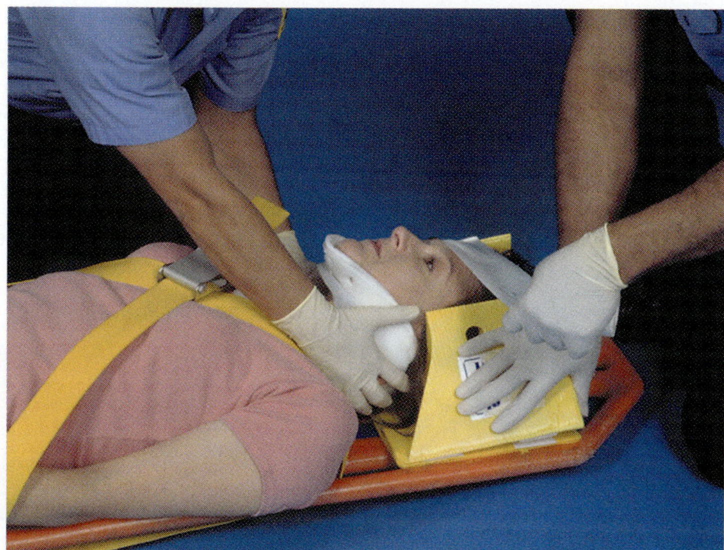

Apply a cervical collar and secure the patient to a long spine board.

4.45 Morgan Lens

1. Remove the patient's contact lenses, if present.
2. Instill topical local anesthetic (tetracaine HCl 0.5% eye drops) to the affected eye(s).
3. Attach the Morgan lens to IV tubing or Morgan lens delivery set.
4. Prime the tubing and lens with irrigation solution.
5. Have the patient look down; insert the Morgan lens under the upper lid.
6. Have the patient look up; retract the lower lid to drop the lens in place.
7. Release the lower lid over the lens.
8. Adjust the flow to the desired rate.
9. Tape the tubing to the patient's forehead to prevent accidental lens removal.
10. Absorb any outflow with towels.

Removal of a Morgan Lens

1. Have the patient look up; retract the lower lid behind the interior border of the lens.
2. Hold this position.
3. Have the patient look down; retract the upper lid and slide the lens out.

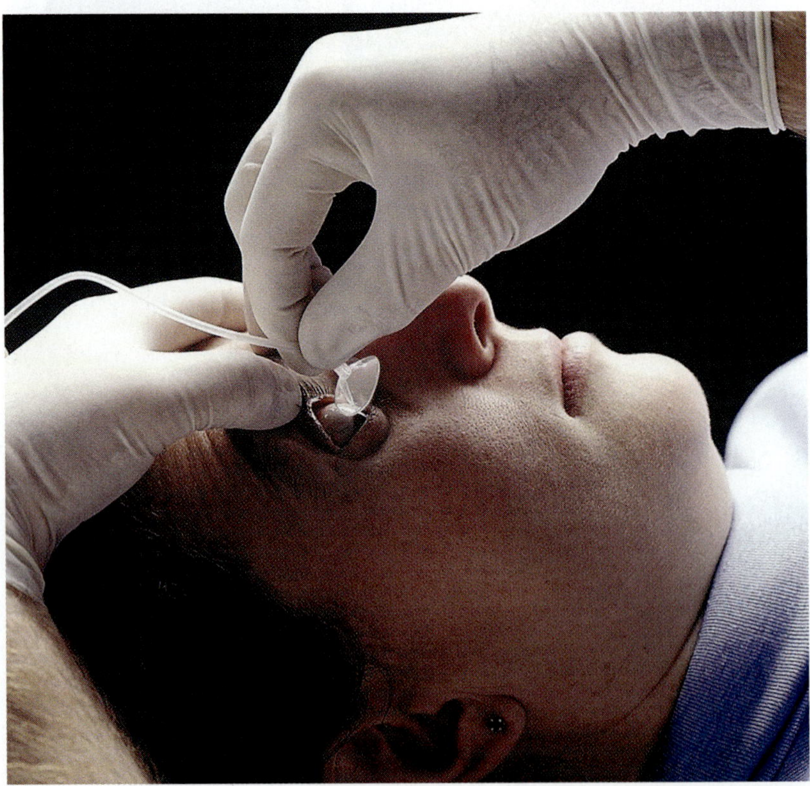

Morgan lens.

4.46 Air Splint

1. Expose the injured area.
2. Evaluate the patient's distal pulse, motor function, and sensory function.
3. Align the extremity, stabilize it, and support the extremity.
   - Do not align a joint injury if resistance is met. Use another device instead.
4. Place your arm through the splint and grasp the patient's hand or foot.
5. Apply gentle traction while sliding the splint into position.
6. Inflate the splint to a point that a slight dent can be made into the plastic when pressed with a finger.
7. Reevaluate the patient's distal pulse, motor function, and sensory function.

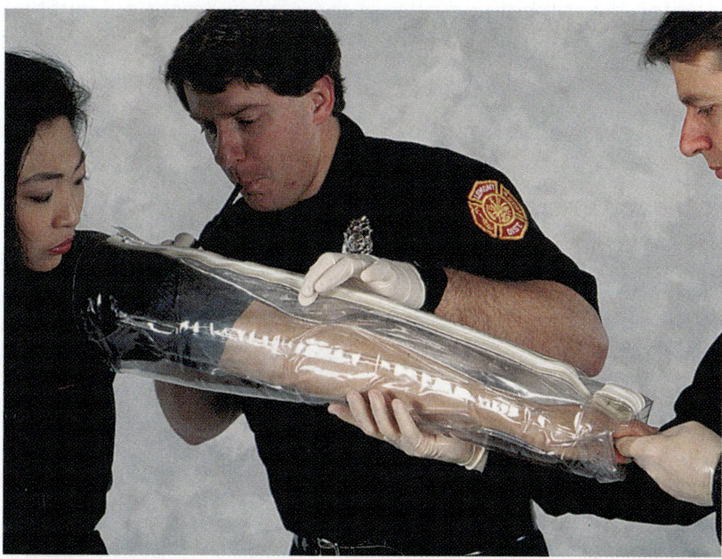

Air splint.

4.47 Hare Traction Splint

1. Expose the injured area.
2. Apply manual traction of the affected leg.
3. Check the patient's distal pulse, motor function, and sensory function.
4. Place the splint next to the uninjured leg. Adjust it to the proper length, from the top of the patient's pelvis to a few inches past the ankle.
5. Attach the ankle hitch about the foot and ankle.
6. Manually apply gentle in-line traction to the ankle hitch.
7. Slide the splint into position under the injured leg.
8. Place the ischial pad against the iliac crest.
9. Fasten the ischial strap.
10. Connect the loops of the ankle hitch to the end of the splint.
11. Tighten the ratchet and release the manual traction. Continue to pull until the patient has relief of pain and muscle spasms.
12. Secure the splint with straps.
13. Reevaluate the patient's distal pulse, motor function, and sensory function.

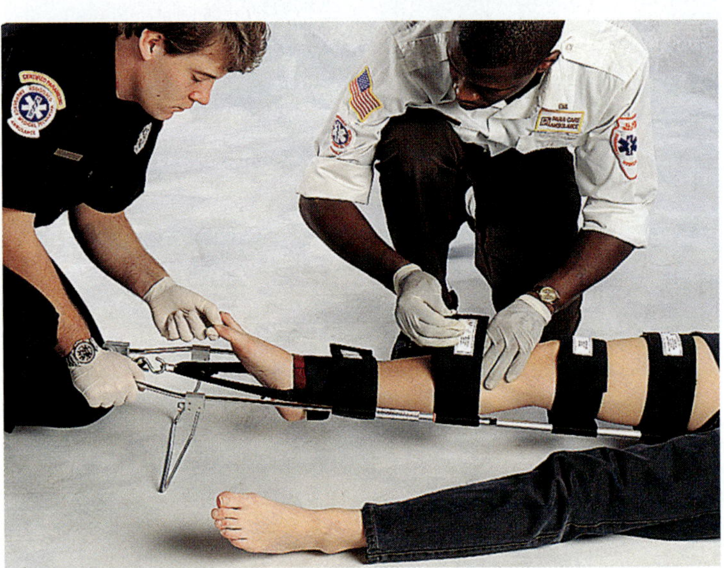

Hare traction splint.

4.48 Pneumatic Anti-Shock Garment for Splinting

1. Expose the wound and evaluate the need to splint the lower extremity or pelvis.
2. Evaluate the distal pulse, motor function, and sensory function of the patient's lower extremities.
3. Apply the garment to the patient.
4. Align the extremity, stabilize it, and support the extremity. Do not align a joint injury if resistance is met.
5. Attach the foot pump to each section of the suit. Open the valves to the sections that require inflation.
6. Inflate the compartments. **Do not inflate the device until the Velcro rips; inflate it only until the device is firm.**
7. Reevaluate the patient's distal pulse, motor function, and sensory function.

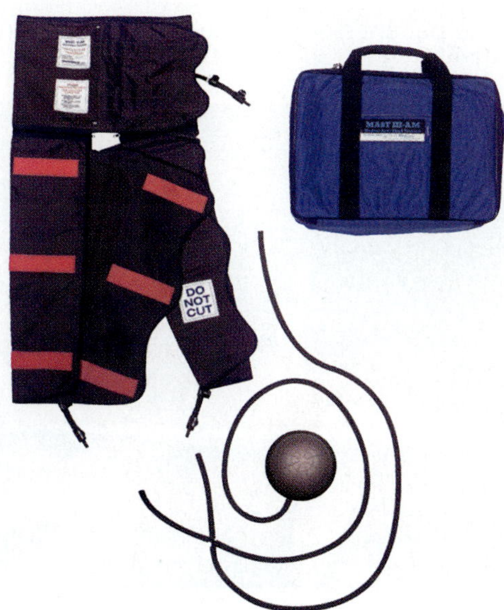

PASG/MAST device.

4.49 Rigid Splint

1. Expose the injured area.
2. Evaluate the patient's distal pulse, motor function, and sensory function.
3. Align the extremity, stabilize it, and support the extremity. Do not align a joint injury if resistance is met.
4. Acquire the appropriate-length wood planks. Provide padding to ensure even contact with the splint.
5. Place the wood on each side of the injury.
6. Secure the extremity to the rigid splint with tape, cling, or Ace wraps.
   - Long bone injury: Immobilize the joint above and joint below the injury.
   - Joint injury: Immobilize the bone above and bone below the injury.
7. Reevaluate the patient's distal pulse, motor function, and sensory function.

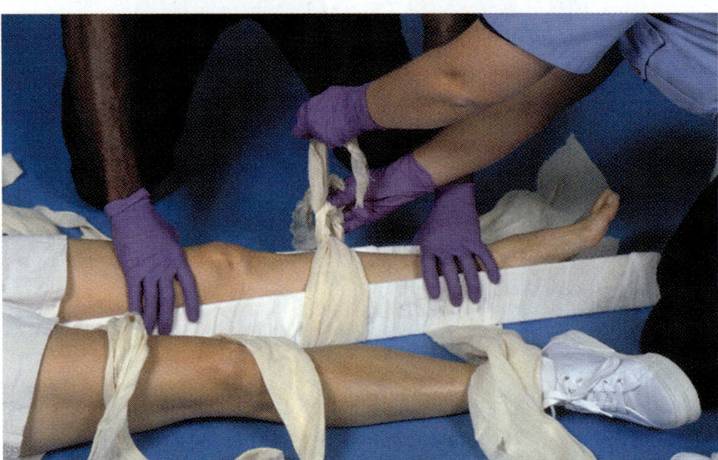

Rigid splint.

4.50 Sager Traction Splint

1. Expose the injured area.
2. Apply manual traction to the affected leg.
3. Check the patient's distal pulse, motor function, and sensory function.
4. Position the Sager traction splint between the patient's legs.
5. Adjust the splint to a distance slightly past the patient's ankle.
6. Apply the abductor bridle (thigh strap) around the upper thigh of the fractured limb.
7. Push the ischial perineal cushion gently down while pulling the thigh strap snugly.
8. Apply the Malleolar Harness (ankle harness) and attach it to the traction handle.
9. Place one hand on the padded shaft and the other hand on the traction handle while gently extending splint.
10. Pull the traction handle and release the manual traction. Continue to pull until one of the following conditions is met:

    - Maximum of 7 kg (15 lb) for one femur fracture.
    - Maximum of 14 kg for bilateral femur fractures.
    - Patient has relief of pain and muscle spasms.

11. Secure the splint with large elastic leg cravats.
12. Reevaluate the patient's distal pulse, motor function, and sensory function.

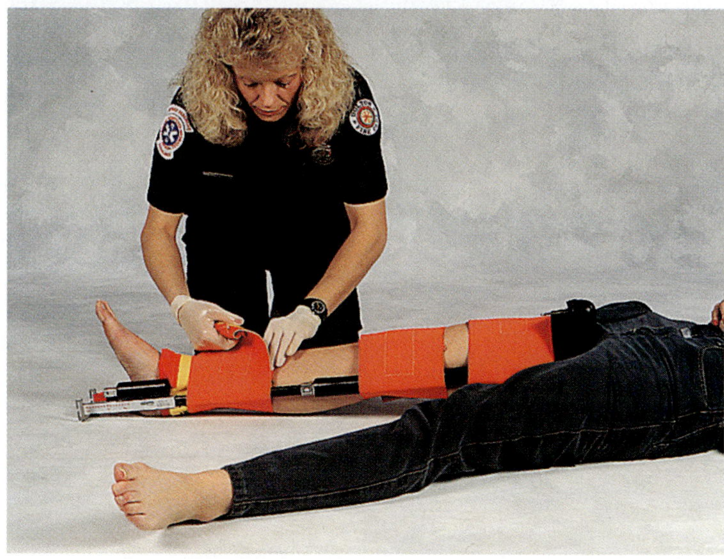

Sager traction splint.

4.51 Vacuum Splint

1. Expose the injured area.
2. Evaluate the patient's distal pulse, motor function, and sensory function.
3. Align the extremity, stabilize it, and support the extremity. Do not align a joint injury if resistance is met.
4. Wrap and secure the vacuum splint around the extremity.
5. Draw the air out of the splint.
6. Reevaluate the patient's distal pulse, motor function, and sensory function.

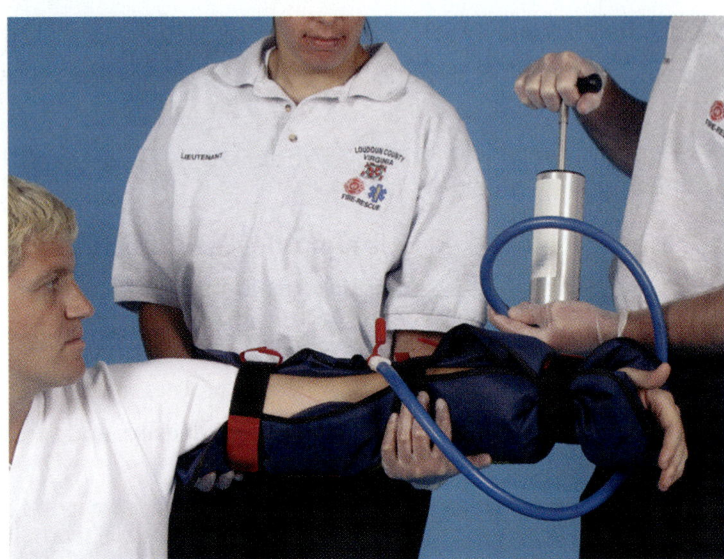

Vacuum splint.

4.52 Spinal Immobilization

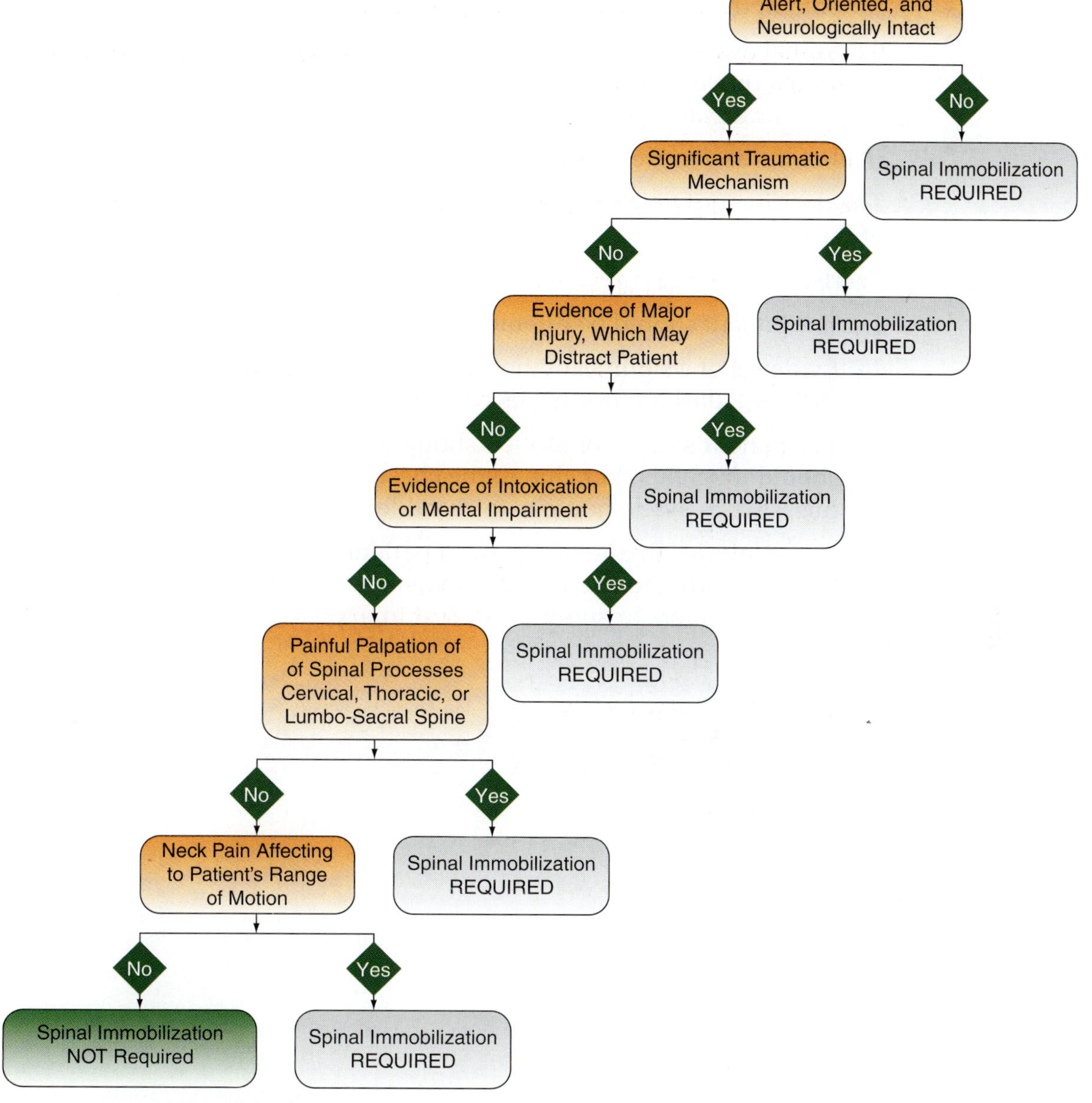

Spinal Immobilization Decision Flowchart.

Spinal Immobilization Decision Assessment

A. Spinal immobilization is **required** if any of the following is present in the trauma patient (remember **NSAIDS**):

1. **N**eurological deficit (e.g., focal deficit, tingling, reduced strength, numbness in extremity).
2. **S**ignificant traumatic mechanism and extremes of age.
3. **A**ltered mental status.
4. **I**ntoxication or mental impairment.

4.52 Spinal Immobilization

5. **D**istracting, painful injury—other painful injury that may distract the patient from the pain of the c-spine injury.
6. **S**pinal exam reveals point tenderness or pain to range of motion of the spinal process (e.g., cervical, thoracic, or lumbar-sacral). This includes any neck pain with or without movement.

B. If all of the above are absent, spinal immobilization is not required.

C. The decision not to implement spinal immobilization is the responsibility of the paramedic.

D. Pearls:

1. The patient should be oriented to person, place, situation, and time.
2. Evidence of a significant mechanism of trauma includes a windshield "spider," dash deformity, ejection, rollover, and space invasion > 1 foot.
3. The patient's range of motion should not be assisted. The patient should touch his/her chin to the chest, extend the neck (look up), and turn side-to-side (shoulder-to-shoulder) without pain.
4. Major injuries that may distract a patient's awareness to pain include pelvic fracture, femur fracture, extensive burns or soft-tissue injury, acute abdomen, or significant chest injury.

4.52.1 Horizontal Spinal Immobilization

1. Manually immobilize the head in a neutral, in-line position. Manual immobilization should be provided without interruption until complete patient immobilization is accomplished.
2. Contraindications to placement in an in-line position:
   - Neck muscle spasm that prohibits neutral alignment.
   - Increased pain.
   - Onset of or increase of a neurological deficit such as numbness, tingling, or loss of motor ability.
   - Compromise of the airway or ventilation.
   - If the patient's injuries are so severe that the head presents with such misalignment that it no longer appears to extend from the midline of the shoulders.
3. Size and apply a cervical collar according to the manufacturer's recommendations.
4. While maintaining manual stabilization with a cervical collar in place:
   - Log-roll the patient.
   - Position the backboard next to the patient so that the head of the backboard is approximately 1–2 feet above the patient's head.
   - Roll the patient onto the backboard in a supine position.
   - Reposition the patient to center him/her on the backboard, by sliding patient in an upward motion (axial) on the board. **Do not slide the patient in a direct lateral position, as this may manipulate the spine.**
5. Secure the patient's body to the board with straps.
   - Immobilize the upper torso to prevent upward sliding of patient's body during movement and transportation. This is accomplished by bringing the straps over the shoulders and across the chest to make an X.
   - Additional straps must be placed to prevent side-to-side movement of the body on the board. This can be accomplished by placing the straps across the iliac crests and mid-to-distal thigh or at the pelvis with groin loops.
   - Arms should be placed at the patient's side to prevent movement of the shoulder girdle.

4.52.1 Horizontal Spinal Immobilization

6. Secure the patient's head with a cervical immobilization device:

   - Commercially available cervical immobilization device: Follow the manufacturer's recommendation.

   or

   - Towel rolls applied to each side of the head: Secure the towels by placing 1- or 2-inch tape directly across the patient's forehead to the underpart of the backboard. Also secure the towels with tape across the surface of the semi-rigid cervical collar to the underpart of the backboard. *Do not* apply tape directly under the patient's chin, as this may create an airway obstruction.

7. Pad the space, as needed, between the back of the patient's head and the back-board to prevent hyperextension of the cervical vertebrae.

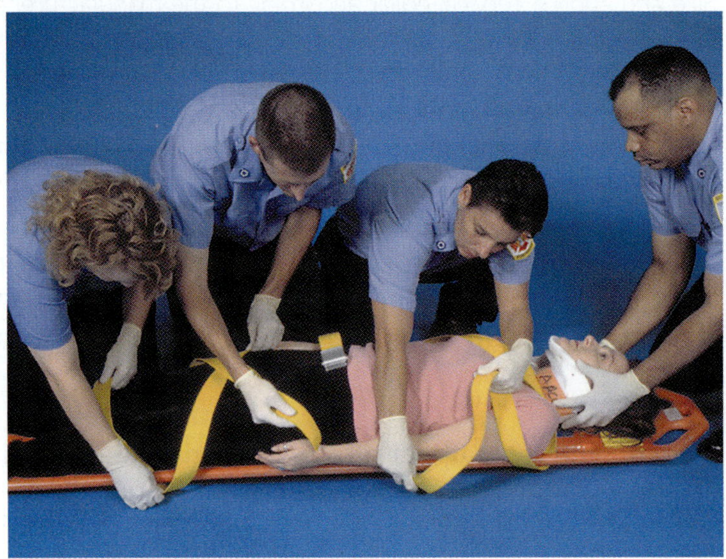

Securing the patient's body to the board.

4.52.2 Pediatric Spinal Immobilization

1. Manually immobilize the patient's head in a neutral, in-line position. Manual immobilization should be provided without interruption until complete patient immobilization is accomplished.
2. Contraindications to placement in an in-line position:
   - Neck muscle spasm that prohibits neutral alignment.
   - Increased pain.
   - Onset of or increase of a neurological deficit such as numbness, tingling, or loss of motor ability.
   - Compromise of the airway or ventilation.
   - If the patient's injuries are so severe that the head presents with such misalignment that it no longer appears to extend from the midline of the shoulders.
3. Size and apply a cervical collar according to the manufacturer's recommendations.
4. While maintaining manual stabilization with a cervical collar in place:
   - Log-roll the patient.
   - Position the pediatric immobilizer next to the patient so that the head of the immobilizer is approximately 6–12 inches above the patient's head.
   - Roll the patient onto the backboard in a supine position.
   - Reposition the patient to center him/her on the immobilizer, by sliding the patient in an upward motion (axial) on the immobilizer. **Do not slide the patient in a direct lateral position, as this may manipulate the spine.**
5. Secure the patient's body to the board with straps.
   - Pediatric immobilizers with integrated strapping design: Secure them according to the manufacturer's recommendation.

   or

   - Immobilize the upper torso to prevent upward sliding of the patient's body during movement and transportation. This is accomplished by bringing the straps over the shoulders and across the chest to make an X.
   - Additional straps must be placed to prevent side-to-side movement of the body on the board. This can be accomplished by placing the straps across the iliac crests and mid-to-distal thigh or at the pelvis with groin loops.

4.52.2 Pediatric Spinal Immobilization

6. If the patient is so small that there is a space left between straps and sides of patient, take up space with pads (e.g., blanket, towel).
7. The patient's arms should be placed at his/her side to prevent movement of the shoulder girdle.
8. Secure the patient's head with a cervical immobilization device.

    - Commercially available cervical immobilization device: Follow the manufacturer's recommendation.

    or

    - Towel rolls applied to each side of the head: Secure the towels by placing 1- or 2-inch tape directly across the patient's forehead to the underpart of the backboard. Also secure the towels with tape across the surface of the semi-rigid cervical collar to the underpart of the backboard. *Do not* apply tape directly under the patient's chin, as this may create an airway obstruction.

9. Pad the space, as needed, between the back of the patient's head and the backboard to prevent hyperextension of the cervical vertebrae.

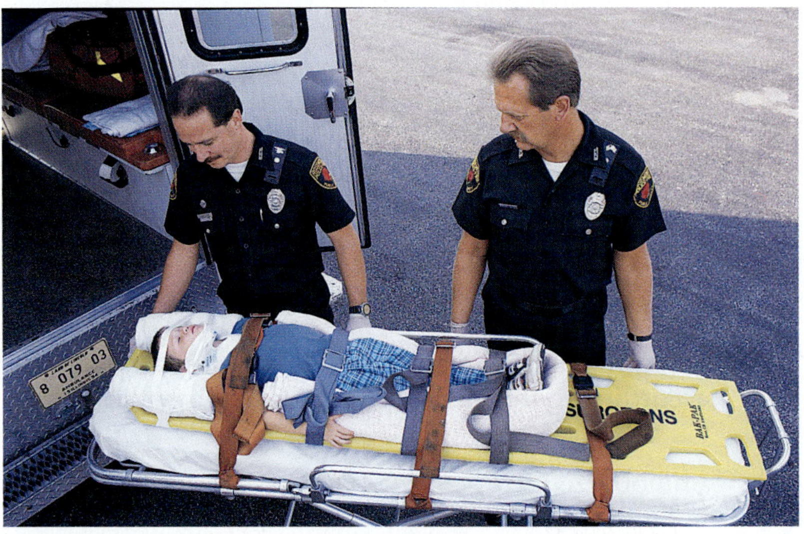

Spinal stabilization must secure the body so that there is no spinal movement.

4.52.3 Standing Spinal Immobilization

1. Manually immobilize the patient's head in a neutral, in-line position from the front to eliminate lateral movements. Manual immobilization should be provided without interruption until complete patient immobilization is accomplished.
2. Contraindications to placement in an in-line position:
    - Neck muscle spasm that prohibits neutral alignment.
    - Increased pain.
    - Onset of or increase of a neurological deficit such as numbness, tingling, or loss of motor ability.
    - Compromise of the airway or ventilation.
    - If the patient's injuries are so severe that the head presents with such misalignment that it no longer appears to extend from the midline of the shoulders.
3. Size and apply a cervical collar according to the manufacturer's recommendations.
4. Position the backboard behind the standing patient.
5. Have the rescuer performing manual stabilization of the head from the front of the patient pass off the stabilization to a second rescuer who will perform manual stabilization of the head from behind the patient, with arms on either side of the standing backboard. The third rescuer can hold the backboard in place during this switch.
6. Have two rescuers on either side of the patient grasp the backboard with one hand and the patient's armpit with the other hand.
7. With one rescuer at each side of the backboard and the third rescuer holding the patient's head, slowly lay the board down. A stop approximately halfway down will be needed to allow the rescuer holding the head to reposition his/her hands.
8. Reposition the patient to center him/her on the backboard, by sliding the patient in an upward motion (axial) on the board. **Do not slide the patient in a direct lateral position, as this may manipulate the spine.**
9. Secure the patient's body to the board with straps.
    - Immobilize the upper torso to prevent upward sliding of patient's body during movement and transportation. This is accomplished by bringing the straps over the shoulders and across the chest to make an X.
    - Additional straps must be placed to prevent side-to-side movement of the patient's body on the board. This can be accomplished by placing the straps across the iliac crests and mid-to-distal thigh or at the pelvis with groin loops.
    - The patient's arms should be placed at his/her side to prevent movement of the shoulder girdle.

4.52.3 Standing Spinal Immobilization

10. Secure the patient's head with a cervical immobilization device:

    - Commercially available cervical immobilization device: Follow the manufacturer's recommendation.

    or

    - Towel rolls applied to each side of the head: Secure the towels by applying 1- or 2-inch tape directly across the patient's forehead to the underpart of the backboard. Also secure the towels with tape across the surface of the semi-rigid cervical collar to the underpart of the backboard. *Do not* apply tape directly under the patient's chin, as this may create an airway obstruction.

11. Pad the space, as needed, between the back of the patient's head and the backboard to prevent hyperextension of the cervical vertebrae.

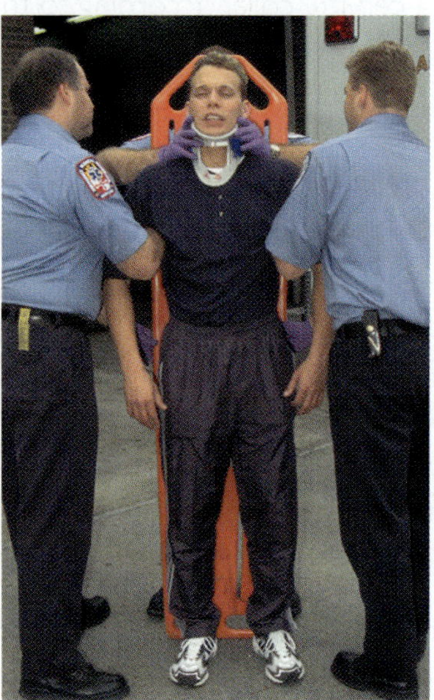

Preparing to lower the board.

4.52.4 Vest-Type Extrication Device (KED)

1. Manually immobilize the patient's head in a neutral, in-line position. Manual immobilization should be provided without interruption until complete patient immobilization is accomplished.
2. Contraindications to placement in an in-line position:
   - Neck muscle spasm that prohibits neutral alignment.
   - Increased pain.
   - Onset of or increase of a neurological deficit such as numbness, tingling, or loss of motor ability.
   - Compromise of the airway or ventilation.
   - If the patient's injuries are so severe that the head presents with such misalignment that it no longer appears to extend from the midline of the shoulders.
3. Size and apply a cervical collar according to the manufacturer's recommendations.
4. Insert the device behind the patient. Try to limit the patient's movement while you are positioning the device.
5. Position the device so that it fits securely under the axilla of the patient. Open the side flaps and place them around the patient's torso. Make sure the device is centered on the patient.
6. Position, connect, and adjust the torso straps. Leave the uppermost strap loose until the patient's head is immobilized.
7. Position and fasten each groin loop. Adjust one side at a time to prevent excess movement of the patient.
8. Place the pad behind the patient's head, filling the void to prevent hyperextension.
9. Position the head flaps. Fasten the forehead strap and apply the chin strap over the cervical collar.

4.53 Auto-Injector EpiPen®

The EMT (or paramedic) may administer prescribed epinephrine via an auto-injector for patients who are exhibiting signs of respiratory distress associated with allergic reaction. These signs may include dyspnea, hives, flushing of the skin, wheezing, edema, and possibly unstable vital signs.

1. Assure the auto-injector is prescribed for the patient: EpiPen® for adult patient and EpiPen Jr.® for pediatric patient.
2. Check the expiration date.
3. Remove the auto-injector's safety cap.
4. Grasp the unit like a pen and position the tip of the EpiPen on the outer thigh mid-way between waist and knee.
5. Push the auto-injector firmly against the site until the injector is activated.
6. Hold the auto-injector in place until the medication is fully injected (minimum of 10 seconds).
7. Record the time.
8. Dispose of the auto-injector in a biohazard puncture-resistant container.
9. Reassess the patient.

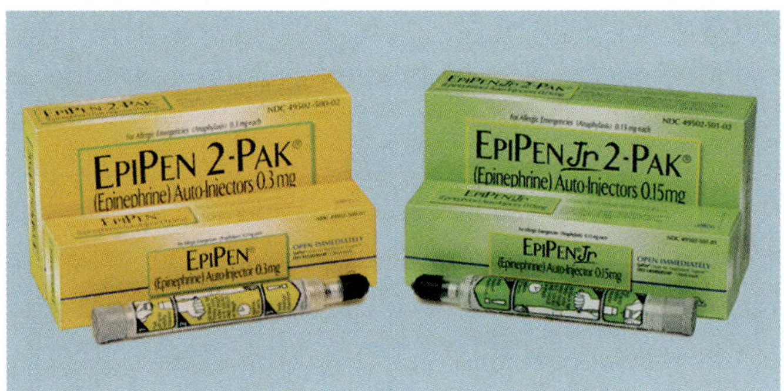

EpiPen® and EpiPen Jr.®

4.54 Auto-Injector Mark I

1. Remove the Mark I from its protective pouch.
2. Hold the unit by the plastic clip.
3. Remove the AtroPen from slot number 1 of the plastic clip. The yellow safety cap will remain in the clip, and the AtroPen will now be armed. ***Do not hold the unit by the green tip:*** The needle is ejected from the green tip.
4. Grasp the unit like a pen and position the green tip of the AtroPen on the outer thigh, midway between waist and knee.
5. Push firmly until the auto-injector fires.
6. Hold the auto-injector in place until the medication is fully injected (minimum of 10 seconds).
7. Remove the 2-PAM Cl ComboPen from slot 2 of the plastic clip. The gray safety cap will remain in the clip and the ComboPen will now be armed. ***Do not hold the unit by the black tip:*** The needle is ejected from the black tip.
8. Grasp the unit like a pen and position the black tip of the ComboPen on the outer thigh, midway between waist and knee.
9. Push firmly until the auto-injector fires.
10. Hold the auto-injector in place until the medication is fully injected (minimum of 10 seconds).
11. Dispose of the unit in a biohazard puncture-resistant container.

4.55 Intramuscular Injection

1. Prepare the equipment. The needle size should be 21–23 gauge and 1–1.5 inches long.
2. Check for proper medication, expiration date, vial integrity, and color and clarity. Draw the medication into the syringe.
3. Cleanse the injection site with alcohol or Betadine in an expanding circular pattern using a firm pressure.
4. With one hand, pull the skin taut and insert the needle at a 90-degree angle into the muscle.
5. Aspirate to ensure that a blood vessel has not been entered. If blood is aspirated, remove the needle and repeat the procedure at a different site.
6. Administer the appropriate dose.
7. Remove the needle from the injection site and dispose of it in a secure sharps container.
8. Monitor the patient.

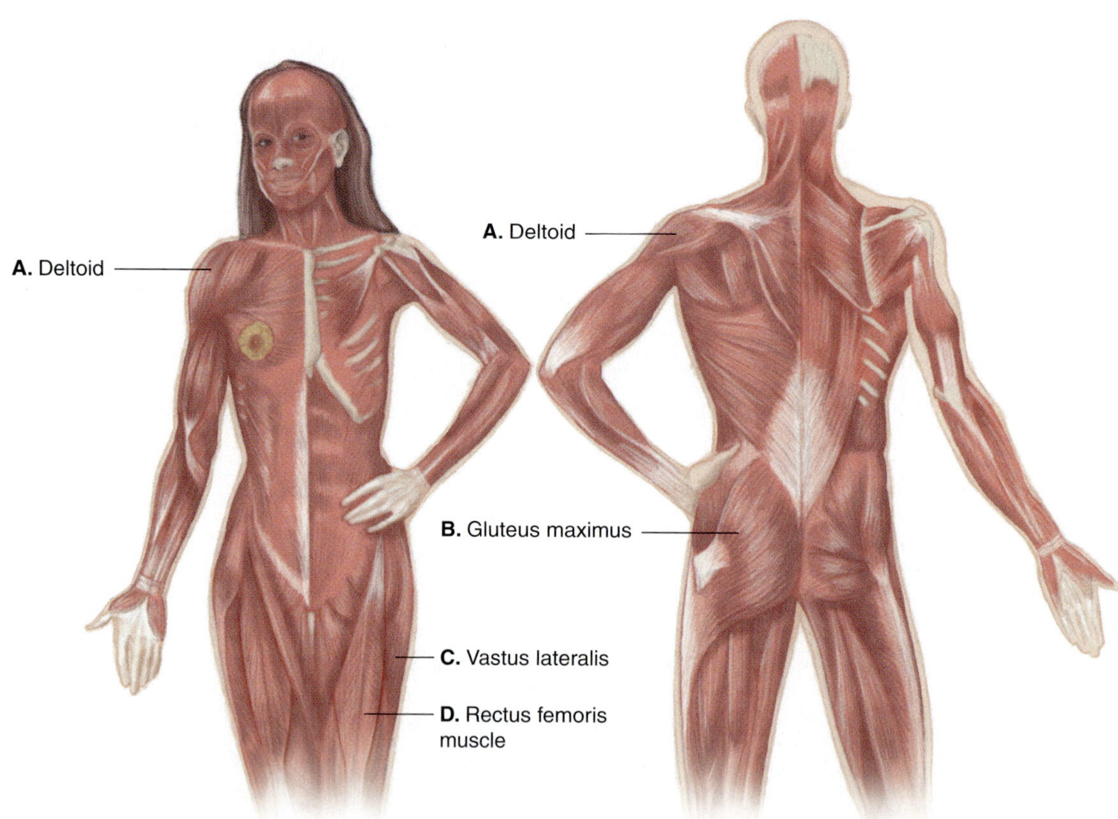

Common sites for intramuscular injections. A. Deltoid muscle. B. Gluteal area. C. Vastus lateralis muscle. D. Rectus femoris muscle.

4.56 BIG (Bone Injection Gun)

Adult

1. Find and mark a penetration site located 2 cm medially and 1 cm proximally to the tibial tuberosity.
2. Clean the area with a povidone-iodine swab.
3. Position the BIG device with one hand to the site and pull out the safety latch with the other hand.
4. Trigger the BIG at a 90-degree angle to the surface.
5. Remove the BIG handle.
6. Pull out the stylet trocar.
7. Fix the cannula with the safety latch.
8. Attach a 10-cc syringe filled with ½ normal saline.
   - Aspirate for bone marrow, then flush with fluid.
   - Observe for any signs of infiltration.
9. If the route is patent, connect it to the drip set tubing.
10. Attach a pressure infuser.
11. Secure the site.

Child

1. Find and mark a penetration site located 1 cm medially and 1 cm proximally to the tibial tuberosity.
2. Clean the area with a povidone-iodine swab.
3. Position the BIG device with one hand to the site and pull out the safety latch with the other hand.
4. Trigger the BIG at a 90-degree angle to the surface.
5. Remove the BIG handle.
6. Pull out the stylet trocar.
7. Fix the cannula with the safety latch.
8. Attach a 10-cc syringe filled with ½ normal saline.
   - Aspirate for bone marrow, then flush with fluid.
   - Observe for any signs of infiltration.
9. If the route is patent, connect it to the drip set tubing.
10. Attach a pressure infuser.
11. Secure the site.

4.57 Cook Pediatric IO

1. Locate the site of cannulation. Palpate the tibial tuberosity, and move 1–3 cm below the tuberosity on the medial surface of the tibia, approximately one finger's width below the tuberosity.
2. Prep the area with antiseptic solution (e.g., povidone-iodine).
3. Grasp the patient's thigh and knee above and lateral to the insertion site palm of the nondominant hand. Wrap your fingers and thumb around the knee to stabilize the proximal tibia. Do not let any portion of your hand rest behind the insertion site.
4. Palpate the landmarks again to confirm the insertion site.
5. Insert the needle through the skin, over the flat anteromedial surface of the tibia.
6. Advance the needle through the bony cortex of the proximal tibia, directing the needle perpendicular (90 degrees) to the long axis of the bone or slightly caudad (toward the toes) to avoid the epiphysial plate, using a gentle back-and-forth twisting or drilling motion.
7. Stop advancing the needle when a sudden decrease in resistance to forward motion of the needle is felt.
8. Unscrew the cap and remove the stylet from the needle.
9. Stabilize the needle and attach a 10-mL syringe filled with normal saline.
10. Aspirate for bone marrow, then flush the needle with normal saline. Check for any signs of increased resistance to injection or swelling of the surrounding tissue.
11. If the test injection is successful, remove syringe and connect the IV tubing.
12. Attach a pressure infuser.
13. Secure the site.

4.58 Fast I Adult IO

1. The following conditions warrant caution when establishing this kind of intraosseous access:

    - Compromised skin or tissue in the area of the manubrium (i.e., trauma, infection, burns).
    - Suspected fracture of the sternum.
    - Previous sternotomy (i.e., open heart surgery).
    - Severe osteoporosis and bone-softening conditions.
    - Extremely small adult.

2. Prepare the insertion site using aseptic technique. The insertion site is located over the manubrium. The iodine and alcohol swabs included in the FAST I package should be used to clean the site; it should be allowed to dry for at least 15 seconds.
3. Remove the top half of the backing (labeled "1") from the target/strain relief patch. Place an index finger in the patient's sternal notch, perpendicular to the manubrium surface, to align the indicator notch in the patch with the patient's sternal notch.
4. Place the target zone (the circular hole in the patch) over the patient's midline. The locating finger must be held perpendicular to the manubrium.
5. Secure the top half of the patch to the body by pressing firmly downward on the patch, engaging the adhesive. Verify its location. Remove the bottom half of backing (labeled "2") and press the patch to the patient's skin.
6. Verify that the indicator notch on the patch matches the patient's sternal notch, and that the target zone is over the patient's midline. If there is error greater than 1 cm (3/8 inch), the patch should be removed and discarded, and a new patch placed. (***Note:*** It may be possible to move and hold the patient's skin so that the patch is correctly positioned for insertion.)
7. Remove the sharps cap from the introducer.
8. Place the bone probe cluster in the target zone, with the vertical axis of the introducer held perpendicular to the skin. It is vital that the introducer is perpendicular (90 degrees) to the skin and manubrium surface at the insertion site. The chest is often rounded; care must be taken to ensure the device is perpendicular to the skin, not to the surface on which the patient rests. Ensure that the entire bone probe cluster is within the target zone.
9. Press the introducer into the target zone with firm and increasing force, until a distinct release of the introducer handle is heard and felt. In some patients, considerable force may be needed to release the introducer. After the release, pull straight back to remove the introducer, exposing the infusion tube. The stylet support sleeves will fall away.
10. Locate the orange sharps plug. Place it on a flat surface with the foam facing up. Keeping both hands behind the needles, push the bone probe cluster straight into the foam. After the sharps plug has been engaged and the sharps are safely covered, reattach the clear cap to the introducer. The cap will fit securely over the plug. This completes the dual sharps protection. Dispose of the introducer using contaminated sharps protocols.

4.58 Fast I Adult IO

11. Attach the right-angle female connector of the patch to the infusion tube.
12. Verify that correct placement has occurred by attaching the enclosed syringe to the straight female connector and withdrawing marrow into the infusion tube.
13. Attach the straight female connector on the patch to a purged source of fluids or drugs. Fluid can now flow to the site and into the bloodstream.
14. Place the protector dome over the patch and press down firmly to engage the Velcro fastening.
15. Attach the unopened remover package to the patient (e.g., on an arm, leg, or pocket, or attached to chart). This package must be transported with the patient. The remover will be needed later to remove the infusion tube from the patient when intraosseous access is no longer required.

Removing the Fast I System

1. Remove the protector dome from the target/strain relief patch.
2. Disconnect the infusion tube from the female connector on the patch.
3. Maintaining aseptic technique, open the remover package.
   - If the remover has been misplaced, obtain a replacement remover.
   - Alternatively, the infusion tube may be removed via a minor surgical procedure performed by a qualified healthcare provider. Through a small incision, grip the stainless steel portal with hemostats and pull straight back. This procedure can be performed wherever the decision to discontinue infusion is made.
4. Remove the tubing protecting the threaded tip, and insert the remover into the infusion tube. The infusion tube should be held straight out (90-degree angle) from the patient; this will ease insertion and prevent the remover stylet from being pushed through the side of the infusion tubing.
5. Advance the remover to engage the threads in the proximal tip of the infusion tube. Turn the remover clockwise until it stops.
6. Pull straight out on the remover to remove the infusion tube.
7. Remove the target/strain relief patch.
8. Apply pressure after removing the patch, and treat the site using aseptic technique and dressing.
9. Dispose of the remover and infusion tube using contaminated sharps protocols. Dispose of the rest of the FAST I system.

4.59 EZ-IO (Adult and Pediatric)

1. Locate an insertion site on the tibia—medial to the tibial tuberosity.
2. Clean the area with a povidone-iodine swab.
3. Select the appropriate needle.
    - Adult needle: weight ≥ 40 kg
    - Pediatric needle: weight = 3–39 kg
4. Remove the needle from the case. Push the needle onto the power driver, and make sure that it is securely seated.
5. Remove and discard the needle set safety cap from the needle.
6. Insert the EZ-IO needle onto the tibial site at a 90-degree angle to the bone surface.
7. Gently power the needle set until it touches bone, and then apply steady downward pressure.
8. Release the driver's trigger until:
    - There is a sudden "give" or "pop."

    or
    - The needle reaches the desired depth at 5 mm, which is indicated on the needle by the black line.
9. Remove the power driver and needle stylet.
10. Confirm that the catheter is stable.
11. Take the syringe containing 10 mL of normal saline and attach the EZ-IO catheter luer lock.
12. Use 5 mL of normal saline to flush the EZ-IO catheter luer lock; attach the luer lock to the needle.
13. Pull back on the syringe to aspirate blood, then flush with 5 mL of normal saline.
14. If the route is patent, connect it to the drip set tubing.
15. Attach a pressure infuser.
16. Secure the site and attach the wrist label to the patient's hand.

4.60 Intravenous Cannulation

1. Locate a suitable venipuncture site. The back of the hand, forearm, and antecubital fossa are preferred sites. The external jugular vein is acceptable if no other suitable site can be found.
2. Place a constricting band to halt venous return without obstructing arterial flow. Leave one end of the slip knot exposed to assure rapid release when the procedure is complete.
3. Inspect the catheter to be sure that catheter hub and primary push-off tab are fully seated to the needle housing assembly.
4. Locate a suitable vein. Palpate one that is well fixed (not rolling) and that does not have valves (firm nubs of tissue) proximal to the intended site of entry.
5. Cleanse the venipuncture site. Employ alcohol or Betadine in an expanding circular pattern, using a firm pressure.
6. Anchor the vein with gentle skin traction.
7. Hold the needle bevel up and insert catheter at a 30- to 45-degree angle until you feel the needle pop into the vein. Flashback of blood should be observed in the catheter/chamber.
8. At this point, the metal stylet is in the vein, but the catheter is not. Advance the cannula approximately 0.5 cm farther. Holding the metal stylet stationary, slide the catheter over the needle into the vein. Place a finger over the vein at the catheter tip and tamponade the vein to prevent blood from flowing out of the catheter.
9. Remove the tourniquet. **Do not reinsert the needle into the catheter at any time.**
10. Secure a luer device to the catheter by following the manufacturer's instructions for that device.
11. Secure the catheter with tape or a commercial device.
12. Dispose of the needle in a secure sharps container.

4.60 Intravenous Cannulation

Troubleshooting a Nonflowing IV

- Has the constricting band been removed? This is the most common cause.
- Is there swelling at the cannulation site? This indicates infiltration into the tissues.
- Are the tubing control valves open?
- Does the cannula need to be repositioned because it is up against a valve or wall of the vein? You may have to remove the securing device to check for this condition.
- Is the IV bag hung high enough?
- Is the drip bag completely filled with solution? If it is, turn bag upside down and squeeze the drip chamber to return some of the fluid to the bag.
- Lower the bag below the level of the insertion site. If blood return is seen in the IV site, the site is patent.
- If problems persist, remove the IV and reestablish it at another site.

4.61 Mucosal Atomization Device

Damaged nasal mucosa may inhibit absorption of the medication. For this reason, contraindications for a mucosal atomization device include the following conditions:

- Facial trauma.
- Epistaxis (nose bleed).
- Nasal congestion or discharge.
- Any recognized nasal mucosal abnormality.

1. Prepare the equipment.
2. Check the medication for proper name, expiration date, vial integrity, and color and clarity.
3. Draw the medication into the syringe.
   - Maximum adult administration: 1 mL per nostril.
   - Maximum pediatric (< 10 years old) administration: 0.5 mL per nostril.
4. Expel all of the air from the syringe.
5. Securely attach the mucosal atomizer to the syringe.
6. The patient should be in a recumbent or supine position. If the patient is sitting, compress the nares after administration.
7. Briskly compress the syringe plunger to properly atomize the medication.
8. Monitor the patient.

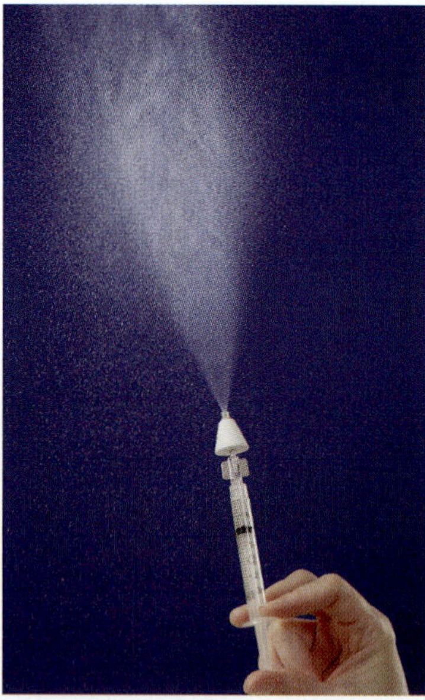

Mucosal atomizer device (MAD).

4.62 Subcutaneous Injection

1. Prepare the equipment. The needle size should be 25–27 gauge and 3/8 to 5/8 inch in length.
2. Check for proper medication, expiration date, vial integrity, and color and clarity. Draw the medication into the syringe.
3. Cleanse the injection site with alcohol or Betadine in an expanding circular pattern, using a firm pressure.
4. With one hand, pinch the skin and insert the needle at a 45-degree angle into the fold.
5. Administer the appropriate dose.
6. Remove the needle from the injection site and dispose of it in a secure sharps container.
7. Monitor the patient.

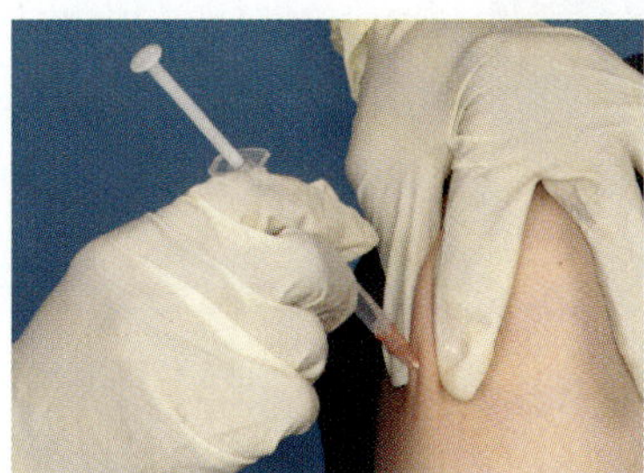

Subcutaneous injection.

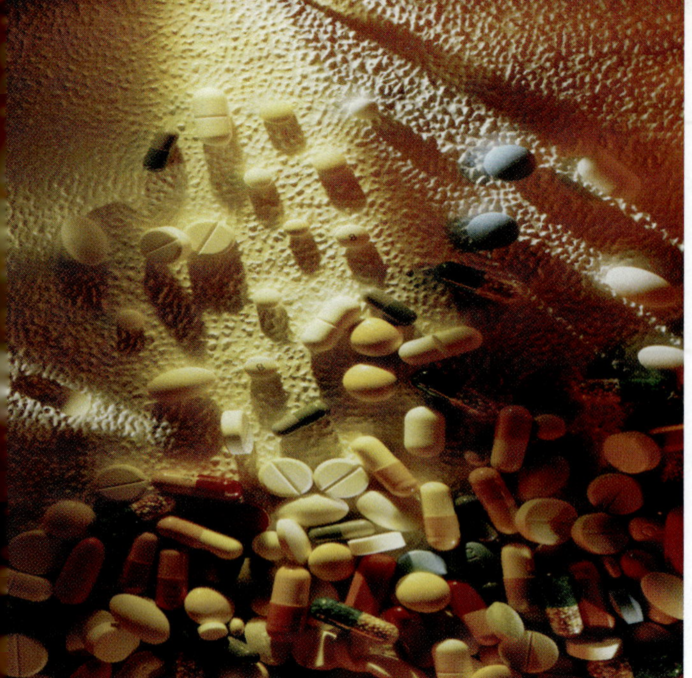

chapter 5

Drug Summaries

5.1 Activated Charcoal (Actidose®)

Actions

Activated charcoal binds and absorbs ingested toxins present in the gastrointestinal tract. Once bound to the activated charcoal, the combined complex is excreted from the body.

Indications

Ingested poisons and medication overdoses after the stomach has been emptied or when vomiting must not occur, but absorption therapy is indicated.

Contraindications

Activated charcoal should not be administered to the patient who has, or has the potential for, an altered level of consciousness unless it is administered by nasogastric tube and the patient's airway is protected by an endotracheal tube. Avoid use in cyanide, methanol, organophosphate toxicity, and/or caustic ingestion.

Precautions

If emesis is to be induced with ipecac, it is often best to wait until the patient has vomited to administer activated charcoal. Activated charcoal given with ipecac will inactivate the ipecac. Contact the Poison Control Center or online medical control prior to administering activated charcoal.

Adverse Reactions and Side Effects

Nausea, vomiting, abdominal cramping/bloating, and constipation (with black stools).

Dosage

Adult: 1 g/kg (average 50–75 g) PO of activated charcoal mixed with a glass of water to form a slurry.

Pediatric: 1 g/kg PO of activated charcoal mixed with a glass of water to form a slurry.

5.2 Adenosine Triphosphate (Adenocard®)

Actions

Adenosine exerts its effects by decreasing conduction through the AV mode. The half-life of Adenocard (adenosine) is less than 10 seconds. Thus its effects—both desired and undesired—are self-limited.

Indications

Adenocard is indicated for supraventricular tachycardia (SVT), including that associated with accessory bypass tracts (Wolff-Parkinson-White syndrome). When clinically advisable, appropriate vagal maneuvers should be attempted prior to Adenocard administration.

Contraindications

Adenocard is contraindicated in second- or third-degree AV block and sick sinus syndrome (except in patients with a functioning artificial pacemaker), and known hypersensitivity to adenosine.

Precautions

The effects of adenosine are antagonized by methylxanthines such as caffeine and theophylline. Thus larger doses may be required for adenosine to be effective in patients who have taken methylxanthines.

Adenosine effects are potentiated by dipyridamole (Persantine™). Thus smaller doses of adenosine may be effective in those who have taken this drug.

Adenosine may produce bronchoconstriction in patients with asthma.

Adverse Reactions and Side Effects

- **Cardiovascular:** Facial flushing, headache, and rarely: sweating, palpitations, chest pain, and hypotension.
- **Respiratory:** Shortness of breath, chest pressure, and rarely: hyperventilating metallic taste, tightness in throat, and head pressure.
- **CNS:** Light headedness and rarely: dizziness, blurred vision, tingling and numbness in extremities, apprehension.

Warnings

Adenocard may produce a short-lasting first-, second-, or third-degree heart block. In extreme cases, transient asystole may result. At the time of conversion to normal sinus rhythm, a variety of new rhythms may appear (PVCs, PACs, sinus bradycardia, sinus tachycardia, skipped beats, and varying degrees of AV block), though they generally last only a few seconds without intervention.

5.2 Adenosine Triphosphate (Adenocard®)

Dosage

Adult: 6 mg rapid IVP immediately followed by 20 mL NS flush.

Repeat in 2 minutes at 12 mg IVP, followed by 20 mL NS flush PRN.

Repeat in 2 minutes at 12 mg IVP, followed by 20 mL NS flush PRN.

Pediatric: 0.1 mg/kg (maximum dose = 6 mg) rapid IVP, immediately followed by 6 mL NS flush.

Repeat in 2 minutes, at 0.2 mg/kg (maximum dose = 12 mg) rapid IVP, followed by 6 mL NS flush PRN.

Repeat in 2 minutes, at 0.2 mg/kg (maximum dose = 12 mg) rapid IVP, followed by 6 mL NS flush PRN.

5.3 Albuterol (Proventil®, Ventolin®)

Actions

Albuterol is primarily a beta$_2$ sympathomimetic and, as such, produces bronchodilation. Because of its greater specificity for beta$_2$-adrenergic receptors, it produces fewer cardiovascular side effects and more prolonged bronchodilation than isoproterenol. Onset of action is within 15 minutes; peak action occurs in 60–90 minutes. Therapeutic effects may be active up to 5 hours.

Indications

The albuterol inhaler is indicated for relief of bronchospasm in patients with reversible obstructive airway disease, including asthma.

Contraindications

Albuterol is contraindicated in patients with a history of hypersensitivity.

Adverse Reactions and Side Effects

- **Cardiovascular:** Tachycardia, hypertension, and angina.
- **CNS:** Nervousness, tremor, headache, dizziness, and insomnia.
- **GI:** Drying of oropharynx, nausea, and vomiting, unusual taste.

Warnings

Use cautiously in patients with coronary artery disease, hypertension, hyperthyroidism, and diabetes. Administer cautiously to patients on MAO inhibitors or tricyclic antidepressants. Beta blockers and albuterol will inhibit each other.

Dosage

If $>$ 1 year or $>$ 10 kg:	Add 2.5 mg of albuterol mixed in 3 mL of NS (0.083%) to the nebulizer and flow oxygen at 6–8 L/min.
If $<$ 1 year or $<$ 10 kg:	Add 1.25 mg of albuterol mixed in 1.5 mL of NS (0.083%) to the nebulizer and flow oxygen at 3 L/min.

Treatment will be delivered over approximately 5–15 minutes.

5.4 Alteplase Recombinant (Activase®)

Actions

Alteplase recombinant is an enzyme (serine protease) that has the property of fibrin-enhanced conversion of plasminogen in plasmin. It produces limited conversion of plasminogen in the absence of fibrin. When introduced into the systemic circulation at pharmacological concentration, alteplase recombinant binds to fibrin in the thrombus and converts the entrapped plasminogen to plasmin. This conversion initiates local fibrinolysis with limited systemic proteolysis.

Indications

Activase is indicated for use in the management of acute myocardial infarction (AMI) in adults for lysis of thrombi obstructing coronary arteries.

Contraindications

- Active internal bleeding
- History of cerebrovascular accident
- Recent (within 2 months) history of intracranial or intraspinal surgery or trauma
- Intracranial neoplasm, arteriovenous malformation, or aneurysm
- Known bleeding diathesis
- Severe uncontrolled hypertension

Precautions

Noncompressible arterial puncture must be avoided (e.g., internal jugular and subclavian punctures). Arterial and venous punctures should be minimized.

Adverse Reactions and Side Effects

Bleeding is the most common adverse reaction, either internal or external, or both. Other adverse reactions include dysrhythmias, nausea/vomiting, hypotension, and fever. Mild hypersensitivity may produce urticaria.

Dosage

Adult: Prehospital bolus of 15 mg IV.

5.5 Amiodarone Hydrochloride (Cordarone®)

Actions

Amiodarone blocks sodium channels at rapid pacing frequencies and exerts a noncompetitive antisympathetic action. One of its main effects, with prolonged administration, is to lengthen the cardiac action potential. In addition, it produces a negative chronotropic effect in nodal tissues. Amiodarone blocks potassium channels, which contributes to slowing of conduction and prolongation of refractoriness. Its vasodilatory action can decrease cardiac workload and consequently myocardial oxygen consumption.

Indications

Amiodarone is indicated for initiation of treatment and prophylaxis of frequently recurring ventricular fibrillation and hemodynamically unstable ventricular tachycardia in patients refractory to other therapy. It may also be used to treat supraventricular tachycardia.

Contraindications

Amiodarone is contraindicated in patients with known hypersensitivity to amiodarone, or in patients with cardiogenic shock, marked sinus bradycardia, and second- or third-degree AV block.

Precautions

Amiodarone may worsen existing or precipitate new dysrhythmias, including torsades de pointes and VF. Use with beta-blocking agents could increase the patient's risk of hypotension and bradycardia. Amiodarone inhibits atrioventricular conduction and decreases myocardial contractility, increasing the risk of AV block with verapamil or diltiazem, or of hypotension with any calcium-channel blocker. Use with caution in pregnant patients and nursing mothers.

Adverse Reactions and Side Effects

Adverse reactions include fever, bradycardia, CHF, cardiac arrest, hypotension, ventricular tachycardia, nausea, and abnormal liver function.

Dosage

Adult: VT with pulse and SVT: 150 mg IV in 50 mL D_5W over 10 minutes. May repeat every 10 minutes PRN.

VF and pulseless VT: 300 mg IV push.

Pediatric: VT with a pulse and SVT: 5 mg/kg in 50 mL D_5W IV/IO over 20 minutes.

VF and pulseless VT: 5 mg/kg IV/IO push.

5.6 Amyl Nitrate

Actions

In cyanide toxicity, nitrite ions combine with hemoglobin to form methemoglobin, which binds with cyanide and assists in cyanide elimination. Amyl nitrate converts hemoglobin (Fe^{2+}) into methemoglobin (Fe^{3+}), which binds with the cyanide.

Indications

Used initially in the management of cyanide toxicity.

Contraindications

- Hypersensitivity to nitrates
- Intracranial pressure/closed head injury
- Cerebral hemorrhage

Adverse Reactions and Side Effects

- **CNS:** Headache, dizziness, weakness.
- **CV:** Orthostatic hypotension, tachycardia.
- **GI:** Nausea and vomiting.
- **Blood:** Methemoglobin.
- **Other:** Flammable, looks similar to ammonia inhalants.

Dosage

Adult: 0.2–0.3 mL inhaled for 15–30 seconds every 3–5 minutes, until sodium nitrite IV solution is available.

5.7 Aspirin (Bayer®, Bufferin®)

Actions

Aspirin is an analgesic, anti-inflammatory, and antipyretic agent, which also appears to inhibit the synthesis and release of prostaglandins. Aspirin also blocks formation of thromboxane A_2 (thromboxane A_2 causes platelets to aggregate and arteries to constrict). Use of aspirin can reduce the overall mortality from acute myocardial infarction.

Indications

Aspirin is indicated in the acute myocardial infarction (AMI) setting to prevent further clotting.

Contraindications

Known allergy to aspirin (e.g., asthma), active GI ulceration or bleeding, hemophilia or other bleeding disorders, during pregnancy, children younger than 2 years of age.

Adverse Reactions and Side Effects

- **GI:** Nausea, vomiting, heartburn, and stomach pain.
- **Otic:** Tinnitus.
- **Hypersensitivity:** Bronchospasm, tightness in chest, angioedema, urticaria, and anaphylaxis.

Dosage

Adult: 162 mg chewable (2 tablets) for AMI. (High doses may interfere with the benefits of aspirin.)

5.8.1 Atropine Sulfate as Cardiac Agent

Actions

Atropine is a potent anticholinergic (parasympathetic blocker, parasympatholytic) agent that reduces vagal tone, thereby increasing automatically the SA node and increasing AV conduction.

Indications

- Sinus bradycardia accompanied by hemodynamic compromise (e.g., hypotension; confusion; frequent PVCs; pale, cold, clammy skin). In infants (< 6 months), bradycardia of less than 80 beats/min should be treated even if BP is normal.
- Asystole.

Contraindications

None in emergency situations.

Adverse Reactions and Side Effects

- **CNS:** Restlessness, agitation, confusion, psychotic reaction, pupil dilation, blurred vision, and headache.
- **Cardiovascular:** Increased heart rate, may worsen ischemia or increase area of infarction, ventricular fibrillation, ventricular tachycardia, angina, flushing of skin.
- **GI:** Dry mouth, difficulty swallowing.
- **Other:** Urinary retention; may worsen preexisting glaucoma.

Warnings

If a too-small dose (< 0.5 mg) is given or if atropine is pushed too slowly, it may initially cause the heart rate to decrease. Antihistamines and antidepressants potentiate the effects of atropine. A maximum dose of 0.04 mg/kg should not be exceeded. For second-degree AV block type II and third-degree AV block, omit atropine and use an external pacer instead.

Dosage

Adult: Bradycardias: 0.5–1 mg IV, or 1–2 mg ET; may repeat every 3–5 minutes until improved or total of 0.04 mg/kg or 3 mg is reached.

Asystole: 1 mg IV or 2 mg ET, repeat every 3–5 minutes to a total dose of 0.04 mg/kg or 3 mg.

Pediatric: 0.02 mg/kg IV or ET (minimum dose = 0.1 mg; maximum single dose = 0.5 mg for a child and 1 mg for an adolescent).

5.8.2 Atropine Sulfate as Antidote for Poisonings

Actions

Atropine is a potent parasympatholytic agent that binds to acetylcholine receptors, thereby diminishing the actions of acetylcholine.

Indications

Anticholinesterase syndrome poisoning, such as with organophosphates (e.g., Parathion, Malathion, Rid-a-Bug) and carbamate (Baygon, Sevin, and many common roach and ant sprays). Signs of organophosphate poisoning are **S**alivation, **L**acrimation, **U**rination, **D**efecation, **G**I distress, **E**mesis—SLUDGE—plus pinpoint pupils, bradycardia, and excessive sweating.

Contraindications

None when used in the management of severe organophosphate poisoning.

Adverse Reactions and Side Effects

Victims of organophosphate poisoning can tolerate large doses (1000 mg) of atropine. Signs of atropinization are the endpoint of treatment: flushing, pupil dilation, dry mouth, and tachycardia.

Warnings

It is important that the patient be adequately oxygenated and ventilated prior to using atropine, as atropine may precipitate ventricular fibrillation in a poorly oxygenated patient. Even after atropine is administered, the patient may require intubation and aggressive ventilatory support.

Dosage

Adult: 0.03 mg/kg IV, repeat q 5–10 minutes until atropinization occurs.

Pediatric: 0.05 mg/kg (maximum dose = 3 mg) IV, repeat q 5–10 minutes until atropinization occurs.

5.9 Calcium Chloride 10%

Actions

Calcium chloride increases the force of myocardial contraction; it may either increase or decrease systemic vascular resistance. In normal hearts, calcium's positive inotropic and vasoconstricting effects produce a predictable rise in systemic arterial pressure.

Indications

Calcium chloride is indicated during resuscitation for the treatment of hypocalcemia and calcium-channel blocker toxicity (e.g., Verapamil or Cardizem overdose) and magnesium sulfate overdose. It also protects the heart from hyperkalemia, which may occur in patients with end-stage renal disease.

Contraindications

Cardiopulmonary arrest not associated with calcium-channel blocker toxicity, hypocalcemia, or hyperkalemia.

Adverse Reactions and Side Effects

If the heart is beating, rapid administration of calcium can produce slowing of the cardiac rate.

Warnings

Calcium chloride should not be administered in the same infusion with sodium bicarbonate, because calcium will combine with sodium bicarbonate to form an insoluble precipitate (calcium carbonate). Calcium chloride should be given with extreme caution, and in reduced dosage, to persons taking digitalis because it increases ventricular irritability and may precipitate digitalis toxicity.

Dosage

Adult: For hypotension following administration of calcium-channel blockers (e.g., Cardizem, Verapamil): 4 mg/kg IV, slowly. If the patient is taking digitalis, 2 mg/kg IV, slowly. Repeat every 10 minutes PRN.

For calcium-channel blocker overdose and hyperkalemia: 8–16 mg/kg IV, slowly.

Pediatric: 5 mg/kg or 0.2 mL/kg IV, slowly, every 10 minutes PRN.

For calcium-channel blocker overdose and hyperkalemia: 20 mg/kg IV, slowly.

5.10 Calcium Gluconate

Actions

Calcium is a basic element that is essential for growth and maintenance of nerve, muscle, and bone tissue. It is necessary for transmission of nerve impulses; contraction of cardiac, smooth, and skeletal muscles; renal function; respirations; and blood clotting. Calcium also plays an important role in the regulation of neurotransmitters, hormones, and amino acid metabolism. Its IV administration improves vascular tone and myocardial contractility in patients in hypocalcemic states. Cardiac output and blood pressure usually increase. In cases of hydrofluoric acid toxicity, calcium binds with fluoride ions, producing calcium fluoride.

Indications

Used in the treatment of hydrofluoric acid burns and magnesium sulfate overdose. Also indicated in the management of black widow spider bites to relieve muscle spasms.

Contraindications

- Absence of hydrofluoric acid burns or magnesium sulfate overdose
- Digitalis toxicity

Adverse Reactions and Side Effects

SQ or IM administration can cause severe tissue necrosis and tissue sloughing. Calcium gluconate can also induce serious cardiac dysrhythmias.

Dosage

Adult: Burns to eyes: Mix calcium gluconate (10%) 50 mL in normal saline 500 mL and wash the eyes with the solution using a Morgan lens.

Burns to skin: Mix calcium gluconate (10%) 10 mL into a 2-oz tube of sterile water-based gel lubricant (KY Jelly). Apply the gel to the burned skin area.

Inhalation: Administer calcium gluconate (10%) 1 mL mixed with normal saline 3 mL via nebulizer. For severe exposure, administer calcium gluconate (10%) 1–2 g via slow IV over 5 minutes.

5.11 Cetacaine® Spray

Actions

Cetacaine produces topical anesthesia rapidly, in approximately 30 seconds.

Indications

Cetacaine is indicated for the production of anesthesia in accessible mucous membranes when control of pain and gagging is needed to facilitate the intubation of a conscious or semiconscious patient.

Contraindications

Cetacaine is not intended for injection. Do not use it on the eyes. Do not apply it to large areas of denuded (open) or inflamed tissue. Do not use Cetacaine under dentures or cotton rolls. Do not use it in cases of known early pregnancy. Do not use it in patients who are known to be hypersensitive to its ingredients (i.e., benzocaine, butyl aminobenzoate, tetracaine hydrochloride, benzalkonium chloride, and cetyl dimethyl ethyl ammonium bromide). Do not spray for more than 2 seconds.

Adverse Reactions and Side Effects

Dehydration of the epithelium or an escharotic effect may result from prolonged contact with Cetacaine. If sprayed longer than 2 seconds, it may cause methemoglobinemia.

Dosage

Cetacaine spray should be applied to the target tissue using a Jelco cannula for approximately 1 second or less. The average expulsion rate of residue from the spray is 200 mg/s. *Do not spray for more than 2 seconds.*

5.12 Dexamethasone (Decadron®)

Actions

Naturally occurring glucocorticoids (hydrocortisone and cortisone), which also have salt-retaining properties, are used as replacement therapy in adrenocortical-deficiency states. Their synthetic analogs, including dexamethasone, are primarily used for their potent anti-inflammatory effects in disorders of many organ systems. Glucocorticoids cause profound and varied metabolic effects. In addition, they modify the body's immune responses to diverse stimuli. At equipotent anti-inflammatory doses, dexamethasone almost completely lacks the sodium-retaining property of hydrocortisone and closely related derivatives of hydrocortisone.

Indications

Control of severe allergic reactions, asthmatic attacks, and bronchospasm associated with COPD.

Contraindications

Known dexamethasone hypersensitivity; neonates; and patients with systemic fungal infections.

Adverse Reactions and Side Effects

- **Cardiovascular:** Fluid retention, hypertension/hypotension, dysrhythmias, CHF electrolyte imbalance.
- **CNS:** Seizures, vertigo, and headache.
- **GI:** Nausea and vomiting, GI bleeding, abdominal distention.

Dosage

Adult: 10 mg IV (or 1–2 mg PO, with a range of 0.75–9 mg total daily dose).

5.13 Dextrose 50% and 25% (Glucose)

Actions

Glucose is a monosaccharide that provides calories for metabolic needs, thereby sparing body proteins and preventing loss of electrolytes. It is readily excreted by the kidneys, producing diuresis. Dextrose is a hypertonic solution.

Indications

Hypoglycemia; coma of unknown origin.

Contraindications

- Intracranial or intraspinal hemorrhage
- DTs with dehydration
- Blood glucose level > 60 mg/dL

Adverse Reactions and Side Effects

- **Cardiovascular:** Thrombosis, sclerosing—if given in a peripheral vein.
- **Local:** Tissue irritation—if infiltration occurs.
- **Other:** Acidosis, alkalosis, hyperglycemia, and hypokalemia.

Warnings

May cause Wernicke-Korsakoff syndrome in acute alcohol intoxication; usually this outcome is prevented by prior administration of thiamine 100 mg IM or IV. Perform a glucose test (if possible) and draw a blood sample (red top tube) prior to administering dextrose.

Dosage

Adult:	(≥ 8 years of age) 50 cc of a 50% solution; (25 g) IV. If conscious, glucose may be given orally (25 g).
Pediatric:	(< 8 years of age) 2 mL/kg slow IV of a 25% solution.
Newborn:	5 mL/kg IV of a 10% solution (dilute D_{50} 4:1 with NS).

5.14 Diazepam Hydrochloride (Valium®)

Actions

A member of the benzodiazepine family, diazepam depresses the limbic system, thalamus, and hypothalamus, resulting in calming effects. Diazepam produces an amnesic effect and is also a muscle relaxant.

Indications

- Status epilepticus
- Premedication prior to cardioversion
- Agitation due to acute alcohol withdrawal
- Short-term relief of acute anxiety
- Cocaine intoxication
- Severe muscle spasm due to acute back strain

Contraindications

- Acute alcohol intoxication
- Pregnancy (except for control of seizures associated with status epilepticus or eclampsia)
- Neonates

Adverse Reactions and Side Effects

- **CNS:** Confusion, muscular weakness, blurred vision, drowsiness, respiratory depression, respiratory arrest, slurred speech.
- **Cardiovascular:** Bradycardia, hypotension, and cardiovascular collapse.
- **GI:** Nausea, vomiting, abdominal discomfort, hiccups.
- **Other:** Potentiates MAOs, barbiturates, tricyclic antidepressants, and phenothiazines; potentiated by cimetidine, ETOH, and other CNS depressants.

Warnings

Do not mix diazepam with any other drug, as it precipitates with almost all medications. When injecting the drug via IV, administer it slowly through the IV tubing, as close as possible to the vein insertion. Do not administer diazepam into small veins such as those on dorsum of the hand, as this causes local irritation and possibly venous thrombosis in small veins.

Dosage

Adult: 5–20 mg IV. The IV route should be administered slowly—no faster than 5 mg/min or 10 mg PR.

Pediatric: For status epilepticus, 0.1–0.2 mg/kg (maximum dose = 10 mg) IV slowly or 0.5 mg/kg (maximum dose = 10 mg) PR.

5.15 Diltiazem Hydrochloride (Cardizem®)

Actions

Diltiazem inhibits the influx of calcium ions during membrane depolarization of cardiac and vascular smooth muscle. The therapeutic benefits of diltiazem in supraventricular tachycardias are related to its ability to slow AV nodal conduction time and prolong AV nodal refractoriness. Diltiazem slows ventricular rates and interrupts the reentry circuit in AV nodal reentrant tachycardias and reciprocating tachycardias (e.g., Wolff-Parkinson-White syndrome). It also prolongs the sinus cycle length and decreases peripheral vascular resistance.

Indications

- Atrial fibrillation or atrial flutter with rapid ventricular response.
- Paroxysmal supraventricular tachycardia. Unless contraindicated, vagal maneuvers should be attempted prior to administration of diltiazem.

Contraindications

- Sick sinus syndrome, except in the presence of a functioning ventricular pacemaker.
- Second- or third-degree AV block, except in the presence of a functioning ventricular pacemaker.
- Severe hypotension or cardiogenic shock.
- Demonstrated hypersensitivity to diltiazem.
- Intravenous diltiazem and intravenous beta blockers should not be administered together or in close proximity (within a few hours).
- Wolff-Parkinson-White syndrome or short PR syndrome.
- Ventricular tachycardia.

Precautions

Diltiazem should be used with caution in patients with impaired liver or renal function. Intravenous diltiazem administered to a patient who is taking oral beta blockers may cause bradycardia, AV block, and/or depression of contractility. Caution should be used when administering diltiazem and anesthetics. Caution should also be used in pregnant females and mothers who are nursing. Use with caution if administered in the presence of CHF.

5.15 Diltiazem Hydrochloride (Cardizem®)

Adverse Reactions and Side Effects

Hypotension, itching or burning at the injection site, flushing of skin, or junctional rhythm. Other side effects are less frequently encountered (e.g., AV blocks, atrial flutter, chest pain).

Dosage

Adult: 0.25 mg/kg IV (over 2 minutes). May repeat at 0.35 mg/kg IV (over 2 minutes), if needed.

5.16 Diphenhydramine Hydrochloride (Benadryl®)

Actions

Diphenhydramine is an antihistamine with anticholinergic (drying) and sedative side effects. Antihistamines appear to compete with histamine for cell receptor sites on effector cells. Diphenhydramine prevents, but does not reverse, histamine-mediated responses—particularly histamine effects on the smooth muscle of the bronchial airways, gastrointestinal tract, uterus, and blood vessels.

Indications

- Allergy symptoms, anaphylaxis (as an adjunct to epinephrine)
- Sedation of a violent patient
- Dystonic reactions from phenothiazine overdose (e.g., Haldol, Compazine, Thorazine, and Stelazine)
- Rhinitis
- Anti-Parkinsonism syndrome
- Nighttime sedation
- Motion sickness

Contraindications

Diphenhydramine is not to be used in newborn or premature infants or in nursing mothers. It is also not to be used in patients with lower respiratory tract symptoms, including asthma.

Adverse Reactions and Side Effects

- **CNS:** Drowsiness, confusion, insomnia, headache, vertigo (all especially in the elderly).
- **Cardiovascular:** Palpitations, tachycardia, PVCs and hypotension.
- **Respiratory:** Thickening of bronchial secretions, tightness of the chest, wheezing, nasal stuffiness.
- **GI:** Nausea, vomiting, diarrhea, dry mouth, and constipation.
- **GU:** Dysuria, urinary retention.

5.16 Diphenhydramine Hydrochloride (Benadryl®)

Warnings

- In infants and children especially, antihistamines in overdose may cause hallucinations, convulsions, or death.
- As in adults, antihistamines may diminish mental alertness in children. In young children, they may produce excitation.
- Diphenhydramine has additive effects with alcohol and other CNS depressants (e.g., hypnotics, sedatives, tranquilizers).
- Antihistamines are more likely to cause dizziness, sedation, and hypotension in elderly patients (60 years or older).

Dosage

Adult: 25–50 mg IV or 50 mg deep IM. The patient may require as much as 100 mg. Do not exceed 400 mg per day.

Pediatric: 1 mg/kg (maximum dose = 50 mg). Dilute with 9 mL NS to equal 50 mg/10 mL. Not to exceed 300 mg per day.

5.17 Dopamine Hydrochloride (Intropin®)

Actions

Dopamine stimulates dopaminergic beta-adrenergic and alpha-adrenergic receptors of the sympathetic nervous system. It exerts an inotropic effect on the myocardium, resulting in an increased cardiac output. Dopamine produces less increase in myocardial oxygen consumption than does isoproterenol, and its use is rarely associated with tachyarrhythmia. Dopamine dilates renal and mesenteric blood vessels at low doses that may not increase heart rate or blood pressure. Therapeutic doses have predominant beta-adrenergic receptor-stimulating actions that result in increases in cardiac output without marked increases in pulmonary occlusive pressure. At high doses, dopamine has alpha-receptor stimulating actions that result in peripheral vasoconstriction and marked increases in pulmonary occlusive pressure.

Indications

To treat shock and correct hemodynamic imbalances, improve perfusion to vital organs, and increase cardiac output.

Contraindications

Dopamine should not be used in patients with pheochromocytoma or hypovolemic shock.

Adverse Reactions and Side Effects

- **CNS:** Headache.
- **Cardiovascular:** Ectopic beats, tachycardia, anginal pain, palpitations, hypotension.
- **GI:** Nausea, vomiting.
- **Local:** Necrosis and tissue sloughing with extravasation.
- **Other:** Piloerection, dyspnea.

5.17 Dopamine Hydrochloride (Intropin®)

Warnings

Do not administer dopamine in the presence of uncorrected tachydysrhythmias or ventricular fibrillation. Do not add dopamine to any alkaline diluent solution, because the drug is inactivated in alkaline solution.

Patients who have been treated with monoamine oxidase (MAO) inhibitors will require substantially reduced dosage. MAO inhibitors include the following agents:

- Furazolidone (Furoxone)
- Isocarboxazid (Marplan)
- Pargyline hydrochloride (Eutonyl)
- Pargyline hydrochloride with methyclothiazide (Eutron)
- Phenelzine sulfate (Nardil)
- Procarbazine hydrochloride (Matulane)
- Tranylcypromine sulfate (Parnate)

Dosage

Adult: Mix dopamine in D_5W to yield a concentration of 800 or 1600 mcg/mL. Begin the infusion at 5 mcg/kg/min and titrate to effect (maximum dose = 20 mcg/kg/min).

no — child dose

5.18.1 Epinephrine 1:1000

Actions

Epinephrine is a sympathomimetic agent that stimulates both alpha- and beta-adrenergic receptors, causing immediate bronchodilation, increase in heart rate, and increase in the force of cardiac contraction. The effects of a subcutaneous dose last 5–15 minutes.

Indications

- Asthma
- Anaphylaxis
- Angioneurotic edema
- Cardiac arrest when high-dose epinephrine is used

Contraindications

Hyperthyroidism, hypertension, cerebral arteriosclerosis in asthma. Epinephrine should not be administered in elderly or debilitated patients with underlying cardiovascular disease. In the setting of anaphylaxis, however, there are no contraindications.

Adverse Reactions and Side Effects

Same as for epinephrine 1:10,000 (see Drug Summary 5.18.2).

Warnings

Same as for epinephrine 1:10,000 (see Drug Summary 5.18.2). Epinephrine 1:1000 also causes hyperglycemia. With the exception of cardiac arrest cases, epinephrine 1:1000 should not be given intravenously; it should be diluted first (1 mg in 9 mL of NS = 1:10,000 or 1 mg/10 mL).

Dosage

Adult: 0.3 (0.3–0.5 cc) subcutaneously; may be repeated every 15 minutes × 3. If the patient in anaphylaxis is hypotensive, start an IV and administer 3 cc of a 1:10,000 solution via slow IV.

Pediatric: 0.01 mg/kg, up to 0.3 mg subcutaneously. Epinephrine (1:1000) is also given in a dosage of 0.1 mg/kg IV or ET as a cardiac agent.

5.18.2 Epinephrine 1:10,000

Actions

Epinephrine is a sympathomimetic agent that stimulates both alpha- and beta-adrenergic receptors. As a result of its effects, myocardial and cerebral blood flows are increased during ventilation and chest compression. Epinephrine increases systemic vascular resistance and, therefore, may enhance defibrillation.

Indications

Asystole, ventricular fibrillation unresponsive to defibrillation, PEA. Other pediatric indications: hypotension in patients with circulatory instability, bradycardia (before use of atropine).

Contraindications

None in the cardiac arrest situation.

Adverse Reactions and Side Effects

- **CNS:** Anxiety, headache, cerebral hemorrhage.
- **Cardiovascular:** Tachycardia, ventricular dysrhythmias, hypertension, angina, palpitations.
- **GI:** Nausea and vomiting.

Warnings

Epinephrine is inactivated by alkaline solutions—never mix it with sodium bicarbonate. Do not mix isoproterenol and epinephrine, as this combination results in exaggerated response. The action of catecholamines is depressed by acidosis; attention to ventilation and circulation is essential. Antidepressants potentiate the effects of epinephrine.

Dosage

Adult: IV push (1:10,000): 1 mg (10 mL) IV; repeat every 3–5 minutes.

ETT (1:1000): 2 mg (2 mL diluted with 8 mL of NS) ET; repeat every 3–5 minutes.

Pressor infusion: 1 mg/250 mL D_5W; start at 1 mcg/min and titrate to effect.

Pediatric: 0.01 mg/kg (0.1 mL/kg IV or IO); repeat every 3–5 minutes.

Use epinephrine (1:1000) 0.1 mg/kg (maximum dose = 2 mL) any time it is given via ET.

5.19 Etomidate (Amidate®)

Actions

Etomidate is a short-acting, nonbarbiturate hypnotic, which lacks the analgesic properties and is used for induction of general anesthesia. Its action occurs at the level of the reticular activating system in the brain stem. Etomidate is generally considered to have minimal adverse effects on cardiac and respiratory function. The duration of action is 3–5 minutes, and excretion occurs through the renal system.

Indications

An **authorized paramedic** may induce general anesthesia to facilitate intubation.

Precautions

Etomidate causes respiratory paralysis; supportive airway control must be continuous and under direct observation at all times. Etomidate can decrease the adrenal gland's production of steroid hormones. Use caution, as this agent may act synergistically with other CNS depressants. Monitoring of vital signs is important.

Adverse Reactions and Side Effects

The most common side effects are nausea and vomiting. Etomidate can also cause uncontrolled skeletal muscle activity. Unstable blood pressures, dyspnea, and chronotropic dysrhythmias are possible as well.

Dosage

Adult and Pediatric (> 10 years of age):	0.2–0.6 mg/kg slow administration (about 1 minute) IV.

5.20 Fentanyl

Actions

Fentanyl is similar to morphine and meperidine in its respiratory effects, except that respiration of healthy individuals returns to normal more quickly after fentanyl. This agent exhibits little hypnotic activity and histamine release rarely occurs.

Indications

For relief of moderate to severe pain.

Contraindications

Patients with known hypersensitivity to hydromorphone, intracranial lesions associated with increased ICP, depressed ventilatory function (e.g., COPD, cor pulmonale, emphysema, kyphoscoliosis, and status asthmaticus).

Adverse Reactions and Side Effects

- **CNS:** Sedation, drowsiness, mental clouding, lethargy, impairment of mental and physical performance, anxiety, fear, dysphoria, dizziness, psychic dependence, and mood changes.
- **Cardiovascular:** Circulatory depression, peripheral circulatory collapse, and cardiac arrest have occurred following rapid administration. Orthostatic hypotension and fainting may occur if the patient stands up following injection.
- **GI:** Nausea and vomiting, constipation.
- **Respiratory:** Respiratory depression.

Warnings

The concomitant use of other CNS depressants—including other opioids, sedatives or hypnotics, general anesthetics, phenolthiazines, tranquilizers, skeletal muscle relaxants, sedating antihistamines, potent inhibitors of P450 (e.g., erythromycin, ketoconazole, and certain protease inhibitors), and alcoholic beverages—may produce increased depressant effects. Hypoventilation, hypotension, and profound sedation may occur.

Dosage

2 mcg/kg via very slow IV. Standing starting dosage is 250 mcg. Maintain systolic BP > 90 mm Hg.

5.21 Furosemide (Lasix®)

Actions

Furosemide is a sulfonamide derivative and potent diuretic that inhibits the reabsorption of sodium and chloride in the proximal and distal renal tubules as well as in the loop of Henle. It has a direct venodilating effect in acute pulmonary edema. With IV administration, onset of venodilation generally occurs within 5–10 minutes; diuresis will usually occur in 20–30 minutes.

Indications

- Pulmonary edema
- Hypertension
- Cerebral edema

Contraindications

Anuria. Furosemide should be used in pregnancy only when its benefits clearly outweigh the risks.

Adverse Reactions and Side Effects

- **CNS:** Dizziness, tinnitus, hearing loss, headache, blurred vision, weakness.
- **GI:** Anorexia, vomiting, nausea.
- **Cardiovascular:** Hypotension.
- **Other:** Pruritus, urticaria, muscle cramping.

Warnings

Furosemide should be protected from light. Dehydration and electrolyte imbalance can result from excessive dosages. Rapid diuresis can lead to hypotension and thromboembolic episodes.

Dosage

Adult: 0.5–1.0 mg/kg IV slowly over 1–2 minutes (40–80 mg).

Pediatric: 0.5–1.0 mg/kg IV slowly over 1–2 minutes.

5.22 Glucagon

Actions

Glucagon, which is produced naturally in the pancreas by the alpha cells of the islets of Langerhans, causes an increase in blood glucose concentrations. It is effective in small doses, and no evidence of toxicity has been reported with its use. Glucagon acts only on liver glycogen, converting it to glucose if the patient has adequate glycogen reserves. Also, glucagon possesses positive inotropic and chronotropic properties.

Indications

Glucagon is indicated for the treatment of hypoglycemia when an IV cannot be established and oral glucose is contraindicated. It may also be effective in symptomatic beta-blocker overdose.

Contraindications

Because glucagon is a protein, hypersensitivity is a possibility.

Adverse Reactions and Side Effects

Occasional nausea and vomiting.

Warnings

Glucagon should be administered with caution in patients with a history of insulinoma and/or pheochromocytoma.

Dosage

Adult: 0.5–1.0 unit (or 0.5–1.0 mg) of glucagon IM (or IV). This can be repeated twice.

If administered via IV: only compatible with D_5W.

Incompatible with normal saline and LR—NaCl, KCl, CaCl.

May require very high IV doses for beta-blocker overdose (8–10 mg IV).

Pediatric: 0.025 unit/kg (mg/kg). Not as effective in children as in adults.

5.23 Haloperidol (Haldol®)

Actions

Haloperidol is a potent, long-acting butyrophenone derivative. It has pharmacologic actions similar to those of piperazine phenothiazines, but is associated with higher incidence of extrapyramidal effects, less hypotension, and relatively low sedative activity. It exerts a strong antiemetic effect; it also impairs central thermoregulation. Haloperidol produces weak central anticholinergic effects and transient orthostatic hypotension. Its actions are thought to be due to blockade of dopamine activity.

Indications

Used for management of manifestations of psychotic disorders and for the treatment of agitated states in acute and chronic psychoses.

Contraindications

Hypersensitivity to haloperidol, Parkinson's disease, seizure disorders, coma, alcoholism, severe mental depression, CNS depression, thyrotoxicosis, and cocaine overdose.

Adverse Reactions and Side Effects

- **CNS:** Parkinson-like symptoms, restlessness, lethargy, headache, exacerbation of psychotic symptoms.
- **Cardiovascular:** Tachycardia, hypotension, hypertension (with overdose).
- **GI:** Nausea, vomiting.
- **Other:** Bronchospasm, laryngospasm, respiratory depression, dry mouth, hypersalivation ("drooling").

Warnings

Use with caution in patients with severe cardiovascular disorders (may cause transient hypotension and/or precipitation of anginal pain), receiving anticonvulsant medication (may lower the convulsive threshold), or with a history of allergic reactions to drugs.

Dosage

Adult: 5–10 mg IM.

5.24 Hydromorphone Hydrochloride

Actions

Hydromorphone hydrochloride is a hydrogenated ketone of morphine, an opiate-type analgesic.

Indications

Indicated for the relief of moderate to severe pain.

Contraindications

Patients with known hypersensitivity to hydromorphone, intracranial lesions associated with increased ICP, depressed ventilatory function (e.g., COPD, cor pulmonale, emphysema, kyphoscoliosis, and status asthmaticus).

Adverse Reactions and Side Effects

- **CNS:** Sedation, drowsiness, mental clouding, lethargy, impairment of mental and physical performance, anxiety, fear, dysphoria, dizziness, psychic dependence and mood changes.
- **Cardiovascular:** Circulatory depressions, peripheral circulatory collapse, and cardiac arrest have occurred following rapid administration. Orthostatic hypotension and fainting may occur if a patient stands up following an injection.
- **GI:** Nausea and vomiting, constipation.
- **Respiratory:** Respiratory depression.

Warnings

Use with caution in elderly patients or patients with impaired renal or hepatic function, hypothyroidism, Addison's disease, prostatic hypertrophy, or urethral stricture. Maintain vigilance for the patient's respirations.

Dosage

1 mg given by very slow IV push; may repeat in 5 minutes and titrate to pain relief. Maintain systolic BP > 90 mm Hg. Can be given IM.

5.25 Hydroxocobalamin (Cyanokit®)

Actions

The action of hydroxocobalamin in the treatment of cyanide poisoning is based on its ability to bind to cyanide ions. Each hydroxocobalamin molecule can bind one cyanide ion by substituting it for the hydroxo ligand linked to the trivalent cobalt ion, thereby forming cyanocobalamin, which is then excreted in urine.

Indications

Hydroxocobalamin is indicated for known or suspected cyanide poisoning. Cyanide poisoning may result from inhalation, ingestion, or dermal exposure to various cyanide-containing compounds, including smoke from closed-space fires. Sources of cyanide poisoning include hydrogen cyanide and its salts, cyanogenic plants, aliphatic nitriles, and prolonged exposure to sodium nitroprusside.

The presence and extent of cyanide poisonings are often initially unknown. There is no widely available, rapid confirmatory cyanide blood test. Treatment decisions must be made on the basis of clinical history and signs and symptoms of cyanide intoxication. If clinical suspicion of cyanide poisoning is high, hydroxocobalamin should be administered without delay.

Common Signs and Symptoms of Cyanide Poisoning

Symptoms	Signs
Headache	Altered mental status (e.g., confusion, disorientation)
Confusion	Seizures or coma
Dyspnea	Mydriasis
Chest tightness	Tachypnea/hyperpnea (early)
Nausea	Bradypnea/apnea (late)
	Hypertension (early) / hypotension (late)
	Cardiovascular collapse
	Vomiting
	Plasma lactate concentration $\geq$ 8 mmol/L

5.25 Hydroxocobalamin (Cyanokit®)

Contraindications

None.

Adverse Reactions and Side Effects

Serious adverse reactions include allergic reactions and increased blood pressure. Other side effects include:

- Red-colored urine
- Red-colored skin and mucous membranes, acne-like rash
- Nausea, vomiting, diarrhea, bloody stools, trouble swallowing, stomach pain
- Throat tightness, dry throat
- Headache, dizziness, memory problems, restlessness
- Infusion site reaction
- Eye swelling, irritation, or redness
- Swelling of feet and ankles
- Irregular heartbeat, increased heart rate
- Fluid in lungs

Warnings

In addition to hydroxocobalamin, treatment of cyanide poisoning must include immediate attention to airway patency, adequacy of oxygenation and hydration, cardiovascular support, and management of any seizure activity. Consideration should be given to decontamination measures based on the route of exposure.

Many patients with cyanide poisoning will be hypotensive; however, elevations in blood pressure have also been observed in known or suspected cyanide poisoning victims.

Dosage

Adult: 5 g (i.e., both 2.5-g vials) administered as an IV infusion over 15 minutes (approximately 15 mL/min)—that is, 7.5 min/vial. Depending on the severity of the poisoning and the clinical response, a second dose of 5 g may be administered by IV infusion for a total dose of 10 g. The rate of infusion for the second dose may range from 15 minutes (for patients in extremis) to 2 hours, as clinically indicated.

Pediatric: The safety and effectiveness of hydroxocobalamin have not been established in this population. In non-U.S. marketing experience, a dose of 70 mg/kg has been used to treat pediatric patients.

5.26 Ipratropium Bromide (Atrovent®)

Actions

Ipratropium bromide is an anticholinergic (parasympatholytic) agent, which causes localized bronchodilation.

Indications

Ipratropium bromide is indicated for relief of bronchospasms associated with asthma and chronic obstructive pulmonary disease, including chronic bronchitis and emphysema that is unresponsive to treatment with albuterol alone.

Contraindications

Hypersensitivity to atropine or its derivatives.

Adverse Reactions and Side Effects

- **Respiratory:** Cough, exacerbation of symptoms.
- **CNS:** Nervousness, dizziness, headache.
- **Cardiovascular:** Palpitations.
- **GI:** Nausea, vomiting, GI distress.
- **Other:** Tremor, dry mouth, blurred vision.

Warnings

Ipratropium bromide is not indicated for the initial treatment of acute episodes of bronchospasms where rapid response is required.

Dosage

Adult: Add 0.5 mg (0.5 mL) of Atrovent to the nebulizer (in addition to the standard dose of albuterol) and flow oxygen at 6–8 L/min.

Pediatric: If patient < 8 years, add 0.25 mg (0.25 mL); if patient > 8 years, add 0.5 mg (0.5 mL) of Atrovent to the nebulizer (in addition to the pediatric dose of albuterol) and flow oxygen at 6–8 L/min.

5.27 Ketorolac Tromethamine (Toradol®)

Actions

Ketorolac tromethamine is a nonsteroidal anti-inflammatory drug (NSAID) with peripheral analgesic, anti-inflammatory, and antipyretic actions. This action is due to inhabitation of prostaglandin synthesis. The drug does not have any known effect on opiate receptors, but has 300 times the analgesic effect of aspirin. A 30-mg IM dose is similar in analgesic efficacy to 8–10 mg of morphine sulfate.

Indications

Relief of moderate to severe pain; useful in renal colic and acute back strain.

Contraindications

- Potential surgical candidate (e.g., trauma patient)
- Known allergy to NSAIDs (e.g., aspirin, ibuprofen)
- History of nasal polyps
- Angioedema
- Bronchospastic reactivity (e.g., asthma)
- Bleeding disorders (e.g., ulcers)
- Kidney dysfunction

Precautions

Ketorolac tromethamine inhibits platelet aggregation and may prolong bleeding time.

Adverse Reactions and Side Effects

Headache, drowsiness, dizziness, nausea, diarrhea, itching, rash, and any side effects common to the NSAID class medications.

Dosage

Adult: With BP > 90 mm Hg, administer 30 mg IV or 60 mg IM.
If patient > 65 years, limit the dose to 15 mg IV or 30 mg IM.

5.28 Labetalol Hydrochloride (Normodyne®, Trandate®)

Actions

Labetalol combines both selective, competitive $alpha_1$-adrenergic blocking and nonselective, competitive beta-adrenergic blocking activity in a single substance. These actions decrease blood pressure without reflex tachycardia and without a significant reduction in heart rate.

Indications

Control of blood pressure in severe hypertension.

Contraindications

- Bronchial asthma
- Overt cardiac failure
- Greater than first-degree heart block
- Cardiogenic shock
- Severe bradycardia

Adverse Reactions and Side Effects

- **Cardiovascular:** Symptomatic postural hypotension, ventricular dysrhythmia, and rarely syncope, bradycardia, and heart block.
- **CNS:** Dizziness, tingling of the scalp/skin, numbness, vertigo.
- **Respiratory:** Wheezing.
- **GI:** Nausea/vomiting.

Dosage

Adult: 20 mg slow (over 2 minutes) IV.

5.29.1 Lidocaine Hydrochloride (Xylocaine®) 1% and 2%

Actions

Decreases ventricular automaticity and raises the ventricular fibrillation threshold.

Indications

- Ventricular tachycardia
- Ventricular fibrillation

Contraindications

- Second-degree AV block, Mobitz II and third-degree AV block.
- Stokes-Adams syndrome.
- If PVCs occur in conjunction with sinus bradycardia, the bradycardia should be treated first.
- Ventricular dysrhythmias associated with tricyclic antidepressant overdose.

Adverse Reactions and Side Effects

- **CNS:** Drowsiness, numbness, dizziness, blurred vision, tinnitus, euphoria, muscle twitching convulsions, tremors.
- **Cardiovascular:** Rare, but with toxic levels, hypotension, widening of QRS complex, bradycardia, and cardiac arrest can occur.
- **Respiratory:** At toxic levels, respiratory depression and/or arrest.

Dosage

Adult: (Use 2%) 1–1.5 mg/kg IV bolus; repeat with 0.5–0.75 mg/kg 5–10 minutes if necessary, to a total of 3 mg/kg; repeat every 3 minutes for ventricular ectopy. Can also be administered ET or IM followed by an infusion at 2–4 mg/min.

Pediatric: (Use 1%) 1 mg/kg IV bolus.

5.29.2 Lidocaine Hydrochloride (Xylocaine®) 4%, 10%, and 20%

Actions

Decreases ventricular automaticity and raises the ventricular fibrillation threshold.

Indications

Same as for 1% and 2% lidocaine (see Drug Summary 5.29.1). Used as a maintenance infusion.

Contraindications

Same as for 1% and 2% lidocaine (see Drug Summary 5.29.1).

Adverse Reactions and Side Effects

Same as for 1% and 2% lidocaine (see Drug Summary 5.29.1).

Warnings

Lidocaine is metabolized in the liver. The maintenance dosage should be cut in half in patients with liver disease and low cardiac output states (e.g., acute MI, shock, congestive heart failure), and in patients older than 70 years.

Dosage

Adult: Mix 1000 mg in 250 mL of D_5W and flow at 1–4 mg/min as follows:

- 1 mg/kg total bolus dose = 2 mg/min (30 gtts/min).
- 1.5–2 mg/kg total bolus dose = 3 mg/min (45 gtts/min).
- 2.5–3 mg/kg total bolus dose = 4 mg/min (60 gtts/min).

Pediatric: Mix 120 mg in 100 mL of D_5W (or 60 mg in 50 mL of D_5W) and flow at 20–50 mcg/kg/min.

5.29.3 Lidocaine Hydrochloride (Xylocaine®) 2% Jelly

Actions

Lubricant and topical anesthetic.

Indications

For lubrication and topical anesthesia as an aid to nasotracheal and orotracheal intubation in the conscious patient.

Contraindications

Same as for 1% and 2% lidocaine (see Drug Summary 5.29.1).

Adverse Reactions and Side Effects

Same as for 1% and 2% lidocaine (see Drug Summary 5.29.1).

Dosage

Apply to the laryngoscope blade and distal end of the endotracheal tube PRN.

5.29.4 Lidocaine Hydrochloride (Xylocaine®) 10% Spray

Actions

Topical anesthetic.

Indications

For topical anesthesia as an aid to nasotracheal and orotracheal intubation in the conscious patient.

Contraindications

Same as for 1% and 2% lidocaine (see Drug Summary 5.29.1).

Adverse Reactions and Side Effects

Same as for 1% and 2% lidocaine (see Drug Summary 5.29.1).

Dosage

Spray in the patient's oropharynx and nasopharynx PRN.

5.30 Lorazepam (Ativan®)

Actions

Lorazepam is a benzodiazepine, so it depresses the central nervous system. It produces sedation, relieves anxiety, causes lack of recall, and provides for relief of skeletal muscle spasms.

Indications

- Adjunct to seizure control
- Control of violent patients

Contraindications

Known sensitivity to benzodiazepines; narrow-angle glaucoma.

Precautions

May cause respiratory depression.

Adverse Reactions and Side Effects

- **CNS:** Excessive CNS depression.
- **Cardiovascular:** Rarely hypotension/hypertension.
- **Respiratory:** Hypoventilation, partial airway obstruction.
- **Local:** Pain, burning, and redness at injection site.
- **General:** Nausea/vomiting and skin rash.

Dosage

Adult: 1–2 mg IV or IM.

5.31 Magnesium Sulfate

Actions

Magnesium is an important cofactor for enzymatic reactions and plays an important role in neurochemical transmission and muscular excitability. Magnesium prevents or controls convulsions by blocking neuromuscular transmission and decreasing the amount of acetylcholine liberated at the end-plate by the motor nerve impulse. It is said to have a depressant effect on the central nervous system, but it does not affect the mother, fetus, or neonate when used as directed in eclampsia and pre-eclampsia. Magnesium acts peripherally to produce vasodilatation.

Indications

- Parenteral anticonvulsant for the prevention and control of seizures in severe toxemia of pregnancy.
- Torsades de pointes.
- Suspected hypomagnesemic state (e.g., chronic alcoholism and chronic use of diuretics).
- Refractory ventricular fibrillation.

Precautions

Because magnesium is removed from the body solely by the kidneys, this drug should be used with caution in patients with renal impairment. Monitoring magnesium serum levels and the patient's clinical status is essential to avoid the consequences of overdose and toxemia. Clinical indications that it is safe to give magnesium to the patient include the presence of a patellar reflex (knee jerk) and the absence of respiratory depression (approximately 16 breaths or more per minute). Calcium chloride should be immediately available to counteract the potential hazards of magnesium intoxication in eclampsia.

5.31 Magnesium Sulfate

Adverse Reactions and Side Effects

Adverse effects of magnesium sulfate IV are usually the result of magnesium intoxication. Signs of hypermagnesemia include flushing, sweating, hypotension, depression of reflexes, flaccid paralysis, hypothermia, circulatory collapse, depression of cardiac function, and central nervous system depression. These symptoms can precede fatal paralysis.

Warnings

Magnesium sulfate should not be given intravenously to mothers with toxemia of pregnancy during the 2 hours immediately preceding delivery. Magnesium sulfate injection USP, 50%, must be diluted to a concentration of 20% or less prior to IV infusion.

Dosage

For eclamptic seizures:	4 gm IV (mixed in 50 mL of D_5W and administered over 5–10 minutes). May repeat once at 2 g IV (mixed in 50 mL of D_5W and administered over 5–10 minutes).
For torsades de pointes and refractory VF:	1–2 g IV (mixed in 50 mL of D_5W and administered over 1–2 minutes), followed by a maintenance infusion (1 g in 250 mL of D_5W administered at 30–60 gtts/min).

5.32 Methylene Blue

Actions

Low concentrations of methylene blue will convert methemoglobin to hemoglobin (methemoglobin is toxic and gives the blood a chocolate-brown color; it does not carry oxygen). High concentrations convert ferrous iron of hemoglobin to ferric iron, thereby forming methemoglobin.

Indications

Initial treatment of methemoglobinemia.

Contraindications

Renal insufficiency (excreted in urine and bile).

Adverse Reactions and Side Effects

Cyanosis, profuse sweating, dizziness, headache, nausea, vomiting, diarrhea (turns urine and stool blue-green). May induce hemolysis in patients deficient in glucose-6-phosphate dehydrogenase.

Dosage

1 mg/kg of a 1% solution. Very slow IV push of 1 mL (10 mg) every 5 minutes.

5.33 Methylprednisolone Sodium Succinate (Solu-Medrol®)

Actions

Methylprednisolone sodium succinate is a potent anti-inflammatory synthetic steroid.

Indications

Control of severe allergic reactions, asthmatic attacks, and bronchospasm associated with COPD that do not respond to other treatments.

Contraindications

Known hypersensitivity, neonates, and patients with systemic fungal infections.

Adverse Reactions and Side Effects

- **Cardiovascular:** Fluid retention, hypertension/hypotension, dysrhythmias, CHF, electrolyte imbalance.
- **CNS:** Seizures, vertigo, headache.
- **GI:** Nausea/vomiting, GI bleeding, abdominal distention.
- **General:** Urticaria, anaphylactic reaction.

Dosage

Adult: Bronchospasm associated with asthma, COPD, or severe allergic reactions: 125 mg IV.

Pediatric: Bronchospasm associated with asthma or severe allergic reaction: 2 mg/kg IV (maximum dose = 125 mg).

5.34 Metoprolol (Lopressor®)

Actions

Metoprolol is a beta-adrenergic receptor-blocking agent.

Indications

Metoprolol tartrate injection is indicated in the treatment of hemodynamically stable patients with definite or suspected acute myocardial infarction to reduce cardiovascular mortality.

Contraindications

Known hypersensitivity; narrow-angle glaucoma. Metoprolol is contraindicated in patients with a heart rate < 45 beats per minute; second- and third-degree heart block; significant first-degree heart block (p-r interval ≥ 0.24 seconds); systolic blood pressure < 100 mm Hg; or moderate to severe cardiac failure.

Precautions

Metoprolol should be used with caution in patients with impaired hepatic function.

Adverse Reactions and Side Effects

- **Respiratory:** Dyspnea has been reported in fewer than 1 of 100 patients.
- **Cardiovascular:** Intensification of AV block.
- **CNS:** Reversable depression, acute reversible disorientation, short term memory loss.
- **GI:** Nausea and abdominal pain has been reported in fewer than 1 of 100 patients.
- **Hypersensitive Reactions:** Fever combined with aching and sore throat, laryngospasm, and respiratory distress.

Dosage

- If ST Elevation MI (STEMI) is identified with signs, symptoms, and history suggestive of AMI and patient has a heart rate > 80 with an SBP > 110 mm Hg, administer Lopressor 5 mg slow IVP. Consider repeating once in 5 minutes if heart rate > 80 and SBP > 110 mm Hg.

5.35 Midazolam (Versed®)

Actions

Midazolam is a short-acting benzodiazepine (a central nervous system depressant) that produces sedation and lack of recall.

Indications

Conscious sedation as an adjunct to cardioversion and intubation.

Contraindications

Known hypersensitivity; narrow-angle glaucoma.

Precautions

Midazolam does not protect against the increase in intracranial pressure and bradycardia associated with multiple intubation attempts.

Adverse Reactions and Side Effects

- **Respiratory:** Respiratory depression, laryngospasm, bronchospasm, dyspnea.
- **Cardiovascular:** PVCs, bradycardia, tachycardia, nodal rhythms, hypotension.
- **CNS:** Retrograde amnesia, altered mental status, dizziness, prolonged emergence from anesthesia.
- **GI:** Nausea/vomiting, hiccoughs, coughing.
- **Local:** Pain, redness, swelling, burning at injection site.

Dosage

Adult: Sedation and seizures: 2 mg (0.03 mg/kg) IV, slowly; may repeat once.

Nonparalytic RSI: 20 mg (0.3 mg/kg) IV, slowly.

5.36 Morphine Sulfate (MS)

Actions

Morphine is a narcotic analgesic. It depresses the central nervous system and decreases sensitivity to pain. It increases venous capacitance, decreases venous return, and produces mild peripheral vasodilatation. Morphine also decreases myocardial oxygen demand.

Indications

- Pain from acute myocardial infarction
- Pulmonary edema
- Pain associated with isolated extremity fracture, renal colic, or burns

Contraindications

- Pain due to trauma or acute abdomen (except isolated extremity trauma or burns)
- Volume depletion or hypotension
- Head trauma
- Acute alcoholism
- Acute asthma
- Known hypersensitivity to MS

Adverse Reactions and Side Effects

- **CNS:** Euphoria, drowsiness, pupillary constriction, respiratory arrest.
- **Cardiovascular:** Bradycardia, hypotension.
- **GI:** Decreased gastric motility, nausea and vomiting.
- **GU:** Urinary retention.
- **Respiratory:** Bronchoconstriction, decreased cough reflex.

5.36 Morphine Sulfate (MS)

Warnings

Morphine is detoxified by the liver. It is potentiated by alcohol, antihistamines, barbiturates, sedatives, and beta blockers.

Dosage

Adult: 2–10 mg IV slowly. Repeat with small increments every 5 minutes until desired response is achieved (maximum dose = 10 mg). Can also be given IM or SC.

Pediatric: 0.1–0.2 mg/kg IV slowly.

Infant: 0.05–0.1 mg/kg IV slowly.

5.37 Naloxone Hydrochloride (Narcan®)

Actions

The mechanism of action for naloxone hydrochloride is not fully understood. It does appear that this agent antagonizes the effects of opiates by competing at the same receptor sites. When given IV, the action is apparent within 2 minutes. Effects appear slightly more slowly with IM or SC administration.

Indications

Naloxone is indicated for the complete or partial reversal of opiate narcotic depression and respiratory depression secondary to opiate narcotics or related drugs:

- Heroin
- Meperidine (Demerol)
- Codeine
- Morphine
- Methadone
- Lomotil
- Hydromorphone (Dilaudid)
- Pentazocine (Talwin)
- Propoxyphene (Darvon)
- Percodan
- Fentanyl (Sublimaze; known on the street as "white china")

Naloxone can also be used for suspected acute opiate overdosage.

Contraindications

Naloxone is contraindicated in patients known to be hypersensitive to it.

Adverse Reactions and Side Effects

- **CNS:** Tremor, agitation, belligerence, pupillary dilation, seizures, increased tear production, sweating, seizures secondary to withdrawal.
- **Cardiovascular:** Hypertension, hypotension, ventricular tachycardia, pulmonary edema, ventricular fibrillation.
- **GI:** Nausea, vomiting.

5.37 Naloxone Hydrochloride (Narcan®)

Warnings

Naloxone should be administered cautiously to persons (including newborns of mothers) who are known or suspected to be physically dependent on opiates; it may precipitate an acute abstinence syndrome in these individuals. Naloxone administration may need to be repeated in this scenario because the duration of action of some narcotics may exceed that of naloxone. Naloxone is not effective against a respiratory depression caused by non-opiate drugs. Use caution during its administration because patients may become violent as their level of consciousness increases.

Dosage

Adult: An initial dose of 2 mg may be administered IV, IM, SC, or ET; may repeat in 2–3 minutes.

If no response after 10 mg, then condition is probably not due to narcotic. Fentanyl may require large doses of naloxone to reverse fentanyl's effects.

Pediatric: 0.1 mg/kg IV, IM, IO, ET, or SC; may repeat with 0.1 mg/kg if no improvement is noted.

5.38.1 Nitroglycerin (Nitrostat®, Nitrolingual® Spray)

Actions

Nitroglycerin is a direct vasodilator that acts principally on the venous system, although it also produces direct coronary artery vasodilation. Its use decreases venous return, which in turn decreases the workload on the heart, and thereby decreases myocardial oxygen demand. Sublingual nitroglycerin is readily absorbed. Pain relief occurs within 1–2 minutes and therapeutic effects can last as long as 30 minutes.

Indications

- Chest pain or discomfort associated with suspected AMI or angina pectoris
- Pulmonary edema with hypertension

Contraindications

Patients with increased intracranial pressure, systolic blood pressure < 100 mm Hg, children younger than 12 years.

Precautions

Tolerance to nitrates easily develops, which necessitates increasing the dosage. Nitroglycerin tablets are inactivated by light, heat, air, and moisture, so they must be kept in amber glass containers with tight-fitting lids. Do not leave cotton in the container. Once the container is opened, nitroglycerin has a shelf life of 3 months. Patients should keep all but a few days' supply of the drug in the refrigerator. Do not shake Nitrolingual spray. Alcohol will accentuate the vasodilating and hypotensive effects of nitroglycerin.

Adverse Reactions and Side Effects

- **CNS:** Headache, dizziness, flushing, nausea and vomiting.
- **Cardiovascular:** Hypotension, reflex tachycardia.

Dosage

Adult: 0.4 mg (1 tablet or 1 spray sublingual); may repeat in 3–5 minutes (maximum dose = 1.2 mg or 3 doses).

5.38.2 Nitroglycerin (Nitro-Bid® Ointment)

Actions

Same as Nitrostat (see Drug Summary 5.38.1).

Indications

Same as for Nitrostat (see Drug Summary 5.38.1). The ointment is used when continued effects of nitroglycerin are desired.

Contraindications

Same as for Nitrostat (see Drug Summary 5.38.1).

Precautions

Same as for Nitrostat (see Drug Summary 5.38.1). In the event that the patient requires cardioversion or pacing, avoid placing the paddles or defibrillator or pacing pads near the nitroglycerin patch. It may be necessary to remove the nitroglycerin patch and wipe off the patient's skin prior to placing paddles or patches for cardioversion or pacing.

Adverse Reactions and Side Effects

Same as for Nitrostat (see Drug Summary 5.38.1).

Dosage

Adult: 1 inch of 2% ointment topically for transdermal absorption.

5.38.3 Nitroglycerin (Nitro-Bid® IV, Tridil®)

Actions

Same as Nitrostat (see Drug Summary 5.38.1).

Indications

Same as for Nitrostat (see Drug Summary 5.38.1). These formulations are used when continued effects of nitroglycerin are desired.

Contraindications

Same as for Nitrostat (see Drug Summary 5.38.1).

Precautions

The nitroglycerin infusion must be protected from light. Cover the IV bag as well as the IV tubing.

Adverse Reactions and Side Effects

Same as for Nitrostat (see Drug Summary 5.38.1).

Dosage

Adult: Mix 5 mg in 100 mL of D_5W (glass bottle); run the infusion at 5–20 mcg/min and titrate to effect.

5.39 Nitrous Oxide 50% Blended in Oxygen (Nitronox®)

Actions

Nitrous oxide is a colorless gas that acts on the central nervous system. When mixed with 50% oxygen and inhaled, it produces an effect similar to a mild intoxicant. The patient laughs and talks but does not go to sleep. When inhaled, nitrous oxide has potent analgesic effects, which dissipate within 2–5 minutes after stopping its administration.

Indications

Moderate to severe pain, as in trauma, burns, renal colic, and labor.

Contraindications

Nitrous oxide is contraindicated in any altered state of consciousness (e.g., head injury, alcohol ingestion, drug overdose). It is also contraindicated in patients with COPD, acute pulmonary edema, pneumothorax, decompression sickness, air embolus, abdominal pain with distention or suspicion of obstruction, and pregnancy (except during delivery), and in patients who are unable to self-administer Nitronox.

Adverse Reactions and Side Effects

Light-headedness, confusion, drowsiness, nausea and vomiting.

Warnings

Because nitrous oxide is heavier than air, it may accumulate on floor of ambulance. During transits lasting more than 15 minutes, nitrous oxide may affect ambulance personnel.

Dosage

Blended mixture of 50% nitrous oxide and 50% oxygen, which is self-administered through inhalation. Also apply O_2 cannula at 4–6 L to maintain O_2 therapy when nitrous oxide is not being administered.

Note

Also see Medical Procedure 4.28, Nitrous Oxide–Nitronox.

5.40 Oxytocin

Actions

This posterior pituitary hormone increases the amplitude and frequency of uterine contractions.

Indications

Postpartum vaginal bleeding, after delivery of the placenta.

Contraindications

It is essential to assure that the placenta has delivered and that there is not another fetus present before administering oxytocin.

Adverse Reactions and Side Effects

Hypotension, dysrhythmias (tachyarrhythmias), seizures, coma, nausea, vomiting.

Dosage

- Place 10 units (1 mL) in 1000 mL of normal saline, which gives a concentration of 10 micro units (mU) per 1 mL.
- IV infusion is titrated to effect, according to uterine response, usually at a rate of 1–2 mL/min. Try not to exceed 20 mU/min.
- Use caution with this agent, as it can be a very fast-acting vasopressor.

5.41 Phenylephrine Hydrochloride (Neo-Synephrine® 1%) Nasal Spray

Actions

Phenylephrine hydrochloride is a powerful postsynaptic alpha-receptor stimulant. It has few effects on the beta receptors of the heart but produces vasoconstriction.

Indications

Vasoconstriction of nasal capillaries prior to nasal intubation or placement of an NG tube.

Contraindications

Severe hypertension, ventricular tachycardia, or known hypersensitivity.

Precautions

Use extreme caution when administering this agent to elderly patients, or patients with hyperthyroidism, bradycardia, partial heart block, myocardial disease, or severe arteriosclerosis.

Adverse Reactions and Side Effects

Headache, reflex bradycardia, excitability, restlessness, and (rarely) dysrhythmias.

Dosage

1 spray in each nostril.

5.42 Pralidoxime (2-PAM®, Protopam Chloride®)

Actions

Pralidoxime reactivates cholinesterase that has been deactivated by organophosphorous pesticides and related products. It inactivates acetylcholine at both muscarinic and nicotinic sites in the periphery.

Indications

Organophosphorous toxicity; used as an adjunct to systemic atropine administration.

Contraindications

- Poisoning with Sevin (a carbamate insecticide); Sevin increases the drug's toxicity.
- Use with extreme caution in patients with a history of asthma, renal insufficiency, and peptic ulcers.

Adverse Reactions and Side Effects

- **CNS:** Dizziness, headache, drowsiness, excitement.
- **Cardiovascular:** Tachycardia.
- **EENT:** Blurred vision, diplopia, impaired accommodation, laryngospasm.
- **GI:** Nausea.
- **Other:** Muscular weakness or rigidity, hyperventilation.

Dosage

Adult:	IV infusion 1–2 g in 100 mL of saline over 30 minutes.
	If pulmonary edema is present, give IVP over 5 minutes.
Pediatric:	20–40 mg/kg in 100 mL of saline over 30 minutes as IV infusion.

Packaged

1 g dry powder: Mix with 20 cc sterile water (50 mg/mL).

5.43 Reteplase

Actions

Reteplase is a recombinant plasminogen activator. It catalyzes the cleavage of endogenous plasminogen to generate plasmin. Plasmin, in turn, degrades the fibrin matrix of the thrombus, thereby producing a thrombolytic action.

Indications

Reteplase is indicated for use in the management of acute myocardial infarction (AMI) in adults for lysis of thrombi obstructing the coronary arteries.

Contraindications

- Active internal bleeding
- History of cerebrovascular accident
- Recent (within 2 months) history of intracranial or intraspinal surgery or trauma
- Intracranial neoplasm, arteriovenous malformation, or aneurysm
- Known bleeding diathesis
- Severe uncontrolled hypertension

Precautions

Noncompressible arterial puncture must be avoided (e.g., internal jugular and subclavian punctures). Arterial and venous punctures should be minimized.

Adverse Reactions and Side Effects

Bleeding is the most common adverse reaction—either internal or external, or both. Other adverse reactions may include dysrhythmias, nausea/vomiting, hypotension, and fever. Mild hypersensitivity may produce urticaria.

Dosage

Adult: Prehospital bolus of 10 units IV over 2 minutes.

5.44 Scopolamine

Actions

Scopolamine is an anticholinergic agent with properties very similar to those of atropine. The eye drops will reduce the eye pain that accompanies organophosphate or anticholinesterase toxicity. Recognize that the miosis resulting from anticholinesterase syndrome may last for weeks.

Indications

Used in acute organophosphate or anticholinesterase syndrome toxicity.

Contraindications

None in acute organophosphate or anticholinesterase toxicity.

Precautions

Use with caution in children. Also use with caution in patients who have a history of urinary retention or glaucoma.

Adverse Reactions and Side Effects

- **CNS:** Delirium, hallucinations, psychiatric or behavioral problems, coma.
- **Cardiovascular:** Tachycardia.
- **Respiratory:** Respiratory depression.
- **Local:** Local irritation.
- **General:** Sweating and flushing.

Dosage

1–2 drops in each eye as needed to reduce pain; may need to repeat multiple times.

5.45 Sodium Bicarbonate 8.4% and 4.2%

Actions

This alkalizing agent is used to buffer acids present in the body during and after severe hypoxia. Bicarbonate combines with excess acids (usually lactic acid) present in the body to form a weak, volatile acid. This acid is broken down into CO_2 and H_2O. Sodium bicarbonate is effective only when administered in patients who have adequate ventilation and oxygenation.

Indications

Metabolic acidosis due to the following causes:

- Salicylate (aspirin) overdose
- Barbiturate overdose
- Tricyclic antidepressant overdose
- Hyperkalemia
- Severe ketoacidosis
- Cardiac arrest
- Shock
- Physostigmine toxicity
- Methanol toxicity
- Ethylene glycol toxicity

Contraindications

Congestive heart failure; alkalotic states.

Adverse Reactions and Side Effects

Metabolic alkalosis; hypernatremia; cerebral acidosis; sodium and H_2O retention, which can cause CHF.

Warnings

Excessive bicarbonate therapy inhibits the release of oxygen. Bicarbonate does not improve the ability to defibrillate. Administration of sodium bicarbonate may inactivate simultaneously administered catecholamines; it will create an insoluble precipitate if mixed with calcium chloride. Administration should be guided by arterial blood gases and pH data, when available.

Dosage

Adult:	1 mEq/kg IV (8.4%). Repeat with 0.5 mEq/kg q 10 minutes.
Pediatric:	1 mEq/kg IV (8.4%). Repeat with 0.5 mEq/kg q 10 minutes.
Infant:	1 mEq/kg IV (4.2%) slowly; may repeat in 10 minutes.

5.46 Sodium Nitrite

Actions

Sodium nitrite produces methemoglobinemia, which combines with the cyanide ion to form cyanmethemoglobin. It dissociates to liberate free cyanide, which is then converted to thiocyanate by sodium thiosulfate. The end product is excreted in the urine.

Indications

- Cyanide toxicity
- Hydrogen sulfide toxicity

Contraindications

- Hypotension: If the patient presents in a hypotensive state, consider skipping this step and proceeding to administration of sodium thiosulfate.
- Pregnancy: Sodium nitrite crosses the placenta and can induce methemoglobinemia in the fetus.

Adverse Reactions and Side Effects

- **Cardiovascular:** Syncope, hypotension.
- **Blood:** Excessive methemoglobinemia is likely to occur with decreased arterial oxygen saturation.

Dosage

Adult: 300 mg IV over 4–5 minutes.

Pediatric: 0.2 mL/kg IV over 4–5 minutes. Use extreme caution because methemoglobin can be fatal in children.

Repeat Dose: For both adults and children, give half the initial dose after 30 minutes.

5.47 Sodium Thiosulfate

Actions

Sodium thiosulfate converts cyanide to the less toxic thiocyanate. The thiocyanate is then excreted in the urine.

Indications

Used in acute cyanide toxicity; not useful in hydrogen sulfide toxicity.

Contraindications

None in acute cyanide toxicity.

Dosage

Adult: 12.5 g (50 mL of 25% solution) given by slow IV over 10 minutes.

5.48 Succinylcholine Chloride (Anectine®)

Actions

Succinylcholine chloride is a short-acting skeletal muscle paralytic. Onset of action occurs in 1–2 minutes, with recovery happening in 5–10 minutes. This agent works by depolarizing the receptors on skeletal muscle. It then blocks the action of acetylcholine, which causes enhanced cholinergic activity, with the face and neck muscles being affected first. These effects are followed by paralysis of the chest, diaphragm, and other skeletal muscles. Use of succinylcholine may trigger histamine release.

Indications

Facilitation of endotracheal intubation.

Contraindications

- Known sensitivity to succinylcholine or other anesthetics
- Preexisting neuromuscular disease (myasthenia gravis)
- Organophosphate or anticholinesterase toxicity
- Severe burns or eye injuries

Adverse Reactions and Side Effects

- Prolonged respiratory depression
- Bradycardia (rare tachycardia or hypertension)
- Hypersalivation and bronchospasm

Dosage

Adult: 1 mg/kg IV

- Preoxygenate the patient and ready the intubation equipment.
- Prepare atropine for bradycardia or hypersecretions.
- Premedicate the awake adult, preferably with midazolam (Versed). If midazolam is unavailable, use diazepam (Valium).
- Consider lidocaine 1–1.5 mg/kg for the patient with a head injury.
- Administer succinylcholine 1 mg/kg IV over 30–60 seconds.
- Using cricoid pressure, intubate the trachea.

5.49 Terbutaline

Actions

Terbutaline is primarily an injectable $beta_2$ sympathomimetic. It produces fewer cardiovascular side effects and more prolonged bronchodilation than some other medications.

Indications

Relief of bronchospasm in patients with reversible obstructive airway disease, including asthma.

Contraindications

Hypersensitivity.

Adverse Reactions and Side Effects

- **CNS:** Headache, nervousness, insomnia, tremor, dizziness.
- **Cardiovascular:** Tachycardia, hypertension, angina.
- **GI:** Nausea and vomiting, dry mouth.

Warnings

Use terbutaline with caution in patients with coronary artery disease, hypertension, hyperthyroidism, and diabetes. Administer cautiously to patients on MAO inhibitors or tricylic antidepressants. Beta blockers and terbutaline will inhibit each other.

Dosage

Adult: 0.25 mg SQ.

Pediatric: 0.01 mg/kg SQ. *Rarely used in pediatric patients younger than 12 years.*

5.50 Tetracaine Hydrochloride 0.5% Eye Drops

Actions

Tetracaine is an ophthalmic solution that anesthetizes the eyes. The onset of anesthesia usually begins within 20 seconds and lasts as long as 15 minutes.

Indications

Tetracaine is intended for use in the patient who is unable to cooperate with the provider in adequately flushing the eye(s) due to discomfort or pain. If flushing can be accomplished easily, tetracaine may not be needed.

Contraindications

Allergy to any topical anesthetic.

Precautions

Do not use the solution if it contains crystals, or if it is cloudy or discolored. Tetracaine eye drops are for topical ophthalmic use only—not for injection. The patient should be advised not to touch or rub the eye(s) until the effect of the anesthesia has worn off.

Dosage

1 or 2 drops in the eye.

5.51 Thiamine Hydrochloride (Vitamin B_1)

Actions

Thiamine is a water-soluble vitamin and a member of the B-complex group. Thiamine functions as an essential coenzyme in carbohydrate metabolism.

Indications

Given along with administration of dextrose 50% to prevent Wernicke and/or Korsakoff syndrome, as seen in acute alcohol intoxication. Indicated when the etiology of coma is unknown or alcohol intoxication or poor nutrition is highly suspected.

Contraindications

Patients with a history of sensitivity to IV administration of thiamine.

Adverse Reactions and Side Effects

Feelings of warmth, weakness, urticaria, pruritus (itching), sweating, nausea, restlessness, tightness of throat, angioneurotic edema, cyanosis, pulmonary edema, cardiovascular collapse, anaphylaxis. Following rapid IV administration, a slight fall in blood pressure may be observed.

Dosage

Adult: 100 mg IV or IM.

5.52 Vasopressin

Actions

Vasopressin is a naturally occurring antidiuretic hormone. In unnaturally high doses—much higher than those needed to produce antidiuretic hormone effects—vasopressin acts as a non-adrenergic peripheral vasoconstrictor. It directly stimulates smooth muscle V1 receptors. In recent studies, after a short duration of ventricular fibrillation, vasopressin during CPR increased coronary perfusion pressure, vital organ blood flow, ventricular fibrillation median frequency, and cerebral oxygen delivery.

Indications

Vasopressin is indicated for patients with shock-refractory VF and VT without a pulse.

Contraindications

None in cardiac arrest.

Precautions

None in cardiac arrest.

Adverse Reactions and Side Effects

None in cardiac arrest.

Dosage

Adult: 40 units IV push or ET.

5.53 Vecuronium Bromide (Norcuron®)

Actions

Vecuronium bromide is a short-acting, nondepolarizing skeletal muscle relaxant. Its binding with cholinergic receptor sites inhibits transmission of nerve impulses, antagonizing the action of acetylcholine. Vecuronium bromide has no analgesic properties, and the patient may be conscious but unable to communicate by any means. The first muscles affected are those of the eyes, face, and neck, followed by the limbs, abdomen, and chest; the diaphragm is affected last. Recovery usually occurs in the reverse order and may take longer than 60 minutes. With IV administration, the onset of action is in 30–60 seconds; peak action occurs in 3–5 minutes and the effects last for 30–60 minutes.

Indications

An **authorized paramedic** may induce general anesthesia to facilitate intubation.

Precautions

Vecuronium bromide causes respiratory paralysis—supportive airway control must be continuous and under direct observation at all times. Myasthenia gravis and other neuromuscular diseases increase sensitivity to the drug.

Adverse Reactions and Side Effects

Hypersensitivity reactions are possible.

Dosage

Adult and Pediatric (> 10 years):	0.08–0.1 mg/kg; slow administration over 30–60 seconds IV. Dose is usually 5–7 mg for an average-size adult.
Pediatric (1–9 years of age):	May require a higher dose.

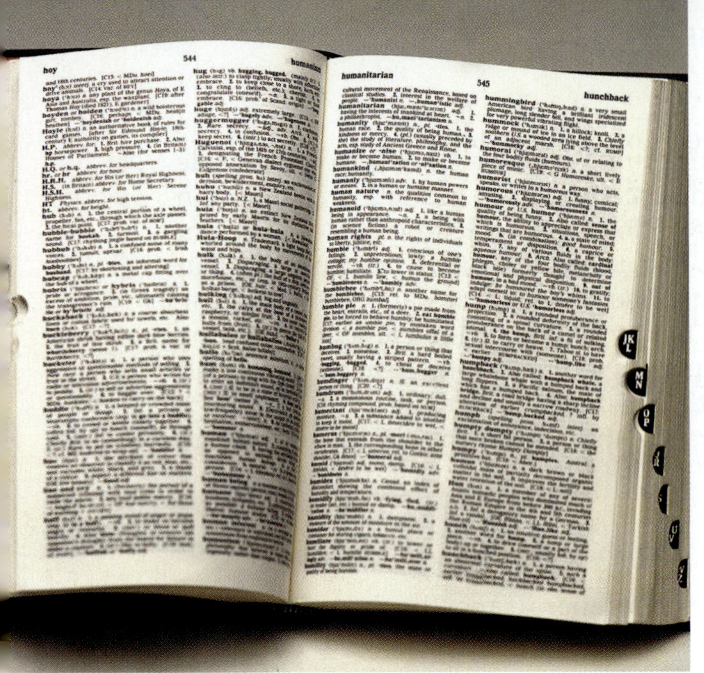

chapter 6
Glossary

6.1 Types of Patients

Adult: A patient who is 16 years of age or older.

Pediatric: A patient who is 15 years of age or younger.

Newborn: A patient who has just been delivered.

Neonate: A patient who is younger than 6 weeks of age.

Infant: A patient who is 1 year of age or younger.

Juvenile: For legal purposes, a patient who is younger than 18 years of age, except in the case of an emancipated minor, a self-sufficient minor, a married minor, or a minor in the military.

6.2 Types of EMS Providers

Paramedic: Being certified by the State of Florida as a Paramedic enables the provider to administer Basic and Advanced Life Support as outlined in these protocols.

EMT-B: Being certified by the State of Florida as an EMT-B enables the provider to administer Basic Life Support as outlined in these protocols.

First Responder: A provider (e.g., fire fighter, lifeguard, police officer) who is not certified as a Paramedic or EMT-B.

6.3 Types of EMS Units

Advanced Life Support Transport: An ambulance (e.g., freightliner rescue) that is licensed by the State of Florida to carry ALS equipment and transport patients in an ALS capacity.

Advanced Life Support Non-transport: An emergency vehicle (e.g., fire engine) that is licensed by the State of Florida to carry ALS equipment, but does not transport patients.

Advanced Life Support Helicopter: An air ambulance (rescue helicopter) that is licensed by the State of Florida to carry ALS equipment and transport patients in an ALS capacity.

6.4 Types of Care

Basic Life Support: All medical care that is classified as BLS by the State of Florida and outlined in these protocols.

Advanced Life Support: All medical care, in addition to BLS care, that is classified as ALS by the State of Florida and outlined in these protocols.

6.5 General Terms

Asthma: Chronic inflammatory disease that can be acutely triggered by many irritants.

Ataxia: Staggered/unsteady gait that may be indicative of neurological impairment.

Baker Act: Florida Statutes, Chapter 394, which relate to the authorization of police, physicians, and the courts to dictate certain medical care for persons who pose a threat to themselves or to others.

Child Abuse: When persons intentionally inflict, or allow to be inflicted, physical or psychological injury to a child, which causes or results in risk of death, disfigurement, or distress.

Child Neglect: When an endangered child's physical, mental, or emotional condition is impaired or because of failure of the legal guardian to supply basic necessities, including adequate food, clothing, shelter, education, or medical care.

CISM: Critical incident stress management. Support and professional intervention provided after a significant traumatic event where personal coping mechanisms may become overwhelmed.

Competent: When individuals are able to understand the nature and consequences of their actions by refusing medical care and/or transportation.

Croup: A viral infection of the upper airway that causes edema/inflammation below the larynx and glottis, with a resultant narrowing of the lumen of the airway.

Decompression Sickness ("Bends"): A disorder resulting from a reduction of surrounding pressure, such as during an ascent from a dive, and attributed to the formation of bubbles from dissolved gas in the body tissues. It is usually characterized by symptoms of pain and neurological dysfunction, which may range from subtle to very acute in nature.

6.5 General Terms

DNRO: Do not resuscitate order; Florida HRS form 1896, provider notification of a patient's/legal guardian's wishes not to be resuscitated.

Epiglottitis: An acute infection and inflammation of the epiglottis that is potentially life-threatening.

Hemiplegia: Weakness on a unilateral side of the body.

Level 1: Actions authorized prior to physician contact.

Level 2: Actions expected or to be requested with physician contact.

Medical Direction: The action of a licensed physician granting authority and accepting responsibility for the care provided by EMS; it includes participation in all aspects of EMS to ensure maintenance of accepted standards of medical practice.

Medication Access Point: Intermittent vascular access site (i.e., saline or heparin lock).

Miosis: Constricted pupils.

Morgan Lens: Ocular irrigation device that is placed on the global surface.

Near Drowning: Submersion in either fresh or saltwater, such that the person may or may not be conscious.

Online Medical Control: The moment-to-moment contemporaneous medical supervision of EMS personnel caring for patients in the field by a licensed physician. It occurs via radio, telephone, or on-scene physicians.

PRN: As needed.

SIDS: "Crib death"; the sudden death of an apparently healthy infant, without observed etiology.

START: **S**imple **T**riage **A**nd **R**apid **T**reatment; A protocol that allows for assessing a large number of victims rapidly and can be used effectively by personnel with limited medical training.

6.6 Infectious Disease Terminology

Aerosolized: In the form of ultramicroscopic solid or liquid particles dispersed or suspended in air or gas.

Amniotic Fluid: The serous liquid in which the embryo is suspended in the uterus.

Antibody: A protein substance produced in the blood or tissues in response to a specific antigen, such as a virus. Antibodies destroy or weaken bacteria and neutralize organic poisons, thereby forming the basis of immunity.

Blood: Human blood, human blood components, and products made from human blood.

Bloodborne Pathogens: Pathogenic microorganisms that are present in human blood and can cause disease in humans. These pathogens include, but are not limited to, hepatitis B, hepatitis C, human immunodeficiency virus (HIV), and syphilis.

Cerebrospinal Fluid: The serum-like liquid that circulates through the ventricles of the brain and the cavity of the spinal cord.

Contraindication: A factor that renders the administration of a drug or the carrying out of a medical procedure inadvisable.

HEPA Mask: A high-efficiency particulate air filter that is used as a personal protective device. It is worn over the nose and mouth to filter/remove bacteria, spores, and viruses whose size is equal to and greater than 0.3 micron. OSHA's standard for respiratory protection requires that employees be trained in the use of respirators and that the mask be fit tested.

Influenza: An acute contagious viral infection characterized by inflammation of the respiratory tract and by fever, chills, and muscular pain.

6.6 Infectious Disease Terminology

Intubation: To insert a tube into a hollow organ or body passage.

Mantoux Test (PPD): A method of assessing whether someone has become infected with *Mycobacterium tuberculosis* complex. The test involves measurement of a subject's immune response to an injection of tuberculin purified protein derivative (PPD) manufactured from killed *M. tuberculosis* bacilli. Also referred to as a tuberculin skin test or PPD test.

Nasopharyngeal Airway: The part of the pharynx above the soft palate that is continuous with the nasal passages.

Percutaneous: Passed, done, or effected through the skin.

Pericardial Fluid: The liquid suspended in the sac surrounding the heart.

Peritoneal Fluid: The liquid suspended in the body cavity that contains most of the abdominal and pelvic organs.

Plasma: The clear yellowish fluid portion of blood, lymph, or intramuscular fluid in which cells are suspended.

Pleural Fluid: The liquid matter contained in and around the body cavity that contains the lungs.

Post-exposure Prophylaxis (PEP, chemoprophylaxis): *Prophylaxis* means disease prevention. *Post-exposure prophylaxis* (PEP) means taking antiviral medications as soon as possible after exposure to a pathogen so that the exposure will not result in an infection.

6.6 Infectious Disease Terminology

Rapid HIV Testing: A laboratory method called Single-Use Diagnostic System (SUDS® HIV-1 Test) that detects and reports HIV antibody test results in the same day.

Seroconversion: Development of antibodies in blood serum as a result of infection or immunization.

Serum: The clear yellowish fluid obtained by separating whole blood into its solid and liquid components.

Sputum: Matter that is coughed up and usually ejected from the mouth, including saliva, foreign material, and substances such as mucus or phlegm from the respiratory tract.

Synovial Fluid: The liquid that lubricates joints and nourishes cartilage.

Titer: A level of concentration of antibodies in a blood sample that shows whether exposure and subsequent immunity to an infectious disease are present.

Triage: The process for sorting and prioritizing injured people into groups based on their need for or likely benefit from immediate medical treatment in a medical setting.

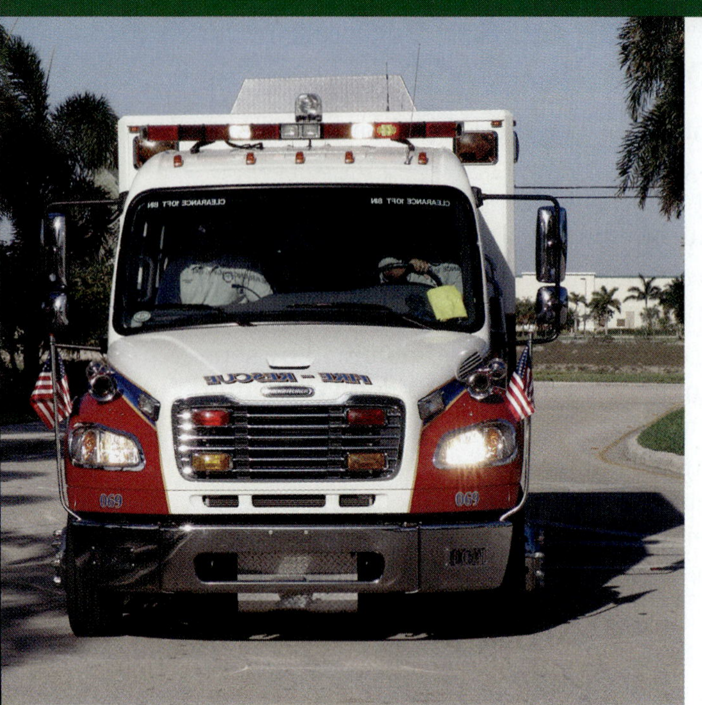

chapter 7
Appendix

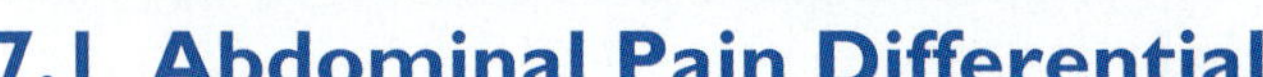

7.1 Abdominal Pain Differential

Upper GI Bleed	Lower GI Bleed	Gynecological
History of peptic ulcer disease; can cause massive hemorrhage	May be occult or bright red; a common cause of orthostatic hypotension and undetected anemia	*Think ectopic!* if the patient is still having menses; diagnosis includes: 1. Lower abdominal pain 2. Hypotension 3. Shoulder pain 4. Vaginal bleeding +/– 5. Syncope

Common Causes Associated with the Different Types of Presenting Pain

Upper GI Bleed	Lower GI Bleed	Gynecological
Esophageal varices (history of cirrhosis, hepatitis)	Diverticulitis	Ectopic pregnancy
Peptic ulcer disease	Hemorrhoids	Pelvic inflammatory disease/STDs
Aspirin, NSAIDs	Cancer	Ovarian cyst
Alcohol	Inflammatory bowel disease	Kidney/urinary tract infection
Ingestion of caustic substances	Chronic diarrhea, overuse of laxatives	Endometriosis

7.1 Abdominal Pain Differential

Back Pain	Colicky Pain	Peritoneal Pain	Vomiting
Every pain presenting with new onset back pain (>60 years) should have an abdominal exam R/O AAA	Spasmodic—usually results from smooth muscle contracting against *obstruction* of hollow organ	Rigid, board-like abdomen, resulting from infection or long-standing rupture	Nonspecific syndrome, can be caused by a wide variety of underlying problems, some of which are serious

Common Causes Associated with the Different Types of Presenting Pain

Back Pain	Colicky Pain	Peritoneal Pain	Vomiting
Abdominal aortic aneurysm	Bowel obstruction	Ruptured appendix	Infection of GI tract
Cholelithiasis	Renal obstruction/"kidney stones"	Ruptured ovarian cyst	Ulcers
Pancreatitis	Gallbladder obstruction	Pelvic inflammatory disease (PID)	Toxic ingestions
Perforated ulcer	Ulcerative colitis Crohn's disease	Perforated ulcer Peritonitis, advanced	Bowel obstruction Stones of the gallbladder or kidney

Reference

Bosker G, MD; Sequeira M, MD, FACED; Weins D, MD, FACEP: *The 60-Second EMT: Rapid BLS/ALS Assessment, Diagnosis, and Triage*, 2nd edition, Mosby, St. Louis, MO, 1996.

7.2 Apgar Score

The Apgar score should be used in newborns at 1 and 5 minutes after birth. If the patient is not immediately improving after birth, see Pediatric Protocol 3.4.1, Newborn Resuscitation.

The Apgar Scoring Chart

Sign	0	1	2	1 Minute	5 Minutes
Appearance (skin color)	Blue, pale	Body pink, hands and feet blue	Completely pink		
Pulse Rate (heart rate)	Absent	Less than 100	More than 100		
Grimace (irritability—response to flick on sole)	No response	Some motion, weak cry	Vigorous cry		
Activity (muscle tone)	Flaccid, limp	Some flexion of extremities	Active motion		
Respiratory (effort)	Absent	Slow, irregular	Good, crying		

7.3 Approved Medical Abbreviations

ABC	Airway, breathing, circulation
A/C	Antecubital fossa
ACLS	Advanced Cardiac Life Support
ALS	Advanced Life Support
a.m.	Morning
AMI	Acute myocardial infarction
ATV	All-terrain vehicle
BLS	Basic Life Support
BP	Blood pressure
BSA	Body surface area (burns)
BSI	Body substance isolation
BVM	Bag-valve mask
CCU	Coronary care unit
CHF	Congestive heart failure
cm	Centimeter
CNS	Central nervous system
CO_2	Carbon dioxide
COPD	Chronic obstructive pulmonary disease
CPR	Cardiopulmonary resuscitation
CSF	Cerebrospinal fluid
C-spine	Cervical spine
CVA	Cerebrovascular accident
D_5W	5% dextrose in water
D_{25}	Dextrose 25%
D_{50}	Dextrose 50%
DCAP-BLS	Deformity, contusions, abrasions, penetrations, burns, lacerations, and swelling
DNR	Do not resuscitate
DNRO	Do not resuscitate order
DOA	Dead on arrival

7.3 Approved Medical Abbreviations

ECG or EKG	Electrocardiogram
EEG	Electroencephalogram
e.g.	For example
EMS	Emergency medical services
EMT	Emergency medical technician
ENT	Ears, nose, and throat
ER	Emergency room
ETA	Estimated time of arrival
ET tube	Endotracheal tube
FBAO	Foreign body airway obstruction
GCS	Glasgow Coma Scale
g, gm	Gram
GU	Genitourinary
GYN	Gynecology
HBP	High blood pressure
HEENT	Head, ears, eyes, nose, and throat
Hgb	Hemoglobin
HIV	Human immuno deficiency virus
HTN	Hypertension
ICU	Intensive care unit
IV	Intravenous
IVP	Intravenous push
JVD	Jugular vein distention
kg	Kilogram
lb	Pound
L&D	Labor and delivery

7.3 Approved Medical Abbreviations

mcg	Microgram
MCI	Mass-casualty incident
mEq	Milliequivalent
mg	Milligram
min	Minute
mL	Milliliter
NG	Nasogastric
NKA	No known allergies
NS	Normal saline
OR	Operating room
$PaCO_2$	Partial pressure of CO_2 in arterial blood
PaO_2	Partial pressure of O_2 in arterial blood
PDR	*Physician's Desk Reference*
per	By
p.m.	Evening
PMD	Private medical doctor
SpO_2	Percentage of oxygen in the blood as measured via pulse oximeter (equal to SaO_2)
TIA	Transient ischemic attack

Miscellaneous

–	Negative
+	Plus/positive
#	Number
%	Percent
@	At

7.4 Burn Severity Categorization

Burn Classification	Characteristics
Minor burn injury	First-degree (1°) burn Second-degree (2°) burn < 15% BSA in adults Second-degree (2°) burn < 5% BSA in children/elderly Third-degree (3°) burn < 2% BSA
Moderate burn injury	Second-degree (2°) burn 16–25% BSA in adults Second-degree (2°) burn 5–20% BSA in children/elderly Third-degree (3°) burn 2–10% BSA
Major burn injury	Second-degree (2°) burn > 25% BSA in adults Second-degree (2°) burn > 20% BSA in children/elderly Third-degree (3°) burn > 10% BSA Burns involving the hands, face, eyes, ears, feet, or perineum Most patients with inhalation injury, electrical injury, concomitant major trauma, or significant preexisting diseases

Reference

American Burn Association, *Burn Severity Categorization.*

7.5 Chest Pain Differential

	Myocardial Infarction	Angina Pectoris	Dissecting Aneurysm	Pericarditis	Peptic Ulcer
Onset	Usually sudden	Exertional/ emotional	Acute	Subacute	Acute/ subacute
Quality	Crushing heaviness, dull pressure, band-like, constricting, squeezing, burning, bursting	Discomfort, choking, pressing, squeezing, strangling, constricting, bursting, burning	Deep tearing, shearing, "knife-like"	Sharp	Burning
Location	Substernal, may vary	Substernal	Substernal	Substernal, more left-sided	Epigastric, substernal
Radiation	Across mid-thorax, anterior arms, shoulder, neck, jaw, teeth, fingers	Same as MI	Back lumbar region	Usually none, occasionally tip of shoulder, neck, flank	Occasionally back
Duration	Usually >30 minutes	5–15 minutes	Hours	Hours	Hours
Provocation	Usually none, see comments	Exercise, excitement, stress, cold, meals	None	Worsened: lying down, breathing, swallowing, coughing, twisting	Alcohol, lack of food, acidic foods
Alleviation	None	Rest, NTG	None	Tripod position, shallow respirations	Antacids, food
Comments	After heavy meals, severe emotional stress, S/S: SOB, N&V, pallor, diaphoresis, impending doom, elderly—atypical	May be nocturnal	Sudden onset, may subside spontaneously or be associated with paralysis	May be associated with URI, flu, Pronestyl, hydralazine, lupus; *may be febrile*	ASA, NSAIDs (e.g., Voltaren, Feldene, Naprosyn, Motrin, Advil) may trigger

7.5 Chest Pain Differential

	Pancreatitis	Esophageal Rupture	Pulmonary Embolism	Esophageal Spasm	Costochondritis
Onset	Acute/ subacute	Acute	Sudden or gradual	Subacute	Sudden or gradual
Quality	Severe or dull	Severe	Sharp or dull	Dull, pressure, colicky	Sharp, superficial
Location	Epigastric	Retrosternal	Multiple	Substernal, epigastric	Anterior/lateral costochondral junction
Radiation	Back	Lateral	None	Jaw, either arm	None
Duration	Hours	Hours	Variable	5–60 minutes	Variable
Provocation	Alcohol, trauma, gallbladder disease	Swallowing	Respirations, cough	Spontaneous, cold liquids, recumbency	Movement, palpation, cough, respirations
Alleviation	Time	None	None	Antacids, occasionally NTG	Time, heat, analgesia
Comments	May be viral (e.g., mumps)	Alcoholics with forceful vomiting; associated with pleural effusion, shock, and hydropneumothorax	May have hemoptysis, signs of peripheral phlebitis, cough, and fever	Mimics angina, may occur after meals, at night with an acid taste, sensation—linear	Signs and symptoms: fever, cough, URI

7.5 Chest Pain Differential

	Cervical Disk	Anxiety	Pneumonia	Pneumothorax	Pleurisy	Gallbladder
Onset	Subacute/ acute	Subacute	Slow	Sudden	Subacute	Acute/ subacute
Quality	Superficial	Occasionally sharp, may be heavy or pressure-like	Sharp or dull ache	Sharp	Sharp	Spasms, colicky, may wax and wane
Location	Arm/neck	Varies in chest, substernal	Frequently lateral or substernal	Lateral	Lateral	Right upper quadrant
Radiation	Along course of nerve being irritated	Usually none	None	None	None	Epigastric, substernal, right thoracic, interscapular
Duration	Variable	2–3 minutes	Variable	Variable	Variable	Hours
Provocation	Motion of head, neck palpation, bending	Emotions, tachypnea	Respirations, cough	Respirations, cough	Respira-tions, cough	Spontaneous or with food
Alleviation	Time, analgesics	Stimulus removal, relaxation	None	None (shallow breathing)	Shallow breath-ing	Time, analgesics
Comments	Not relieved by rest	Paraesthesia—facial, circumoral, finger or toe, spasms	Signs and symptoms: fever, cough, URI	More common in tall, thin people	Usually associ-ated with flu-like symptoms	1–2 hours after meals, usually nausea and vomiting

Reference

The University of Miami School of Medicine.

7: appendix

7.6 Dive Accident Checklists

DIVE HISTORY/PROFILE

Complete as much as possible.

1. Type of Dive: Rescue ____ Commercial ____ Recreational ____
2. Type of Gas Used: Compressed Air ____ Nitrox ____ Heliox ____ Other ____________
3. Water Type: Contaminated ____ Fresh ____ Salt ____
4. Water Temperature: ___________
5. Number of Dives in the Past Several Days: _______

   List Each Dive with:

Maximum Depth	Bottom Time	Surface Interval
____________	____________	____________
____________	____________	____________
____________	____________	____________
____________	____________	____________

6. Time of Last Ascent: ____________
7. Did Diver: Panic? ____ Emergency Ascend? ____ Run Out of Air? ____

   Hold Breath Upon Ascent? ____ Miss a Decompression Stop(s)? ____
8. Problems During Dive (e.g., Buoyancy, Clearing Ears, Equipment):

   ____

   ____
9. Possible Contact with Dangerous Marine Life: _______
10. Fly After Diving: ______ How Long After: ____________
11. Alcohol Ingestion: _____ When: _____ Quantity: __________________________
12. Dive Workload (e.g., Currents, Hard Work, Over-weighted):

    ____

    ____
13. Any Post-dive Physical Activity: ____
14. Dive Buddy: _____ Is He/She Present? _____ Name and Phone Number:

    ____
15. Other Witnesses (Names and Phone Numbers):

    ____

    ____
16. Statements and Other Information:

    ____

    ____

    ____

    ____

    ____

    ____

7.6 Dive Accident Checklists

DIVE ACCIDENT: SIGNS AND SYMPTOMS

Enter "Y" (yes) or "N" (no). Explain where needed.

1a. Joint Pain _____ 1b. Location______________________________

2a. Head Pain ____ 2b. Location ______________________________

3a. Chest Pain ____ 3b. Location ______________________________

3c. Increase with Inspiration or Cough _____ 3d. Radiates _____

3e. Location ____

4a. Abdominal Pain _____ 4b. Encircling Pain _____

5a. Unconsciousness _____ 5b. When ______________________________

6a. Difficulty Breathing _____ 6b. Rapid Respirations _____

7. Convulsions _____

8. Confused/Disoriented _____

9. Extremity Edema _____

10a. Rash _____ 10b. Blotching _____ 10c. Itching _____

11. Shock _____

12. Weakness/Fatigue _____

13a. Numbness _____ 13b. Tingling _____ 13c. Decreased Sensation _____

13d. Location ____

14a. Faintness _____ 14b. Dizziness _____

15a. Difficulty Urinating _____

15b. Difficulty Moving Bowels _____

16a. Difficulty Hearing _____ 16b. Which Ear? __________

17a. Difficulty Speaking _____ 17b. Facial Droop _____ 17c. Which Side? _____

18a. Staggering _____ 18b. Paralysis _____ 18c. Location ______________________

19. Visual Disturbances _____

20a. Apnea _____ 20b. Bloody Froth from Mouth _____ 20c. Cough _____

21a. Cyanosis _____ 21b. Location ______________________________

22a. Feeling of Blow to Chest During Dive _____ 22b. When? ____________________

7.6 Dive Accident Checklists

DIVE ACCIDENT: RAPID FIELD NEUROLOGIC EXAM RECORD

Answer yes or no.

Mental Status: Does He/She Know

1a. His/her name?_______
1b. Where he/she is?_______
1c. Time of day?_______
1d. Most recent activity?_______
1e. Speech is clear, correct?_______

Sight

2a. Correctly counts fingers?_______
2b. Vision clear?_______

Eye Movement

3a. Move all four directions?_______
3b. Nystagmus absent?_______

Facial Movements

4a. Teeth clench okay?_______
4b. Able to wrinkle forehead?_______
4c. Tongue moves all directions?_______
4d. Smile symmetrical?_______

Head/Shoulder Movements

5a. Adam's apple moves?_______
5b. Shoulder shrug normal, equal?_______
5c. Head movements normal, equal?_______

Hearing

6a. Normal for that diver?_______
6b. Equal in both ears?_______

Sensations: Present, Normal, and Symmetrical Across

7a. Face?_______
7b. Chest?_______
7c. Abdomen?_______
7d. Arms (front)?_______
7e. Hands?_______
7f. Legs (front)?_______
7g. Feet?_______
7h. Back?_______
7i. Arms (back)?_______
7j. Buttocks?_______
7k. Legs (back)?_______

Muscle Tone: Present, Normal, and Symmetrical for

8a. Arms?_______
8b. Legs?_______
8c. Hand grips?_______
8d. Feet?_______

Balance and Coordination

9a. Romberg okay?_______
9b. If supine, heel–shin slide okay?_______
9c. Alternating hand movements okay?_______

7.7 Glasgow Coma Scale Score

Eye Opening

4 Spontaneous: At this point, with no further stimulation, the patient has eyes open.

3 To Voice: If the patient's eyes are unopened, a request to "open your eyes" should be spoken, and if necessary, should be shouted.

2 To Pain: If verbal stimulation is unsuccessful in eliciting eye opening, the standard painful stimulus is applied. NOTE: Document if eyes are closed due to swelling, facial injuries, or other causes.

1 None: No eye opening.

Best Verbal Response

5 Oriented: After the patient is aroused, he/she is asked who he/she is, where he/she is, and what the year and month are. If accurate answers are obtained, this is recorded as oriented.

4 Confused: Although the patient is unable to give correct answers to previous questions, he/she is capable of producing complete phrases, sentences, and even conversational exchange.

3 Inappropriate Words: The patient speaks or exclaims only a word or two. Such a response is usually obtained only by physical stimulation rather than a verbal stimulus, although occasionally a patient will shout obscenities or call relatives names for no apparent reasons.

2 Incomprehensible Words: The patient's response consists of groans, moans, or indistinct mumbling and does not contain any intelligible words.

1 No Verbal Response: Prolonged and, if necessary, repeated stimulation does not produce any phonation.

7.7 Glasgow Coma Scale Score

Best Motor Response

6 Obeys Command: This requires an ability to comprehend instructions, usually given in some form of verbal commands but sometimes by gestures and writing. The patient is required to perform the specific movements requested. The command is given to hold up two fingers (if physically feasible); the patient should respond appropriately.

5 Localizes Pain: If the patient does not obey commands, a painful stimulus may be applied as firm pressure to the sternum or nail bed for 5 seconds. The patient should reach to and/or try to remove source of pain

4 Withdrawals: After painful stimulus:
- Elbow flexes
- Rapid movement
- No muscle stiffness
- Arm is drawn away from the torso

3 Flexion Response: After painful stimulation:
- Slow movement
- Accompanied by stiffness
- Forearm and head held against the body
- Limbs assume hemiplegic position

2 Extension Response: After painful stimulation:
- Legs and arms extend
- Accompanied by stiffness
- Internal rotation of shoulder and forearm

1 None: No motor response.

Note

The Glasgow Coma Scale measures cognitive ability. Therefore, if injury (chronic or acute) has caused paraplegia or quadraplegia, alternate methods of assessing motor response must be used (e.g., ability to blink eyes = obeys commands).

7.8 Pediatric Glasgow Coma Scale

		>1 Year	<1 Year
Eye Opening	4	Spontaneously	Spontaneously
	3	To verbal command	To verbal command
	2	To pain	To pain
	1	No response	No response

		>1 Year	< 1 Year
Best Motor Response	6	Obeys	
	5	Localizes pain	Localizes pain
	4	Flexion—withdrawal	Flexion—normal
	3	Flexion—abnormal (decorticate rigidity)	Flexion—abnormal (decorticate rigidity)
	2	Extension (decerebrate rigidity)	Extension (decerebrate rigidity)
	1	No response	No response

		>5 Years	<2–5 Years	0–23 Months
Best Verbal Response	5	Oriented and converses	Appropriate words and phrases	Smiles, coos, cries appropriately
	4	Disoriented and converses	Inappropriate words	Cries
	3	Inappropriate words	Cries and/or screams	Inappropriate crying and/or screaming
	2	Incomprehensible	Grunts	Grunts
	1	No response	No response	No response

7.9 Hospital Capabilities

All hospitals licensed under Chapter 395, Florida Statutes, are required to accept patients via their emergency departments in accordance with Chapter 395.1041, Florida Statutes, and other state and federal laws. However, some patients may require specialized treatment not available at every hospital. It is these specialized care capabilities that should be considered when determining a transport destination. In most cases, patients with medical needs that do not require specialized care would be transported to the closest hospital emergency room. For those patients who require specialized care, the following hospital capabilities should be considered.

Trauma Center

These hospitals are able to provide specialized trauma care and have been designated as a Trauma Center as defined in Chapter 395.4001, Florida Statutes.

Adult trauma patients who meet Adult Trauma Alert Criteria must be transported to a Level 1 or Level 2 Trauma Center, if available (see General Protocol 1.10).

Pediatric patients who meet Pediatric Trauma Alert Criteria must be transported to a Pediatric Trauma Referral Center, if available (see General Protocol 1.10).

Maternity (OB) Hospital

These hospitals are able to provide specialized obstetric care, including labor and delivery services in accordance with the guidelines established by the Joint Commission on Accreditation of Healthcare Organizations (JCAHO) and Agency for Health Care Administration (AHCA).

Primary Stroke Center

These hospitals are able to provide specialized care to stroke patients in accordance with the standards outlined by the American Stroke Association (ASA) or JCAHO and AHCA, and have been designated by the State of Florida as Stroke Centers.

Psychiatric Treatment Center

These hospitals are able to provide specialized care to psychiatric patients in accordance with Chapter 394, Florida Statute. All patients who have been "Baker Acted" (see General Protocol 1.2) should be transported to the closest hospital, as defined in Chapter 395, Florida Statutes, for medical clearance prior to transport to a mental health facility that does not meet the requirement for a hospital in Chapter 395, Florida Statutes.

7.9 Hospital Capabilities

Interventional Cardiovascular Center

These hospitals are able to provide specialized cardiac care and have been designated as Interventional Cardiac Centers by JCAHO or AHCA. These hospitals will be able to provide the following services:

1. An Emergency Department with dedicated chest pain triage, treatment, interventional beds, and staffing. Must have immediate 12-lead ECG capabilities available in the ED.
2. 24 hour/day, 7 day/week committed receiving station (fax machine and/or electronic receiving station) in the ED for transmission of prehospital ECGs.
3. 24 hour/day, 7 day/week interventional cardiology catheterization lab availability within 30 minutes of prehospital field notification and ED confirmation via 12-lead ECG transmission.
    a. Documented track record of at least 20 acute coronary non-elective (from ED to cath lab) interventions per year.
    b. 24 hour/day emergency cardiac surgery availability, which does not have to be "in-house."
    c. 24 hour/day left ventricular (LV) assist capabilities, including intra-aortic balloon pump (IABP) insertion and maintenance.
    d. One on-call interventional team per participating interventional facility that will respond upon ED notification.
4. An interventional cardiologist on call, 24 hour/day, 7 day/week. Must have a track record that meets all ACC guidelines, with optimal outcomes and acceptable complication rates, and must be signed off by the Cath Medical Director.
5. Documented volume of at least 200 acute MI patients admitted to the hospital per year.
6. Dedicated coronary care unit with sufficient beds and staff to accommodate acute MI and sudden death patients with ROSC.
7. Identification of a research coordinator/administrator to track and release treatment and patient outcomes of patients transported to the facility by Fire/Rescue personnel.

7.10 IV Drip Calculations

Dopamine

Mix 400 mg in 250 mL of D_5W
Concentration = 1600 mcg/mL
Dosage: 5–15 mcg/kg/min

Using a microdrip (60 gtt/mL):
15 gtt/min = 400 mcg/min
30 gtt/min = 800 mcg/min
45 gtt/min = 1200 mcg/min
60 gtt/min = 1600 mcg/min

Alternative: Mix 400 mg in 500 mL of D_5W
Concentration = 800 mcg/mL

Using a microdrip (60 gtt/mL):
30 gtt/min = 400 mcg/min
60 gtt/min = 800 mcg/min
90 gtt/min = 1200 mcg/min
120 gtt/min = 1600 mcg/min

Quick Calculation:

Take the patient's weight in pounds, drop the last number, and then subtract 2. This will give you the starting drip rate at 5 mcg/kg/min. For every change in micrograms, add or subtract 3 drops.

Example:

Patient weighs 175 lb.
Drop last number (5) from 175 = 17
17 – 2 = 15
5 mcg/kg/min = 15 gtt/min
6 mcg/kg/min = 15 + 3 = 18 gtt/min

(This quick calculation gives a very close approximate dose.)

Epinephrine

Mix 1 mg of 1:10,000 in 250 mL D_5W
Concentration = 4 mcg/mL
Dosage: 2–10 mcg/min

Using a microdrip (60 gtt/mL):
15 gtt/min = 1 mcg/min
30 gtt/min = 2 mcg/min
45 gtt/min = 3 mcg/min
60 gtt/min = 4 mcg/min
75 gtt/min = 5 mcg/min
90 gtt/min = 6 mcg/min
105 gtt/min = 7 mcg/min
120 gtt/min = 8 mcg/min
135 gtt/min = 9 mcg/min
150 gtt/min = 10 mcg/min

Lidocaine

Maintenance:
Mix 1 g (4%, 10%, or 20%) in 250 mL of D_5W
Concentration = 4 mg/mL
Dosage: 1–4 mg/min

Using a minidrip (60 gtt/min):
15 gtt/min = 1 mg/min
30 gtt/min = 2 mg/min
45 gtt/min = 3 mg/min
60 gtt/min = 4 mg/min

7.10 IV Drip Calculations

Magnesium Sulfate

Eclamptic Seizures:

Mix 4 g in 50 mL of D_5W
Concentration = 80 mg/mL
Dosage: 4 g over 5–10 min

Using a macrodrip (10 gtt/min):
Run at 58–116 gtt/min

Torsades de Pointes and VF:

Mix 1–2 g in 50 mL of D_5W
Concentration = 20–40 mg/mL
Dosage: 1–2 g over 5–10 min

Using a macrodrip (10 gtt/min):
Run at 270 gtt/min

Maintenance:

Mix 1 g in 250 mL of D_5W
Concentration = 4 mg/mL
Dosage: 2–4 mg/min

Using a microdrip (60 gtt/mL):
30 gtt/min = 2 mg/min
45 gtt/min = 3 mg/min
60 gtt/min = 4 mg/min

Nitroglycerin

Mix 5 mg in 100 mL of D_5W (glass bottle)
Concentration = 50 mcg/mL
Dosage: 5–20 mcg/min

Using a microdrip (60 gtt/mL):
6 gtt/min = 5 mcg/min
7 gtt/min = 6 mcg/min
8 gtt/min = 7 mcg/min
10 gtt/min = 8 mcg/min
11 gtt/min = 9 mcg/min
12 gtt/min = 10 mcg/min
13 gtt/min = 11 mcg/min
14 gtt/min = 12 mcg/min
16 gtt/min = 13 mcg/min
17 gtt/min = 14 mcg/min
18 gtt/min = 15 mcg/min
19 gtt/min = 16 mcg/min
20 gtt/min = 17 mcg/min
22 gtt/min = 18 mcg/min
23 gtt/min = 19 mcg/min
24 gtt/min = 20 mcg/min

7.10 IV Drip Calculations

Amiodarone

SVT/VT with a Pulse:

Mix 150 mg in 50 mL of D_5W
Dosage: 150 mg over 8–10 min

Using a macrodrip (10 gtt/mL):
Run at 60–75 gtt/min

VF/Pulseless VT:

Mix 300 mg in 50 mL of D_5W
Dosage: 300 mg over 8–10 min

Using a macrodrip (10 gtt/mL):
Run at 60–75 gtt/min

Pediatric:

Mix 5 mg/kg in 50 mL of D_5W
Dosage: 5 mg/kg over 8-10 min

Using a macrodrip (10 gtt/mL):
Run at 60–75 gtt/min

7.11 Pediatric Vital Signs

Age	Weight (kg)	Minimum Systolic BP	Normal Heart Rate	Normal Respiratory Rate
Premature	<2.5	40	120–170	40–60
Term	3.5	60	100–170	40–60
3 months	6	60	100–170	30–50
6 months	8	60	100–170	30–50
1 year	10	72	100–170	30–40
2 years	13	74	100–160	20–30
4 years	15	78	80–130	20
6 years	20	82	70–115	16
8 years	25	86	70–110	16
10 years	30	90	60–105	16
12 years	40	94	60–100	16

Typical blood pressure in children 1 to 10 years of age:
80 mm Hg + (child's age in years × 2)

Lower limits of systolic blood pressure in children 1 to 10 years of age:
70 mm Hg + (child's age in years × 2)

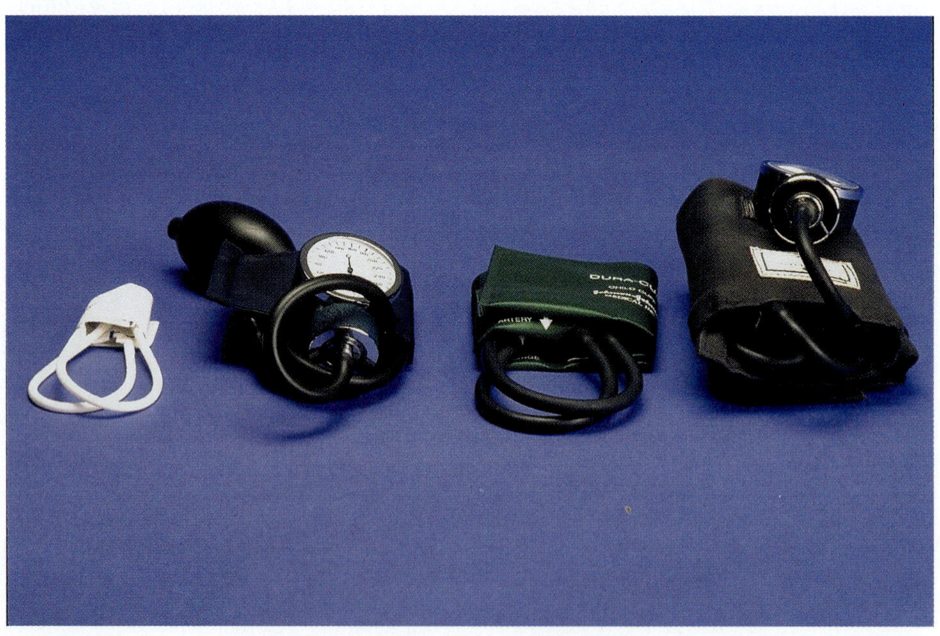

To obtain an accurate BP reading, use a cuff that is two-thirds the length of the child's upper arm.

7.12 Phone Numbers

Other Resource Numbers

Agency for Toxic Substance and Disease Registry (ATSDR)	(404) 639-0615
Chemtrec	(800) 424-9300
Diver's Alert Network (Duke University)	(919) 684-4326
Domestic Abuse Hotline	(800) 550-1119
Florida Abuse Hotline	(800) 962-2873
Florida Department of Health—Bureau of EMS	(904) 226-1911
Poison Information Center	(800) 222-1222
Runaway Hotline	(800) 231-6946

7.13 Oxygen Tolerance in COPD

It is common to find protocols that caution against the use of high concentrations of supplemental oxygen for patients with COPD (emphysema). Such protocols may restrict supplemental oxygen for a spontaneously breathing COPD patient at 2 liters/minute by nasal cannula. The intent is to avoid inhibition of their spontaneous respiratory efforts. However, it is desirable to minimize how long a patient, including those with COPD or serious hypoxia, must endure. Shock from hypoxia is life threatening. All patients should receive supplemental oxygen as quickly and as high a concentration as their systems will tolerate when serious hypoxia is present. The clinical problem in the field is determining how much supplementary oxygen a COPD patient can safely tolerate.

COPD patients regulate their spontaneous ventilation by internal measurement of the oxygen content in their blood. This is different from normal patients who use CO_2 content to guide ventilation. When a COPD patient is hypoxic, ventilation is overstimulated. If the COPD patient has a large surplus of oxygen, as may occur with inappropriate use of high concentrations of supplemental oxygen, spontaneous ventilation decreases or becomes apneic. An understanding of this simple physiologic control mechanism can be used to safely titrate oxygen administration with COPD patients.

When COPD patients have acute respiratory distress, oxygen may be given in high concentrations until the rapid respiratory rate begins to slow down towards normal. This shows that hypoxia is becoming less severe and respiratory drive is starting to return to normal. The supplemental oxygen dosage may then be reduced in a titrated manner as the respiratory rate returns to normal. This approach allows oxygenation to be restored as quickly as possibly and reduces the potential harm of extended hypoxia.

If spontaneous ventilation becomes severely compromised, perform bag-mask ventilations without supplemental oxygen until adequate spontaneous ventilations resume. If the spontaneous ventilation becomes further compromised from an acute respiratory emergency, and not from excessive oxygen, assist ventilations with supplemental oxygen. These two situations may be distinguished from one another by signs of severe hypoxia such as cyanosis, pallor, or diaphoresis. These would indicate acute respiratory distress. If there is uncertainty about whether or not to give oxygen, always give the oxygen and be ready to assist ventilations as needed. This will be less dangerous than withholding oxygen from a patient who may be in desperate need of it.

7.14 Report of Abuse

Florida Abuse Hotline: (800) 962-2873

State Substantive Laws (Crimes)

Chapter 415: Protection from Abuse, Neglect, and Exploitation
415.102 Definitions of terms used in FS 415.101–415.113.

(1) "Abuse" means the non-accidental infliction of physical or psychological injury or sexual abuse upon a disabled adult or an elderly person by a relative, caregiver, or household member, or an action by any of those persons which could reasonably be expected to result in physical or psychological injury, or sexual abuse of a disabled adult or an elderly person by any person. "Abuse" also means the active encouragement of any person by a relative, caregiver, or household member to commit an act that inflicts or could reasonably be expected to result in physical or psychological injury to a disabled adult or an elderly person.

(10) "Disabled adult" means a person 18 years of age or older who suffers from a condition of physical or mental incapacitation due to a developmental disability, organic brain damage, or mental illness, or who has one or more physical or mental limitations that substantially restrict ability to perform the normal activities of daily living.

(11) "Elderly person" means a person 60 years of age or older who is suffering from the infirmities of aging as manifested by advanced age or organic brain damage, or other physical, mental, or emotional dysfunctioning to the extent that the ability of the person to provide adequately for the persons' own care or protection is impaired.

415.111 Criminal penalties.

(1) A person who knowingly and willfully fails to report a case of known or suspected abuse, neglect, or exploitation of a disabled adult or an elderly person or who knowingly and willfully prevents another person from doing so, commits a misdemeanor of the second degree, . . .

415.503 Definitions of terms used in FS 415.502–415.514.

(1) "Abused or neglected child" means a child whose physical or mental health or welfare is harmed, or threatened with harm, by the acts or omissions of the parent or other person responsible for the child's welfare or, for the purposes of reporting requirements, by any person.

(2) "Child abuse or neglect" means harm or threatened harm to a child's physical or mental health or welfare by the acts or omissions of a parent, adult household member, or other person responsible for the child's welfare, or, for purposes of reporting requirements, by any person.

7.14 Report of Abuse

415.504 Mandatory reports of child abuse or neglect; mandatory reports of death; central abuse hotline.

(1) Any person, . . . who knows, or has reasonable cause to suspect, that a child is an abused, abandoned, or neglected child shall report such knowledge or suspicion to the department . . .

415.511 Immunity from liability in cases of child abuse or neglect.

(1)(a) Any person, official, or institution participating in good faith in any act authorized or required by FS 415.502–415.514, or reporting in good faith any instance of child abuse to any law enforcement officer shall be immune from any civil or criminal liability which might otherwise result by reason of such action.

415.513 Penalties relating to abuse reporting.

(1) A person who is required by FS 415.504 to report known or suspected child abuse or neglect; and who knowingly and willfully fails to do so, or who knowingly or willfully prevents another person from doing so, is guilty of a misdemeanor of the second degree . . .

7.15 Rule of Nines

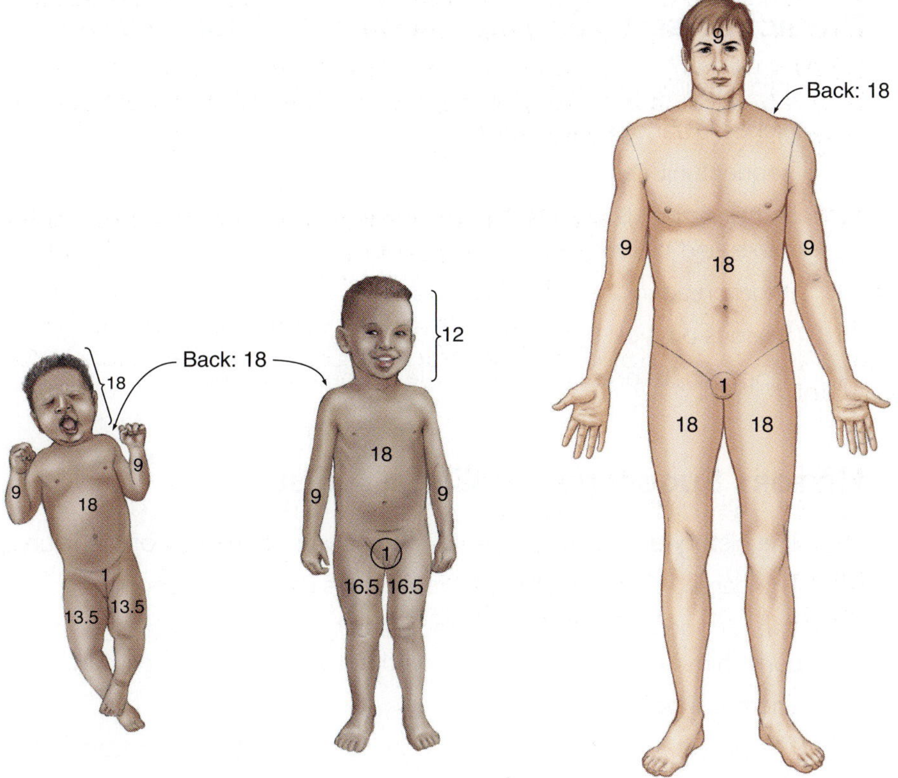

Rule of Nines.

7.16 Signs of Child Abuse

Physical Assessment Suggestive of Child Abuse

1. Fractures in children younger than 2 years of age.
2. Injuries in various stages of healing.
3. Frequent injuries.
4. Bruises or burns in patterns (e.g., iron or cigarette burns, cord marks, bite or pinch marks, and bruises to head, neck, back, or buttocks).
5. Widespread injuries over the body.
6. Obvious physical neglect (malnutrition, lack of cleanliness).
7. Inappropriate dress (e.g., very little clothes in winter).

History Suggestive of Child Abuse

1. The history does not match with the nature or severity of the injury.
2. The parents' and/or caregivers' account is vague or changes.
3. The "accident" is beyond the capabilities of the child (e.g., a 12-month-old who burns himself/herself by turning on the hot water in the bathtub).
4. There is a delay in seeking help.
5. The parent and/or caregiver may be inappropriately unconcerned about the child's injury.

Characteristics of the Abused Child

1. If younger than 5 years old, is likely to be passive.
2. If older than 5 years of age, is likely to be aggressive.
3. Does not look to the parent (the abuser) for support, comfort, or reassurance.
4. May cry without any expectation of receiving help.
5. May be quiet and withdrawn.
6. May be fearful of the parent (the abuser).

Characteristics of the Abuser

1. Crosses all religious, ethnic, occupational, educational, and socioeconomic boundaries.
2. May resent or reject the child.
3. May have feelings of worthlessness about self or about the child.
4. May have unrealistic expectations of what the child is capable of doing.
5. May be very critical of the child.
6. Oftentimes is repeating what the abuser learned as a child (the abuser was more than likely abused as a child).
7. May be overly defensive rather than concerned.

7.17 Sudden Infant Death Syndrome

Sudden infant death syndrome (SIDS), also known as "crib death," is the sudden and unexpected death of an apparently healthy infant, usually younger than 1 year of age, which remains unexplained after a complete medical history, death scene investigation, and postmortem examination.

The majority of SIDS deaths (90%) occur in infants younger than 6 months of age. SIDS is more common in males (60%) than in females (40%). SIDS almost always occurs when the infant is asleep or thought to be asleep. It is more prevalent in winter months and in infants with low birth weights. SIDS occurs in all socioeconomic, racial, and ethnic groups. Occasionally, a mild upper respiratory infection may be present prior to death.

Physical examination of a SIDS infant may reveal lividity or settling of blood, which produces mottled, blue, or gray skin. The lividity may give the appearance of "bruising." There may also be a froth, consisting of blood-tinged mucus draining from the infant's mouth and nostrils. In addition, cooling and rigor mortis may be present. The SIDS infant usually appears well developed and does not exhibit any signs of external injury.

SIDS should not be confused with child abuse (see Appendix 7.16, Signs of Child Abuse). Initially, it is difficult to distinguish a SIDS death from other causes of death in infants. SIDS is the leading cause of death between 1 week and 1 year of age in the United States.

For specific treatment for SIDS, see Pediatric Protocol 3.4.2.

7.18 Consent for the Care of a Minor

Emancipation: Florida Statute 326

Freedom of a child from legal subjection to parents/guardians and having the right to labor for himself/herself and collect and control the person's own wages is called "emancipation."

- Emancipation of a child may be in writing.
- Emancipation of a child may be by parol (word of mouth).
- Emancipation of a child may be expressed or implied from the parents' conduct, which makes further obedience of the child difficult.
- Emancipation cannot result merely from a minor child giving birth and becoming a parent.

Emancipation becomes a matter of law when a minor leaves home permanently, secures his/her own living quarters, and becomes completely self-supporting, with the parents paying none of his/her bills. Once emancipation is established, the parent is no longer liable for the child's debts, including those for "necessities" such as medical treatment.

Removal of Disabilities of Non-age (Court-Ordered Emancipation): Florida Statute 743.075

The court may determine that the removal of disability of non-age (minor), at least 16 years of age, is in the child's best interest and shall enter an order to that effect. This order shall give a minor the status of an adult for purposes of all criminal and civil laws of the state. The judgment is recorded in the county where the minor resides, and a certified copy shall be issued as proof.

Married Minors

Any minor who is married, even if divorced or widowed, may give consent.

Unwed Pregnant Minor or Minor Mother—Consent to Medical Care: Florida Statute 743.065

- An unwed pregnant minor may consent to care relating to her pregnancy.
- An unwed minor mother may consent to care for her child.

7.18 Consent for the Care of a Minor

Emergency Medical Care to Minors Without Parental Consent: Florida Statute 743.064

Emergency medical care may be given to a minor who has been injured in an accident or is suffering from acute illness if, within a reasonable degree of medical certainty, delay of treatment would endanger the health or physical well-being of the minor.

This applies only when parental consent cannot be obtained for the following reasons:

- The minor's condition causes him/her to be unable to reveal the identity of parents/guardian and that information is also unknown to anyone who is with the minor.
- The parents/guardian cannot be located.
- Notification must be made as soon as possible after emergency medical care is administered.

The EMS Run Report must indicate the reason consent was not obtained.

Other Persons Who May Consent to Medical Care of a Minor: Florida Statute 743.0645

Any of the following persons, *in order of priority listed,* may consent to the medical care of a minor:

1. A person who possesses a power of attorney to provide medical consent for the child.
2. Stepparent.
3. Grandparent.
4. Adult brother or sister.
5. Adult aunt or uncle.

The EMS Run Report should reflect that a reasonable attempt was made to contact the person who has power to consent. "Medical care and treatment" means ordinary and necessary medical and dental examination and treatment, including blood testing, immunization, and TB testing. It does *not* include surgery, anesthesia, psychotropic medications, or other extraordinary procedures.

7.19 Recommended Guidelines for Occupational Exposures to Infectious Diseases

I. Prevention

A. **Purpose.** Emergency medical and public safety employees ("workers") are at risk for exposure to and possible transmission of vaccine preventable diseases. Maintenance of immunity is, therefore, an essential part of prevention and infection control programs.

B. **At-Risk Workers.** Workers who are exposed to blood, body fluids, feces, and/or respiratory secretions should have on record before employment or should be offered during employment all immunizations currently recommended by the U.S. Public Health Service.

C. **Low-Risk Workers.** Timely post-exposure prophylaxis rather than pre-exposure vaccination may be considered for other workers whose exposure to infectious agents is infrequent.

D. **Special-Risk Groups.** Periodic evaluations may be done as indicated for job reassignment, for ongoing programs (e.g., TB screening), or for evaluation of work-related problems.

E. **History of Immunity.** A medical evaluation that includes childhood immunity or immunization history for measles, mumps, rubella, and varicella zoster (chickenpox) should be obtained from and recorded for all new workers at the time of hire or as part of a catch-up program (CDC MMWR 1997;46[No. RR-18]) (NFPA 1581, 2-5.2.2).

II. Baseline and Annual Screening

A. **Baseline Screening.** Baseline screening for TB and hepatitis A, B, and C is indicated for presumptive law requirements (FS 112.181 6(a)(b)).

B. **TB Screening.** Tuberculin skin test shall be performed for all workers who do not have a history of a positive skin test result. A two-step Mantoux skin testing shall be used for the initial screening of workers who have not been tested. The two-step procedure should be performed only once (CDC MMWR 1994;43[RR-13]). After that, only a PPD skin test should be administered annually. Workers with a new positive PPD should have a baseline chest X-ray performed with one follow-up chest X-ray a year later.

C. **Hepatitis Screening.** If baseline screening for hepatitis A and B shows that immunity is absent, the employer should offer vaccination to the worker. Hepatitis C screening is performed for baseline and post-exposure only.

D. **Test Result Maintenance.** Baseline and annual screening test results shall be maintained according to applicable laws governing medical confidentiality, and released strictly by and between the medical provider conducting the tests and the worker. The employer may maintain a sealed copy of baseline, titer, and/or annual test results in the worker's infection control file and may not cause to open said result(s) without the specific written consent from the worker (29 CFR 1910.1030 (h)).

7.19 Recommended Guidelines for Occupational Exposures to Infectious Diseases

III. Immunization

A. **Education.** Workers shall have bloodborne/airborne pathogen training prior to immunization (29 CFR 1910.1030(f)(2)). Medical providers and/or designated infection control officers should offer upon request vaccine product and safety information to workers considering or undergoing vaccination. Educational materials need to be appropriate in content and vocabulary to the educational level and literacy of the worker.

B. **Declination.** Workers who waive vaccination shall sign a Declination Form. If the worker initially declines vaccination(s) but at a later date decides to accept the vaccination(s), the employer shall make the vaccination(s) available (29 CFR 1910.1030(f)).

C. **Hepatitis Vaccination.** Hepatitis B vaccination shall be offered to at-risk workers within 10 days of initial assignment, unless the worker has documentation of previously complete vaccination series, documentation of immunity, or physician's documentation of medical contraindication for the vaccine (29 CFR 1910.1030(f)(2)). Hepatitis A vaccination may be offered if specific local conditions dictate (NFPA 1581, 2-5.2.2).

1. **Post-vaccination Screening for Hepatitis A.** Post-vaccination screening for immunity to hepatitis A is not indicated if the vaccine series is completed, because of the high rate of adult vaccine response.
2. **Post-vaccination Screening for Hepatitis B.** Post-vaccination screening for immunity to hepatitis B is indicated. If vaccinated workers fail to develop a protective hepatitis B antibody level, the entire HBV vaccination series should be repeated only once.
3. **Periodic Serologic Screening and Booster Doses.** Any periodic post-vaccination screening is not recommended. Booster doses are not currently recommended. If the U.S. Public Health Service recommends a routine booster dose(s) of hepatitis vaccine at a future date, such booster dose(s) shall be made available (29 CFR 1910.1030(f)(1)(ii)).

D. **Influenza.** Workers are considered to be at significant risk for acquiring or transmitting influenza (the common flu). Influenza vaccine should be made available to workers from October through February annually (CDC MMWR 1997;46[No. RR-18]).

7.20 Infectious Exposure Reference Sheet

Airborne	Transmission	Prevention	Post-exposure	Follow-up
Tuberculosis (TB)	Droplets: coughing, sneezing, intubation, suctioning.	Initial two-step test, then annual PPD. HEPA mask.	Source = PPD. Employee = PPD, unless PPD tested within prior 12 weeks or previously PPD reactive.	PPD at week 12 post-exposure. If new positive: chest X-ray and treatment with isoniazid for 6 months.
Meningitis (bacterial/viral)	Droplets: coughing, sneezing, intubation, suctioning.	HEPA mask.	Antibiotic: Cipro, rocephin, rifampin.	Seek medical care if symptoms of meningitis develop: fever, stiff neck, severe headache.
Influenza	Close contact, drop-lets: coughing, sneezing, intubation, suctioning. Also direct contact with vesicle fluid.	Flu shot.	Treatment: analgesics, rimantadine, Tamiflu, Relenza.	As determined by medical professional.
Varicella zoster (Chick-enpox)	Close contact, droplets: coughing, sneezing, intubation, suctioning. Also direct contact with vesicle fluid.	Vaccine = one-shot (Varivax). HEPA mask.	Treatment: varicella zoster immune globulin (VZIG) within 96 hours of exposure.	As determined by medical professional.
Other	**Transmission**	**Prevention**	**Post-exposure**	**Follow-up**
Tetanus	Soiled object causing open wound.	Vaccine good for 10 years.	If no vaccine, administer at this time. If more than 7 years from last vaccination and sustained open wound, booster dose.	Seek medical care if symptoms of tetanus develop: lockjaw, rigid muscles.
Lyme disease	Tickborne: tick attached 24 hours.	Avoid tick-infested areas. Vaccine = three-shot series for prone areas.	Antibiotics: amoxicillin, doxycycline.	As determined by medical professional.
Scabies	Direct contact: mite-infested areas, bedding/clothing, nursing homes.	Avoid infected areas.	Lindane and Kwell applied to the whole body for 24 hours.	Close supervision of treatment, including bathing.
Rabies	Virus-laden saliva of infected animal: animal bites.	Avoid animal bites.	Wash infected areas. Administer rabies antiserum injection and first dose of rabies vaccine. Contact animal control; monitor animal for presence of infection.	If animal is positive, continue to treat employee with vaccine.
HAV	Fecal/oral.	Vaccine = two-shot series.	Source = acute hep panel. Employee = acute hep panel. If source positive, employee not immune: administer immune globulin and consider HAV vaccine series.	Periodic screening: 12 weeks after exposure or if symptoms occur.

7.20 Infectious Exposure Reference Sheet

Blood-borne	Transmission	Prevention	Post-exposure	Follow-up
HIV	Blood to blood, to non-intact skin and mucous membranes.	No vaccine.	See Post-exposure Management (General Protocol 1.12).	Periodic screening: 6, 12, 26 weeks after exposure.
Syphilis	Blood and/or open sores/lesions.	No vaccine.	Source = RPR. Employee = RPR. Penicillin. Repeat test at 3 and 6 months; if positive, refer to FTA.	As determined by medical professional.
HBV	Blood to blood, to non-intact skin and mucous membranes.	Vaccine = three-shot series. Titer and reimmunize if necessary.	Source = acute hep panel. Employee = acute hep panel. If source positive, employee not immune: administer immune globulin and consider HBV vaccine series.	Periodic screening: 6, 12, 26 weeks after exposure.
HCV	Blood to blood, to non-intact skin and mucous membranes.	No vaccine.	Source = acute hep panel. Employee = acute hep panel.	Periodic screening: 6, 12, 26 weeks after exposure. If source positive, consider employee qualitative HCV RNA and ALT testing 6 weeks after exposure. If employee becomes HCV RNA positive, treat with interferon/ ribavirin × 6 months.

Terminology	
HEPA mask	A personal protective device worn on the face to remove particles equal to and greater than 0.3 micron in size (which essentially includes all bacteria, spores, and viruses) with an efficiency of 99.97%.
PPD	A method of assessing whether someone has become infected with *Mycobacterium tuberculosis* complex. The test involves measurement of a subject's immune response to an injection of tuberculin purified protein derivative (PPD) manufactured from killed *M. tuberculosis* bacilli. Also referred to as tuberculin skin tests or PPD tests.
Vesicle fluid	The serum from the blister formed during a varicella zoster infection.
VZIG	Varicella zoster immune globulin.
Qualitative HCV-RNA	Blood test to detect the presence of hepatitis C virus.
ALT	Blood test to measure a liver-specific enzyme that indicates liver cell death or inflammation.

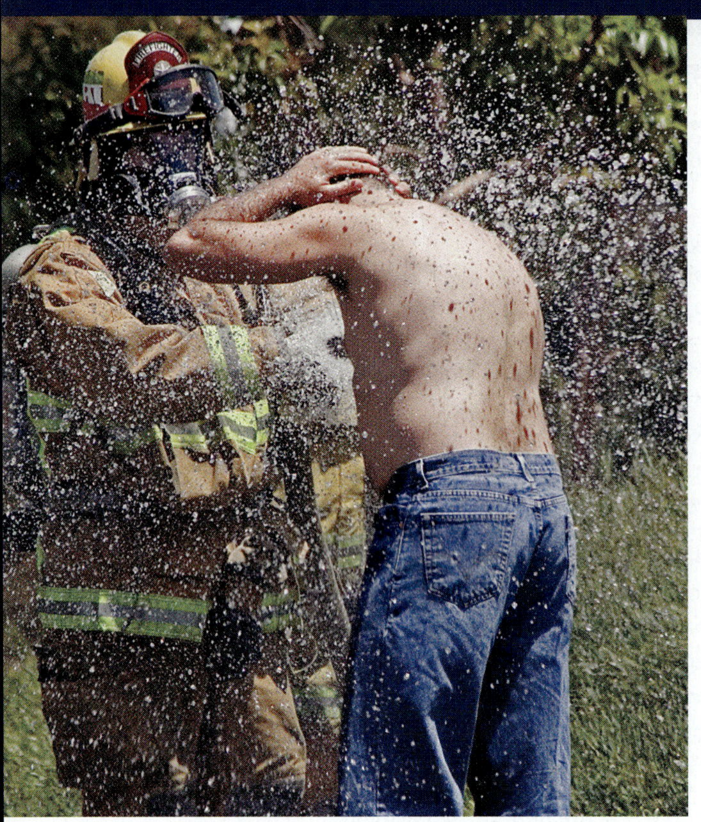

chapter 8

Hazardous Materials Exposure

Introduction

These protocols have been developed to address the specialized treatment of patients exposed to hazardous materials. Some of the agents covered in these protocols may be used as a weapon of mass destruction (WMD) in a terrorist attack. In these instances, **scene safety and a need to stage at a safe distance from the scene should be a primary concern for all personnel.** The protocols cover exposure to chemical (8.1), biological (8.2), and radiological (8.3) agents. A color code is assigned to each protocol in the Chemical section (8.1), which coincides with the chemical treatment guide and color-coded chemical antidote drug box. **The Chemical Treatment Guides are divided into adult and pediatric sections.**

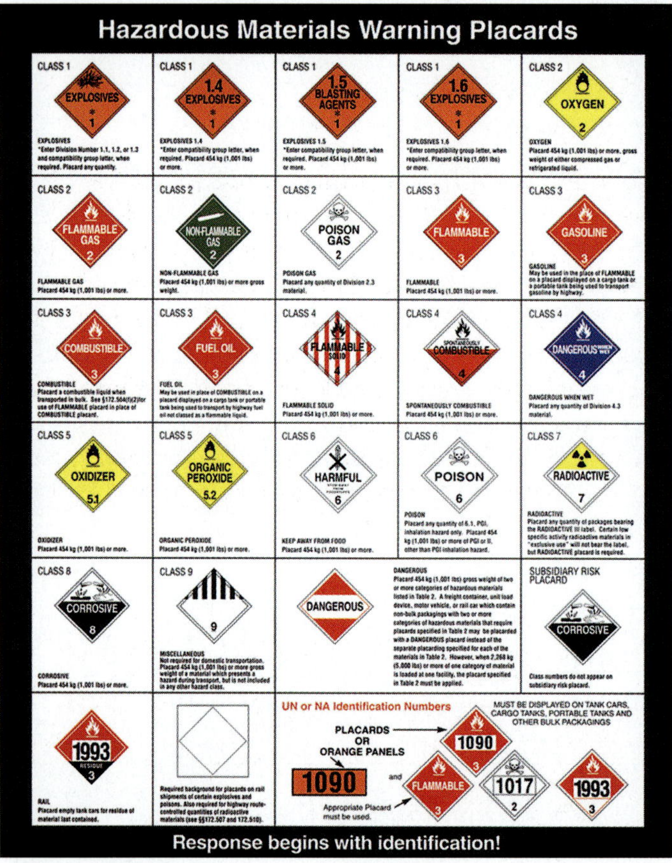

Hazardous materials warning placards.

8.1 Adult Hazardous Material Exposure (Chemicals)

This protocol is to be used for those patients suspected of exposure to hazardous materials via any route of exposure (e.g., inhalation, absorption). The protocols give specific considerations for each type of exposure as well as general treatment guidelines. Scene safety should be of primary concern, with special attention being paid to the need for personal protective equipment. Additional assistance may be necessary in certain cases (e.g., hazardous materials team for toxic exposure, police for scene control, including a violent and/or impaired patient—see Adult Protocol 2.5.2).

A history of the events leading to the illness or injury should be obtained from the patient and bystanders, to include the following information:

1. To which poison or other substances was the patient exposed?
2. When and how much?
3. Duration of symptoms?
4. Is there any pertinent medical history?
5. Accidental? Nature of accident?
6. Duration of exposure (if applicable)?

If risk of exposure from fumes is high, call the hazardous materials team. In this instance, refer to the appropriate hazardous materials PPE protocol, as the risk of secondary contamination is very high. All patients who have been exposed to hazardous materials must be properly decontaminated prior to initiation of extensive medical treatment and transportation to the hospital.

Contact the Poison Information Center (1-800-222-1222) for consultation regarding specific therapy, and then contact the receiving emergency department for confirmation of Level 2 orders.

It is imperative that the emergency department be made aware early that a contaminated patient is being transported so that the proper preparations can be made to receive the patient.

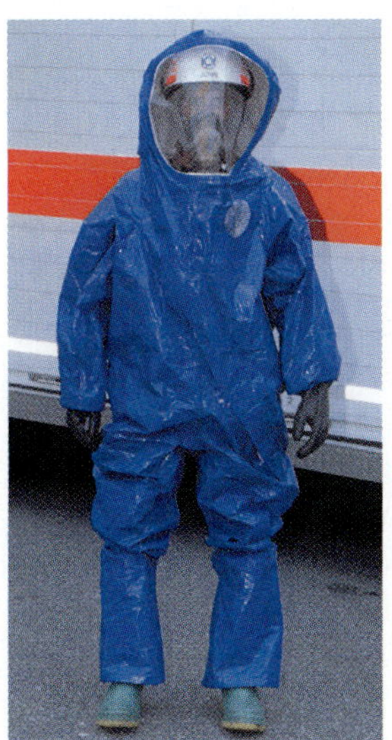
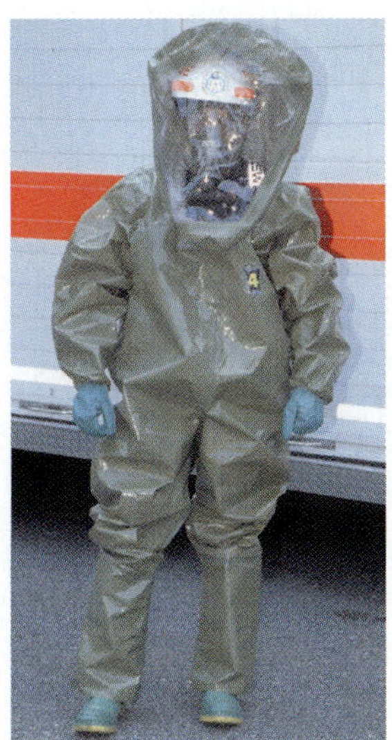
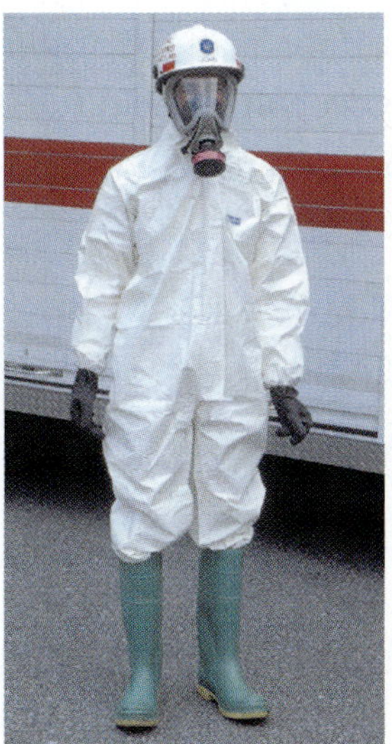
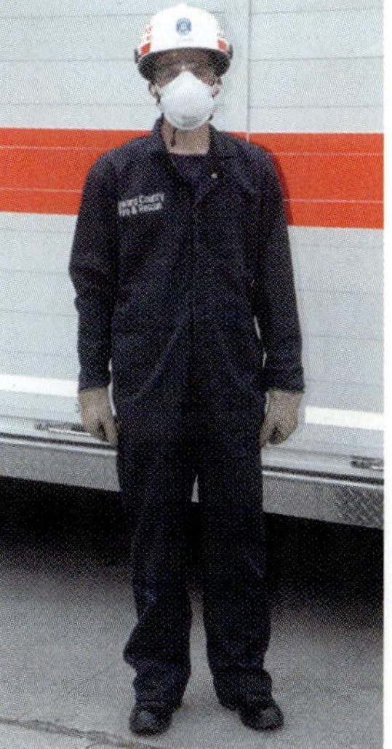

Four levels of protection. A. Level A protection. B. Level B protection. C. Level C protection. D. Level D protection.

8.1.1 Acids and Acid Mists

Treatment

Chemical Treatment Guide 1: *YELLOW*

Description

Acids are colorless to yellow liquids with strong irritating odors. Some acids may be **flammable** agents. Acids act as direct irritants and corrosive agents to moist membranes and to intact skin to a lesser extent.

Signs and Symptoms

Low concentrations of airborne acids can produce rapid onset of eye, nose, and throat irritation.

Higher concentrations can produce cough, stridor, wheezing, chemical pneumonia, and non-cardiogenic pulmonary edema. Ingestion of acids can result in severe injury to the upper airway, esophagus, and stomach. In addition, there may be circulatory collapse, as well as partial- or full-thickness burns.

End-stage symptoms may resemble organophosphate poisoning. However, patients will have **normal or dilated pupils** (patients *will not* have pinpoint pupils). These patients *should not* be given atropine or 2-PAM.

Note

This protocol does *not* include hydrofluoric acid (see Adult Protocol 8.1.13).

Examples

- Sulfuric acid (battery acid)
- Muriatic acid (pool cleaner)
- Hydrochloric acid (HCl)
- Some drain cleaners

8.1.2 Alkaline Compounds

Treatment

Chemical Treatment Guide 1: *YELLOW* ☐

Description

Most alkaline compounds are solids. Alkalis will impart a soapy texture to aqueous solutions. Alkalis act as direct irritants and corrosive agents to moist membranes and to intact skin to a lesser extent. The extent of tissue penetration and severity of injury is usually greater with alkalis than with acids.

Signs and Symptoms

Low concentrations of airborne alkalis can produce rapid onset of eye, nose, and throat irritation.

Higher concentrations can produce cough, stridor, wheezing, chemical pneumonia, and non-cardiogenic pulmonary edema. Ingestion of alkalis can result in severe injury to the upper airway, esophagus, and stomach. In addition, there may be circulatory collapse, as well as partial- or full-thickness burns.

End-stage symptoms may resemble organophosphate poisoning. However, patients will have **normal or dilated pupils** (patients *will not* have pinpoint pupils). These patients *should not* be given atropine or 2-PAM.

Examples

- Lye (baseball field line chalk)
- Cement
- Some drain cleaners
- Sodium hydroxide

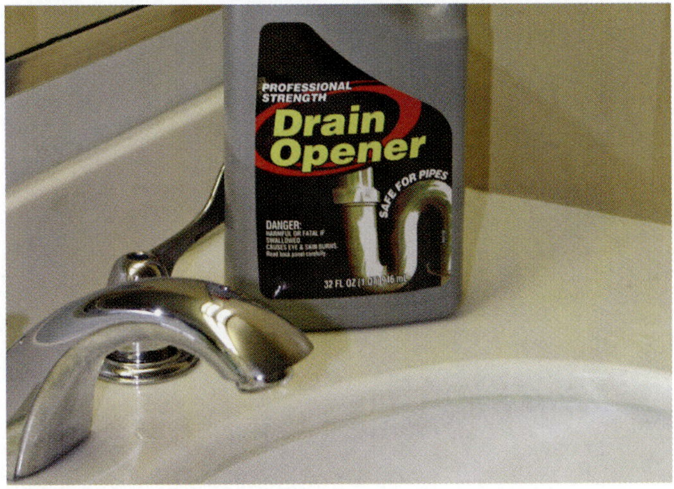

Plumbing agents used in the home.

8.1.3 Ammonia (Liquid and Gas)

Treatment

Chemical Treatment Guide 1: *YELLOW* □

Description

Ammonia is a colorless gas having an extremely pungent odor, which may be in an aqueous solution or gaseous state. Liquefied compressed gas may produce a cryogenic (freezing) hazard as it is released into the atmosphere. Common household ammonia contains 5–10% ammonia. It is a direct irritant and, in much higher concentrations, an alkaline corrosive agent to moist mucous membranes and, to a lesser extent, to intact skin. A chloramine gas can be liberated when household ammonia is mixed with a hypochlorite solution (bleach), which may injure the airway.

Signs and Symptoms

Low concentrations of airborne ammonia can produce cough, stridor, wheezing, and chemical pneumonia (non-cardiogenic pulmonary edema).

Ingestion of concentrated ammonia (e.g., >5%) may cause corrosive injury to the esophagus, stomach, and eye.

End-stage symptoms may resemble organophosphate poisoning. However, patients will have **normal or dilated pupils** (patients *will not* have pinpoint pupils). These patients *should not* be given atropine or 2-PAM.

Examples

- Component of household cleaners
- Refrigerant gases
- Used in manufacture of plastics, explosives, and pesticides
- Corrosion inhibitor
- Used in water purification process
- Component of fertilizers

8.1.4 Aromatic Hydrocarbons (Benzene, Toluene, Xylene) and Ketones

Treatment

Chemical Treatment Guide 2: *BLUE* ■

Description

Aromatic hydrocarbons may be found as colorless liquids or in a solid form with an ether-like or pleasant odor. These compounds may be highly **flammable.**

Ketones are organic compounds derived from secondary alcohols by oxidation. They generally have low viscosity, low to moderate boiling points, moderate vapor pressures, and high evaporation rates. Most ketones are chemically stable liquids. Routes of exposure include absorption through the skin and eyes, inhalation, and ingestion.

Signs and Symptoms

Mild exposure: cough, hoarseness, headache, drowsiness, dizziness, weakness, tremors, transient euphoria, vision and hearing disturbances, nausea/vomiting, salivation, and stomach pain.

Moderate to severe exposure: cardiovascular collapse, tachydysrhythmias (especially ventricular fibrillation), chest pain, pulmonary edema, dyspnea, tachypnea, respiratory failure, paralysis, altered mental status, seizures, excessive salivation, and delayed carcinogenic effects.

Halogenated hydrocarbons (chloride, bromide, iodide, fluoride) may present with ventricular tachycardia, ventricular fibrillation, and supraventricular tachycardias.

Aromated hydrocarbons may present with altered mental status.

End-stage symptoms may resemble organophosphate poisoning. However, patients will have **normal or dilated pupils** (patients *will not* have pinpoint pupils). These patients *should not* be given atropine or 2-PAM.

Examples

- Components of gasoline
- Methyl benzene
- Methyl benzol
- Phenyl methane

8.1.5 Arsenic Compounds (Heavy Metal Poisoning)

Treatment

Chemical Treatment Guide 2: *BLUE* ■

Description

Arsenic compounds may be found as white, transparent, or colorless crystals; colorless liquids; or colorless gas (e.g., ant poison). They are either odorless or have a garlic-like odor. Some are **flammable.** Exposure can be fatal or cause severe injury at concentrations too low to detect.

Lewisite is a blistering agent made from arsenic that causes immediate pain, irritation, and blistering of skin and mucous membranes. It is very similar in action to mustard and may be treated as mustard (see Protocol 8.1.17).

Arsine gas is made from arsenic and causes renal failure and destruction of red blood cells. Most exposures commonly occur when arsine gas is used to extract precious metals from ore.

Signs and Symptoms

Severe gastrointestinal fluid loss, burning abdominal pain, watery or bloody diarrhea, muscle spasm, seizures, cardiovascular collapse, tachycardia, hypotension, ventricular dysrhythmias, shock, and coma. There may be respiratory or cardiac arrest, and acute renal failure may occur with bronze urine within a few minutes.

Examples

- Component of wood preservatives, insecticides, and herbicides
- Arsine gas: used to extract precious metals from ore

8.1.6 Carbamate (Insecticide Poisoning)

Treatment

Chemical Treatment Guide 4: *GREEN* ■

Description

Carbamate may be found in a solid, powder, or liquid form; it has a white or gray color and a weak odor. This reversible acetyl cholinesterase inhibitor is found in insecticides, herbicides, and some medicinal products.

Many carbamates are well absorbed through intact skin, so they pose a serious exposure risk to rescuers. Simple water washing may be sufficient to remove oily compounds. Carbamates affect both the parasympathetic nervous system (muscarinic effects) and the sympathetic nervous system (nicotinic effects). Although the muscarinic effects may be reversed with atropine, the nicotinic effects may cause respiratory paralysis and require intubation and aggressive ventilatory support.

Carbamates may be incorporated in a **flammable** base.

Signs and Symptoms

Muscarinic effects are the same as seen with organophosphates, which are described as the classic **SLUDGE** syndrome (excessive **S**alivation, **L**acrimation, **U**rination, **D**iarrhea, **G**astrointestinal distress, and **E**mesis). Additional muscarinic effect include bronchorrhea, bronchospasm, and bradycardia. The patient will have **constricted pupils** (miosis) with inhalation or skin exposure. Ingestion may or may not cause miosis; however, stimulation of nicotinic receptors will produce tachycardia, muscle paralysis (apnea), muscle twitching/fasiculations, and seizures.

Examples

Insecticides used for house tenting: Temic, Metical, Isolan, Furadan, Lannae, Zectran, Mesurol Dimetialn, Bagon

Note

PPE (usually Level A) with SCBA must be worn in the hazardous area when carbamates are present. PPE with a minimum of Level C protection must be worn for treatment outside the hazardous area.

8.1.7 Carbon Monoxide Poisoning

Treatment

Chemical Treatment Guide 2: *BLUE* ■

Description

Carbon monoxide (CO) poisoning should be suspected when the patient has been exposed to the products of combustion (e.g., smoke, automobile exhaust, exhaust fumes from fuel-powered machinery) and is experiencing symptoms. These symptoms may vary with the level of CO exposure.

Signs and Symptoms

Mild CO exposure: headache, nausea/vomiting, poor concentration, irritability, agitation, and anxiety. May resemble flu-type symptoms. Suspect CO exposure during a cold snap with use of charcoal heaters and other types of furnaces, and where there are multiple victims in the same house or building.

Moderate to severe CO exposure: altered mental status, chest pain, cardiac dysrhythmias, pale skin, cyanosis, seizures, and rarely cherry-red skin.

Examples

- Suspect CO poisoning when multiple victims in same building exhibit symptoms.
- Use of petroleum-fueled heaters, machinery, and other devices inside a building (especially with improper ventilation).
- Incomplete burning of natural gas, LP gas, gasoline, kerosene, oil, coal, wood, or any other material containing carbon.
- Fire fighters working at a fire scene, especially during overhaul operations.

8.1.8 Chlorinated Hydrocarbons

Treatment

Chemical Treatment Guide 2: *BLUE* ■

Description

Methylene chloride is a volatile liquid that yields heavy vapors. At room temperature, it is a clear, colorless liquid with a pleasant (ether-like) odor. Exposure can occur through skin absorption, eye contact, inhalation, and ingestion. Methylene chloride is converted inside the body to carbon monoxide.

Signs and Symptoms

Cardiovascular collapse, ventricular dysrhythmias, respiratory arrest, pulmonary edema, dyspnea and tachypnea, headache, drowsiness, dizziness, altered mental status, seizures, nausea/vomiting, diarrhea, abdominal cramps, and chemical burns.

Examples

- Component (solvent) in paint, varnish strippers, and degreasing agents
- Used in production of photographic films, synthetic fibers, pharmaceuticals, adhesives, inks, and printed circuit boards
- Employed as a blowing agent for polyurethane foams, as a propellant for insecticides, in air fresheners, and in paint

8.1.9 Chlorine Gas and Phosgene (CG)

Treatment

Chemical Treatment Guide 1: *YELLOW* ☐

Description

Chlorine is either a colorless to amber-colored liquid (aqueous chlorine is usually in the form of hypochlorite [bleach] in variable concentrations) or a greenish-yellow gas (anhydrous) with a characteristic odor. The liquid hypochlorite solutions are very unstable and react with acids to release chlorine gas (e.g., bleach mixed with vinegar or a toilet bowl cleaner containing HCl). Liquefied compressed chlorine gas may produce a cryogenic (freezing) hazard as it is released into the atmosphere. Clothing that has been soaked in a hypochlorite solution can be a hazard to rescuers. A chloramine gas may be liberated when a hypochlorite solution (bleach) is mixed with household ammonia, which may cause injury to the airway.

Phosgene (CG) is a chemical warfare agent. Phosgene gas can be liberated when Freon or chlorinated compounds (e.g., bleach mixed with ammonia) are heated. Phosgene has similar effects on the body as chlorine; however, symptoms from phosgene may be delayed for several hours.

Signs and Symptoms

Both agents: dyspnea, tachypnea, cough, choking sensation, rhinorrhea, acute or delayed chemical pneumonia (non-cardiogenic pulmonary edema), ventricular dysrhythmias, cardiovascular collapse, severe irritation and burns of the mucous membranes and lungs, headache, dizziness, altered mental status, nausea/vomiting, and severe irritation and burns to the eyes and skin.

Examples

- Chlorine gas is used in water purification processes at water plants and sewage treatment plants, as well as in pesticides, refrigerants, and solvents.
- Hypochlorite solutions are used in cleaning solutions and as disinfectants for water (drinking, waste, and swimming pools).
- Phosgene is used in paint removers, dry cleaning fluid, dyes, and pesticides.

8.1.10 Cyanide: Hydrogen Cyanide, Hydrocyanic Acid (AC), Cyanogen Chloride (CK), Potassium Cyanide, Sodium Cyanide

Treatment

Chemical Treatment Guide 5: *RED*

Description

Cyanide can be found in a liquid (solutions of cyanide salts), solid (cyanide salts), or gaseous (hydrogen cyanide) form. In solid form, it is white and has a faint almond odor (20% of the population is genetically unable to detect the odor). Hydrogen cyanide gas may be formed when acid is added to cyanide salt or a nitrite or when plastics burn. If a large amount of liquid or solid cyanide material is present on the victim's clothing or skin, it poses a significant risk of exposure to rescuers. Exposure can occur through skin absorption, eye contact, inhalation, and ingestion. If the patient is unconscious and is being rescued from a fire, there is a high probability of concurrent carbon monoxide and cyanide poisoning; both conditions must be treated (also see Chemical Treatment Guide 2: *Blue* for these patients).

Signs and Symptoms

Cardiovascular: initially, pulse decreases and BP rises; in later stages, dysrhythmias and cardiovascular collapse can occur. There may also be palpitations and/or chest tightness.

Respiratory: can cause immediate respiratory arrest. Initially, there is usually an increase in the rate and depth of respirations, which later become slow and gasping.

CNS: can cause immediate coma. Initially there is usually weakness, headache, and confusion; seizures are common.

GI: nausea/vomiting, salivation.

Skin: pale, cyanotic, or reddish color. Death is caused by an inhibitory action on the cytochrome oxidase system, preventing tissue usage of oxygen.

Note

- PPE (usually Level A) with SCBA must be worn in the hazardous area when cyanide compounds are present. PPE with a minimum of Level C protection must be worn for treatment outside the hazardous areas.
- Good medical supportive care, including airway management, is paramount and should precede the use of the cyanide antidote kit. However, the rapid administration of the cyanide antidote kit will be the only therapy that will reverse the **life-threatening symptoms** of cyanide poisoning.

8.1.10 Cyanide: Hydrogen Cyanide, Hydrocyanic Acid (AC), Cyanogen Chloride (CK), Potassium Cyanide, Sodium Cyanide

Examples

- Hydrogen cyanide is used in the production of organic chemicals (it may be called nitrile).
- Potassium and sodium cyanide are used primarily in electroplating and metal treatment.
- Cyanides may be present in smoldering fires (e.g., wool, foams).

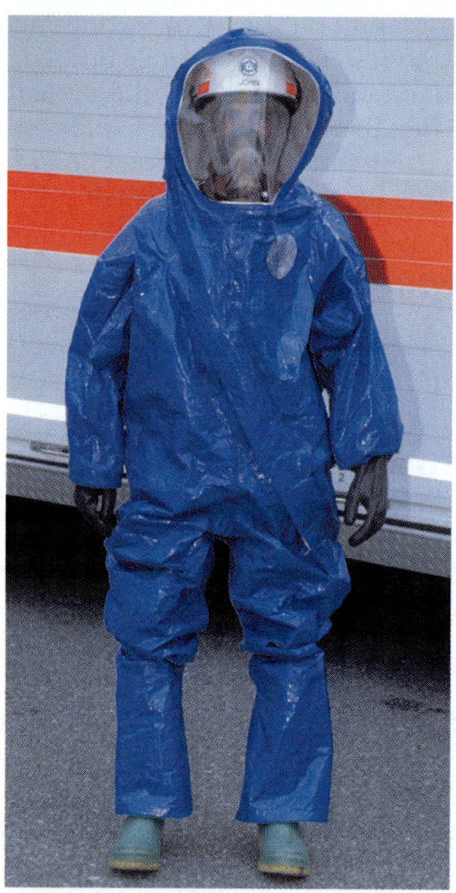

PPE (usually level A) with SCBA must be worn in hazardous areas where cyanide compounds are present.

8.1.11 Dinitrobenzene (DNB)

Treatment

Chemical Treatment Guide 3: *GRAY* ■

Description

DNB is a colorless, oily liquid with a characteristic and peculiar sweet odor. It can also be found as a solid. DNB causes methemoglobinemia, resulting in a state of relative hypoxia due to the inability of RBCs to carry oxygen. **DNB is *explosive;* it is detonated by heat or shock.**

Signs and Symptoms

Signs and symptoms of the methemoglobinemia caused by this exposure include chocolate-brown-colored blood, headache, ataxia, vertigo, tinnitus, dyspnea, CNS depression, hypotension, heart blocks, ventricular dysrhythmias, seizures (rare), cyanosis, and cardiovascular collapse.

8.1.12 Ethylene Glycol

Treatment

Chemical Treatment Guide 6: *PINK*

Description

Ethylene glycol is an odorless, colorless, syrupy liquid found in antifreeze, brake fluid, and other industrial products. Because it is readily available and relatively inexpensive, it is often used in suicide attempts. Ingestion is the primary route of exposure. The potential lethal dose is reported to be 100 mL (1.0–1.5 mL/kg) in adults. It is the toxic metabolites—not the parent compound—that are responsible for the associated toxic effects. These effects include metabolic acidosis, tetany, QT interval prolongation on the ECG, and irreversible kidney failure. Ethylene glycol poisoning can be fatal, and quick diagnosis and intervention are imperative to prevent the damaging effects of the metabolites. If the patient has concurrently ingested ethanol, symptoms of ethylene glycol toxicity may be delayed.

Signs and Symptoms

The clinical manifestations of ethylene glycol poisoning occur in three phases:

- **Phase I (30 minutes to 12 hours):** ethanol-like inebriation, metabolic acidosis, seizures, and coma.
- **Phase 2 (12 to 36 hours):** tachycardia, tachypnea, hypertension, pulmonary edema.
- **Phase 3 (36 to 48 hours):** crystalluria, acute tubular necrosis with oliguria—renal failure.

Examples

- Component of antifreeze (including new-generation-type antifreeze)
- Brake fluids
- Inks in stamp pads and ballpoint pens
- Paints and plastics

8.1.13 Hydrofluoric Acid (HF)

Treatment

Chemical Treatment Guide 7: *ORANGE*

Description

Hydrofluoric acid is a colorless to yellow liquid with a strong, irritating odor. Because the boiling point of HF is 67°F, when exposed to air, HF will readily change to a gaseous state. When HF comes in contact with metals, it forms hydrogen gas, which is extremely **flammable.** Once HF is absorbed into the tissues, it binds to calcium and magnesium. This form of fluoride poisoning can be fatal, even if exposure is due to a dilute solution (<3%). Contact with as little as 7 mL of 100% solution can cause death.

Signs and Symptoms

Hypovolemic shock and collapse, tachycardia with weak pulse, acute pulmonary edema, asphyxia, chemical pneumonitits, upper airway obstruction with stridor, pain and cough, decreased LOC, nausea/vomiting, diarrhea, possible GI bleeding, and possible blindness. HF also causes severe skin burns. The damage may be severe with no outward signs, except that the patient will complain of severe pain.

Examples

- Rust removers
- Metal plating
- Glass etching
- Computer manufacturing

8.1.14 Hydrogen Sulfide, Sulfides, and Mercaptans

Treatment

Chemical Treatment Guide 5: *RED* ■

Description

Members of this class of gases are colorless but have a strong offensive odor, like rotten eggs or sewer gas. When they are present at high levels, however, the olfactory senses will be overwhelmed, making the gas odorless. These chemicals may be found in a liquid form at low temperatures or high pressures. Clothing that has become soaked in sulfide solutions or mercaptans may pose a risk to rescuers. These types of chemicals can cause severe respiratory irritation, including pulmonary edema and respiratory paralysis (especially likely with hydrogen sulfide).

Signs and Symptoms

Cardiovascular collapse, tachycardia, dysrhythmias, irritation of the respiratory tract, cough, dyspnea, tachypnea, respiratory arrest, pulmonary edema, headache, altered mental status, garlic taste in mouth, seizures, nausea/vomiting, diarrhea, profuse salivation, dermatitis, sweating, and possible cyanosis.

Examples

- Found in sewers, septic tanks, livestock waste pits, manholes, well pits, and similar settings
- Found in chemical wastes, petroleum, and natural gas (28%)
- Produced in industrial processes that work with sulfur compounds

8.1.15 Methanol

Treatment

Chemical Treatment Guide 6: *PINK*

Description

Methanol is found as a highly volatile clear liquid and in mixtures. It is used in solvents, additives, and emulsifiers. It is a frequent ingredient in windshield washer fluid. Routes of exposure include skin absorption, eye contact, inhalation, and ingestion. Methanol has CNS depressant properties that are highly toxic upon aspiration and can cause respiratory failure and cardiac dysrhythmias. The metabolites that are formed following the metabolism of methanol—formaldehyde and formic acid—can cause a severe delayed toxicity.

Signs and Symptoms

Cardiovascular: dysrhythmias and hypotension.

Respiratory: respiratory insufficiency or arrest, pulmonary edema, chemical pneumonitis, and bronchitis.

CNS: CNS depression and coma, seizures, headache, muscle weakness, and delirium.

GI: GI bleeding, nausea/vomiting, and diarrhea.

Eye: chemical conjunctivitis.

Skin: problems ranging from irritation to full-thickness burns.

Examples

- Sterno

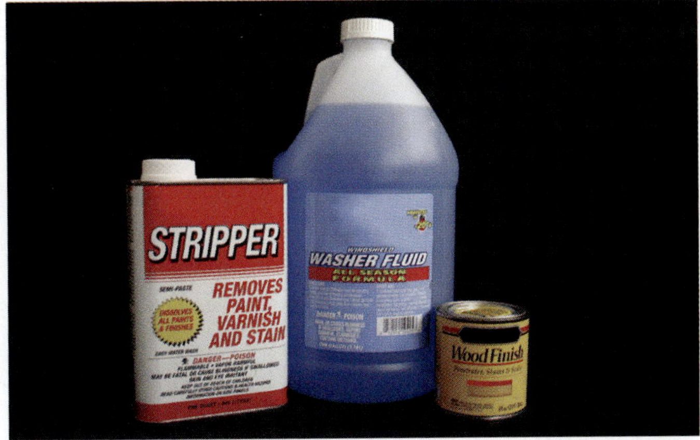

Methanol is found in solvents and windshield washer fluid, as well as varnishes.

8.1.16 Methylene Biphenyl Isocyanate, Ethyl Isocyanate, and Methylene DiIsocyanate (MDI)

Treatment

Chemical Treatment Guide 1: *YELLOW* ☐

Description

MDI is found as a solid, whose color ranges from white to yellow flakes. Various liquid solutions are also used for industrial purposes. There is no odor to the solid or liquid solutions. The vapor is approximately eight times heavier than air.

This chemical is a strong irritant to the eyes, mucous membranes, skin, and respiratory tract. MDI is also a very potent respiratory sensitizer. Various industrial processes utilize MDI in production and usage of (poly)urethane foams, lacquers, and sealants; MDI is also used in the production of insecticides and laminating materials. These chemicals are not cyanide compounds.

Signs and Symptoms

Irritation to the eyes, mucous membranes, skin, and respiratory tract (cough, dyspnea, and pulmonary edema).

Examples

- Component of smoke in plastic fires

8.1.17 Mustard (Sulfur Mustard): Lewisite, Blister Agents (H, HD, HS)

Treatment

Chemical Treatment Guide 1: *YELLOW* □

Description

Mustard is a "blister agent" that causes cell damage and destruction. It is a colorless to light yellow to dark brown oily liquid with the odor of garlic, onion, or mustard. It does not evaporate readily, but may pose a vapor hazard in warm weather. Mustard is a vapor and liquid hazard to skin and eyes, and a vapor hazard to airways. Its vapor is five times heavier than air.

Sulfur mustard has been used as a research tool to study DNA damage and repair. A variety of military munitions are filled with mustard, including projectiles, mortars, and bombs. Mustard damages DNA in cells, which leads to cellular damage and death. It penetrates the skin and mucous membranes very quickly, and cellular damage begins within minutes.

Lewisite is a "blister agent" that has the same effect on the body as mustard, with the exception that onset of symptoms begins immediately.

Signs and Symptoms

Mustard: Clinical effects begin within 2 to 24 hours. The initial effects include the following issues: (1) eyes: itching or burning, redness, corneal damage; (2) skin: erythema with itching and burning, blisters; and (3) respiratory tract: epistaxis, hoarseness, sinus pain, dyspnea, and cough.

Lewisite: same effect on the body as mustard, with the exception that onset of symptoms begins immediately.

Examples

- Chemical warfare agents

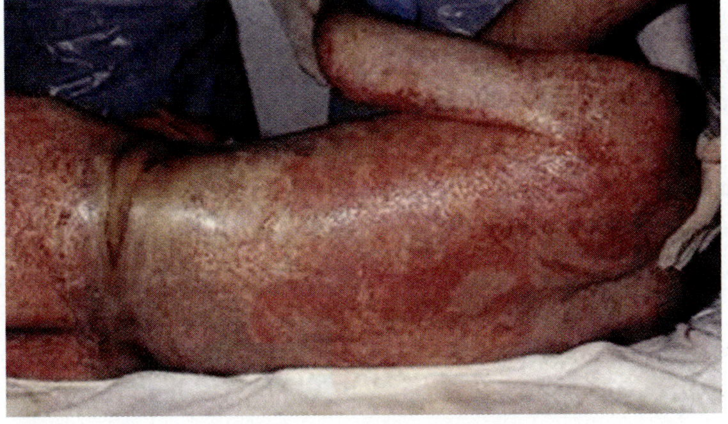

Skin damage resulting from exposure to sulfer mustard (agent H).

8.1.18 Nitrogen Products and Other Products Causing Methemoglobinemia

Treatment

Chemical Treatment Guide 3: *GRAY* ■

Descriptions

These products can be found in a gas, liquid, or solid form. They are released from the combustion or decomposition of substances that contain nitrogen. Depending on the individual compound, these agents may pose a significant health hazard for rescuers. Many are well absorbed through intact skin. Simple water washing may be sufficient to remove oil compounds. Other routes of exposure include eye contact, inhalation, and ingestion. These products are respiratory tract irritants that can cause a severe, delayed pulmonary edema or immediate upper airway irritation and edema. They also change Fe^2 to Fe^3 (methemoglobinemia), which does not bind to oxygen.

Signs and Symptoms

Cardiovascular: cardiovascular collapse with weak and rapid pulse.

Respiratory: a mild, transient cough and tachypnea (only symptoms at the time of exposure to most agents). A delayed onset of dyspnea, tachypnea, violent coughing, cyanosis, and pulmonary edema follows. Some agents work immediately on the upper airway, resulting in pain and choking, spasm of the glottis, temporary reflex arrest of breathing, and possibly upper airway obstruction spasm or edema of the glottis.

CNS: headache, dizziness, vertigo, fatigue, restlessness, and decreased LOC (usually delayed signs).

GI: burning of the mucous membranes, nausea/vomiting, and abdominal pain.

Eye: chemical conjunctivitis.

Skin: irritation of moist skin areas, pallor, and cyanosis with normal SpO_2.

Note

Symptoms may be immediate or may be delayed for 5 to 72 hours.

Examples

- Propellant fuels and agricultural fumigants
- Also used in laboratory research solvents, bleaching agents, and refrigerants
- Found in grain silos (silo filler's disease)
- Product of combustion in most fires (e.g., structure fires)

8.1.19 Organophosphates: Insecticide Poisoning and Nerve Agents (GA, GB, GD, GF, VX)

Treatment

Chemical Treatment Guide 4: *GREEN* ■

Description

Organophosphate compounds are used as insecticides in residential applications as well as commercial agriculture. They are found as liquids, dusts, wettable powders, concentrates, and aerosols. **Chemical nerve agents include Tabun (GA), Sarin (GB), Soman (GD), GF, and VX.** Many are well absorbed through intact skin, so they pose a serious hazard to rescuers. Simple water washing may be sufficient to remove oily compounds. Routes of exposure include skin absorption, eye contact, inhalation, and ingestion.

Organophosphates affect both the parasympathetic nervous system (muscarinic effects) and the sympathetic nervous system (nicotinic effects). Although the muscarinic effects may be reversed with atropine, the nicotinic effects may cause respiratory paralysis and require intubation and aggressive ventilatory support. Organophosphates may be incorporated in a **flammable** base.

Signs and Symptoms

Exposure may produce the classic **SLUDGE** syndrome (excessive **S**alivation, **L**acrimation, **U**rination, **D**iarrhea, **G**astrointestinal distress, and **E**mesis). Additional muscarinic effects include bronchorrhea, bronchospasm, and bradycardia. The patient will have **constricted pupils** (miosis, which may last as long as 2 months) with inhalation or skin exposure. Ingestion may or may not cause miosis. However, stimulation of nicotinic receptors will produce tachycardia, muscle paralysis (apnea), muscle twitching/fasiculations, and seizures.

Examples

- Pesticides (e.g., Chlorthion, Diazinon, Dipterex, Di-Syton, Malathion, Parathion, Phosdrin)
- Chemical warfare agents (e.g., VX, Sarin, Tabun, Soman)

Note

PPE (usually Level A) with SCBA must be worn in the hazardous area when organophosphates are present. PPE with a minimum of Level C protection must be worn for treatment outside the hazardous areas.

8.1.20 Phenol

Treatment

Chemical Treatment Guide 9: *WHITE* ☐

Description

Phenol (**carbolic acid**), at room temperature, is a translucent, colorless, crystalline mass; white powder; or thick, syrupy liquid. The crystals turn pink to red in air. Phenol has a sweet, tar-like odor that is readily detected at low concentrations. It is soluble in alcohol, glycerol, petrolatum, and, to a lesser extent, water.

Phenol is absorbed rapidly by all routes; however, the inhalation hazard is limited. In dilute concentrations (1% to 2%), phenol may cause severe burns. Systemic toxicity can rapidly lead to death.

Phenol is mainly used in the manufacture of phenolic resins and plastics. It is also used as a disinfectant and has some medicinal applications (e.g., Campho Phenique®).

Signs and Symptoms

Nausea/vomiting, diarrhea, excessive sweating, headache, dizziness, ringing in the ears, seizures, loss of consciousness, coma, respiratory depression, inflammation of the respiratory tract, shock, and death. Exposure to skin can result in severe burns, which will cause the skin to have a white, red, or brown appearance. Failure to decontaminate the skin may allow the phenol to be absorbed systemically, resulting in death.

Examples

- Used in the manufacture of phenolic resins and plastics
- Used as a disinfectant
- Campho Phenique®

8.1.21 Phosphine

Treatment

Chemical Treatment Guide 8: *PURPLE* ■

Description

Phosphine can be found in a gas, liquid, or solid form. Most gases are colorless to brown, and have a sharp odor. Phosphine is used as a chemical warfare and protection agent, as a propellant fuel, and as an agricultural fumigant. Some compounds are used in laboratory research, solvents, and pesticides. They are released from the combustion or decomposition of substances that contain nitrogen. A toxic exposure can result from working on or in grain silos.

Very small amounts of phosphine can be trapped in a victim's clothing after an overwhelming exposure, posing a risk to rescuers. Routes of exposure include skin absorption, eye contact, inhalation, and ingestion. Phosphine is a respiratory tract irritant that can cause a severe, delayed pulmonary edema or immediate upper airway irritation and edema.

Signs and Symptoms

Cardiovascular: cardiovascular collapse with weak and rapid pulse. Patients may present with a reflex bradycardia.

Respiratory: mild and transient cough (only symptom at the time of exposure to most agents). A delayed onset of dyspnea, tachypnea, violent coughing, and pulmonary edema follows. Some agents work immediately on the upper airway, resulting in pain and choking, spasm of the glottis, temporary reflex arrest of breathing, and possibly upper airway obstruction spasm or edema of the glottis.

CNS: fatigue, restlessness, and decreased LOC (usually delayed signs).

GI: burning of the mucous membranes, nausea/vomiting, and abdominal pain.

Eye: chemical conjunctivitis.

Skin: irritation of moist skin areas, pallor, and cyanosis.

Note

Symptoms may be immediate or may be delayed for 5 to 72 hours.

Examples

- Pesticides (especially rodenticides). Also see description.

Note

PPE (usually Level A) with SCBA must be worn in the hazardous area where phosphine is present. PPE with a minimum of Level C protection must be worn for treatment outside the hazardous areas.

8.1.G Chemical Treatment Guide Index

Chemical Name or Group Name	Treatment Guide
Acids and acid mists	Guide 1—YELLOW
Alkaline compounds	Guide 1—YELLOW
Ammonia (liquid and gas)	Guide 1—YELLOW
Aromatic hydrocarbons (benzene, toluene, xylene)	Guide 2—BLUE
Arsenic compounds (heavy metal poisoning)	Guide 2—BLUE
Blister agents (H, HD, HS)	Guide 1—YELLOW
Carbamates: insecticide poisoning	Guide 4—GREEN
Carbon monoxide poisoning	Guide 2—BLUE
Chlorinated hydrocarbons (methylene chloride)	Guide 2—BLUE
Chlorine gas	Guide 1—YELLOW
Cyanide	Guide 5—RED
Cyanogen chloride (CK)	Guide 5—RED
Methylene biphenyl isocyanate	Guide 1—YELLOW
Dinitrobenzene (DNB)	Guide 3—GRAY
Ethylene glycol	Guide 6—PINK
Ethyl isocyanate	Guide 1—YELLOW
Hydrocyanic acid (AC)	Guide 5—RED
Hydrogen cyanide	Guide 5—RED
Hydrofluoric acid (HF)	Guide 7—ORANGE
Hydrogen sulfide, sulfides	Guide 5—RED
Ketones	Guide 8—PURPLE
Lewisite	Guide 1—YELLOW
Mercaptans	Guide 5—RED
Methanol	Guide 6—PINK
Methylene biphenyl isocyanate	Guide 1—YELLOW
Methylene dilsocyanate (MDI)	Guide 1—YELLOW
Mustard (sulfur mustard)	Guide 1—YELLOW
Nerve agents (GA, GB, GD, GF, VX)	Guide 4—GREEN
Nitrogen products and other products causing methemoglobinemia	Guide 3—GRAY
Organophosphate insecticide poisoning	Guide 4—GREEN
Phenol (carbolic acid)	Guide 9—WHITE
Phosgene (CG)	Guide 1—YELLOW
Phosphine	Guide 8—PURPLE
Potassium cyanide	Guide 5—RED
Sodium cyanide	Guide 5—RED
Sulfur mustard (mustard)	Guide 1—YELLOW

Chemical Treatment Guide 1A: *YELLOW*

- **Acids and acid mists**
- **Alkaline compounds**
- **Ammonia (liquid and gas)**
- **Chlorine gas and phosgene (CG)**
- **Methylene biphenyl isocyanate, ethyl isocyanate, and methylene dilsocyanate (MDI)**
- **Mustard (sulfur mustard): Lewisite, blister agents (H, HD, HS)**

Signs and Symptoms

Low concentrations of airborne acids and alkalis can produce rapid onset of eye, nose, and throat irritation. Higher concentrations (low concentrations of ammonia) can produce cough, stridor, wheezing, and chemical pneumonia (non-cardiogenic pulmonary edema). Ingestion of acids and alkalis can result in severe injury to the upper airway, esophagus, and stomach. In addition, there may be circulatory collapse, as well as partial- or full-thickness burns.

End-stage symptoms may resemble organophosphate poisoning. However, patients will have **normal or dilated pupils** (patients *will not* have pinpoint pupils). These patients *should not* be given atropine or 2-PAM.

Supportive Care

- Remove the patient from the hazardous area (a).
- If the patient was exposed externally, remove his/her clothing and jewelry and decontaminate with copious amounts of water. Provide ocular irrigation with normal saline (do not attempt to neutralize with another solution) (see Medical Procedure 4.45, Morgan Lens).
- If the patient has external burns, see Adult Protocol 2.10.8, Burn Injuries.
- Medical Supportive Care Protocol 2.1.3. (Ipecac, charcoal, and NG tube are contraindicated; avoid oral airways.)
- Contact the Poison Information Center (1-800-222-1222).
- If the patient has pulmonary edema, maintain adequate ventilation and oxygenation, and provide pulmonary suction to remove fluid. Non-cardiogenic pulmonary edema should not be treated with Lasix, but with positive end-expiratory pressure (PEEP) or a CPAP mask (see Medical Procedure 4.24).

ALS Level 1

- If the patient has bronchospasm:
  - Albuterol (Ventolin®): 1 nebulizer treatment containing 2.5 mg of albuterol pre-mixed with 2.5 mL normal saline (see Medical Procedure 4.27). May repeat twice PRN (b)(c).
  - May give terbutaline (Brethine®) 0.25 mg SQ, if available.
- If bronchodilators are administered, may add ipratropium bromide (Atrovent®) 0.5 mg (0.5 mL) to either albuterol or levalbuterol nebulizer treatment **on first nebulizer treatment only** (b)(c).
- If the patient has inhaled chlorine or hydrochloric acid (HCl) and has significant respiratory distress, administer sodium bicarbonate via nebulizer (8.4% 3 mL mixed with normal saline 3 mL or 4.2% 6 mL).

Chemical Treatment Guide 1A: *YELLOW* ☐

- If the patient is seizing, administer one of the following benzodiazepines:
  - Diazepam (Valium®) 5 mg IV. If unable to start an IV, administer diazepam 5 mg intranasally or 10 mg per rectum. May repeat PRN up to 20 mg maximum dose (d)(e).

  or

  - Lorazepam (Ativan®) 2 mg IV. If unable to start an IV, administer lorazepam 2 mg IM. May repeat once PRN (maximum dose = 4 mg) (d).

  or

  - Midazolam (Versed®) 2 mg IV. If unable to start an IV, administer midazolam 2 mg intranasally. May repeat once PRN (maximum dose = 4 mg) (d).
- If hypotension persists, treat PRN (see Adult Protocol 2.4.1).

ALS Level 2

None.

Note

(a) If risk of exposure from fumes is high, call for a hazardous materials team. Refer to the appropriate hazardous materials PPE protocol, as the risk of secondary contamination is very high.

(b) Do not give albuterol or ipratropium bromide if the patient's heart rate ≥ 140.

(c) Caution should be used when the patient is older than 40 years of age or has a history of hypertension or heart disease.

(d) Intranasal administration of benzodiazepines requires the use of a mucosal atomization device.

(e) Use a tuberculin or 3–5 mL syringe *without the needle* to administer diazepam (Valium®). Position the patient in a decubitus knee position or supine, with the legs held apart, and insert the lubricated syringe approximately 5 cm (approximately 2 inches) into the rectum. Inject the diazepam, remove the syringe, and tape the patient's buttocks closed.

Chemical Treatment Guide 2A: *BLUE* ■

- **Aromatic hydrocarbons (benzene, toluene, xylene)**
- **Arsenic compounds (heavy metal poisoning)**
- **Carbon monoxide poisoning**
- **Chlorinated hydrocarbons (methylene chloride)**

Signs and Symptoms

Mild exposure signs and symptoms: Cough, hoarseness, headache, poor concentration, irritability, agitation, anxiety, drowsiness, dizziness, weakness, tremors, transient euphoria, vision and hearing disturbances, nausea/vomiting, salivation, diarrhea, stomach pain, and chemical burns with chlorinated hydrocarbons. (For arsenic signs and symptoms, see below.)

Moderate to severe exposure signs and symptoms: Cardiovascular collapse, tachydysrhythmias (especially ventricular fibrillation), chest pain, pulmonary edema, dyspnea, tachypnea, respiratory failure, paralysis, altered mental status, seizures, excessive salivation, pale skin, cyanosis, rarely cherry-red skin with carbon monoxide, and delayed carcinogenic effects. (For arsenic signs and symptoms, see below.)

Signs and symptoms of arsenic exposure: Severe gastrointestinal fluid loss, burning abdominal pain, watery or bloody diarrhea, muscle spasm, seizures, cardiovascular collapse, tachycardia, hypotension, ventricular dysrhythmias, shock, and coma. There may be respiratory or cardiac arrest, and acute renal failure may occur with bronze urine within a few minutes.

End-stage symptoms may resemble organophosphate poisoning. However, patients will have **normal or dilated pupils** (patients *will not* have pinpoint pupils). These patients *should not* be given atropine or 2-PAM.

Products may be **flammable.**

Supportive Care

- Remove the patient from the hazardous area (a).
- Medical Supportive Care Protocol 2.1.3. (Ipecac and an NG tube are contraindicated. Avoid oral airways.)
- If the patient was exposed externally, remove his/her clothing and jewelry and decontaminate as appropriate. Provide ocular irrigation with normal saline (see Medical Procedure 4.45, Morgan Lens).
- Administer high-flow oxygen (100%) (b).
- Contact the Poison Information Center (1-800-222-1222).
- If the patient has pulmonary edema, maintain adequate ventilation and oxygenation, and provide pulmonary suction to remove fluid. Non-cardiogenic pulmonary edema should not be treated with Lasix, but with positive end-expiratory pressure (PEEP) or a CPAP mask (see Medical Procedure 4.24).

Chemical Treatment Guide 2A: *BLUE*

ALS Level 1

- If the patient has dysrhythmias, treat PRN (see Adult Protocol 2.3) (c).
- If the patient is seizing, administer one of the following benzodiazepines:
  - Diazepam (Valium®) 5 mg IV. If unable to start an IV, administer diazepam 5 mg intranasally or 10 mg per rectum. May repeat PRN up to 20 mg maximum dose (d)(e).

  or

  - Lorazepam (Ativan®) 2 mg IV. If unable to start an IV, administer lorazepam 2 mg IM. May repeat once PRN (maximum dose = 4 mg) (d).

  or

  - Midazolam (Versed®) 2 mg IV. If unable to start an IV, administer midazolam 2 mg intranasally. May repeat once PRN (maximum dose = 4 mg) (d).
- If hypotension persists, treat PRN (see Adult Protocol 2.4.1) (c).

ALS Level 2

None.

Note

(a) If risk of exposure from fumes is high, call for a hazardous materials team. Refer to the appropriate hazardous materials PPE protocol, as the risk of secondary contamination is very high.

(b) Document the duration of exposure to CO and when oxygen therapy was started (this information is needed to assist in making HBO decisions).

(c) Administration of epinephrine to patients in a pre-code status may not be desirable for this group of patients. A physician or the Poison Information Center should guide the administration of epinephrine in these cases.

(d) Intranasal administration of benzodiazepines requires the use of a mucosal atomization device.

(e) Use a tuberculin or 3–5 mL syringe *without the needle* to administer diazepam (Valium®). Position the patient in a decubitus knee position or supine, with the legs held apart, and insert the lubricated syringe approximately 5 cm (approximately 2 inches) into the rectum. Inject the diazepam, remove the syringe, and tape the patient's buttocks closed.

Chemical Treatment Guide 3A: *GRAY* ■

- **Dinitrobenzene (DNB)**
- **Nitrogen products and other products causing methemoglobinemia**

Signs and Symptoms

Methemoglobinemia characterized by chocolate-brown-colored blood, CNS depression, headache, dizziness, ataxia, vertigo, tinnitus, dyspnea, tachypnea, violent coughing, choking, possibly upper airway obstruction spasm or edema of the glottis, abdominal pain, hypotension, heart blocks, ventricular dysrhythmias, seizures (rare), pallor, cyanosis, and cardiovascular collapse.

Note

Symptoms may be immediate or may be delayed for 5 to 72 hours.

Supportive Care

- Remove the patient from the hazardous area (a).
- Medical Supportive Care Protocol 2.1.3.
- If the patient was exposed externally, remove his/her clothing and decontaminate as appropriate.
- Administer high-flow oxygen (100%).
- Contact the Poison Information Center (1-800-222-1222).
- If nitrogen product ingestion occurred, administer activated charcoal 50 g PO.

ALS Level I

- If the patient is dyspneic, is cyanotic, has normal SpO_2, and has chocolate-brown-colored blood, administer methylene blue (1%) 1–2 mg/kg slow IV over 5 minutes, followed by a normal saline 30 mL flush to decrease pain at the IV site.
- If the patient has dysrhythmias, treat PRN (see Adult Protocol 2.3).
- If the patient is seizing, administer one of the following benzodiazepines:
  - Diazepam (Valium®) 5 mg IV. If unable to start an IV, administer diazepam 5 mg intranasally or 10 mg per rectum. May repeat PRN up to 20 mg maximum dose (b)(c).

  or

  - Lorazepam (Ativan®) 2 mg IV. If unable to start an IV, administer lorazepam 2 mg IM. May repeat once PRN (maximum dose = 4 mg) (b).

  or

  - Midazolam (Versed®) 2 mg IV. If unable to start an IV, administer midazolam 2 mg intranasally. May repeat once PRN (maximum dose = 4 mg) (b).
- If hypotension persists, treat PRN (see Adult Protocol 2.4.1).
- Do *not* induce vomiting.

Chemical Treatment Guide 3A: *GRAY*

ALS Level 2

- If cyanosis persists, administer methylene blue (1%) 1–2 mg/kg slow IV over 5 minutes, followed by a 30 mL flush of normal saline to decrease pain at the IV site.

NOTE

(a) If risk of exposure from fumes is high, call for a hazardous materials team. Refer to the appropriate hazardous materials PPE protocol, as the risk of secondary contamination is very high.

(b) Intranasal administration of benzodiazepines requires the use of a mucosal atomization device.

(c) Use a tuberculin or 3–5 mL syringe *without the needle* to administer diazepam (Valium®). Position the patient in a decubitus knee position or supine, with the legs held apart, and insert the lubricated syringe approximately 5 cm (approximately 2 inches) into the rectum. Inject the diazepam, remove the syringe, and tape the patient's buttocks closed.

Chemical Treatment Guide 4A: *GREEN*

- **Carbamates: insecticide poisoning**
- **Organophosphates: insecticide poisoning and nerve agents (GA, GB, GD, GF, VX)**

Signs and Symptoms

The muscarinic effects are described as the classic **SLUDGE** syndrome (excessive **S**alivation, **L**acrimation, **U**rination, **D**iarrhea, **G**astrointestinal distress, and **E**mesis). Additional muscarinic effects include bronchorrhea, bronchospasm, and bradycardia. The patient will have constricted pupils (miosis, which may last as long as 2 months despite appropriate treatment) with inhalation or skin exposure. Ingestion may or may not cause miosis. Stimulation of nicotinic receptors will produce tachycardia, muscle paralysis (apnea), muscle twitching/fasiculations, and seizures.

Supportive Care

- Remove the patient from the hazardous area (a).
- Avoid exposure to the patient's sweat, vomit, stool, and vapors emitting from soaked clothes.
- Medical Supportive Care Protocol 2.1.3. Administer high-flow O_2.
- If the patient was exposed externally, remove his/her clothing and decontaminate as appropriate (place the patient's clothes in sealed bag).
- Contact the Poison Information Center (1-800-222-1222).

ALS Level I

If treating 1–4 patients:

- If the patient is bradycardic (patient is usually tachycardic) or has excessive pulmonary secretions, administer atropine 0.03 mg/kg IV (2 mg/70 kg). Repeat every 5 minutes until secretions are inhibited (b)(c).
- In case of organophosphate poisoning, consider pralidoxime (Protopam®, 2-PAM®) 1–2 g mixed in 100 mL NS IV drip over 30 minutes. In severe cases, 2-PAM® may be given via IV at a maximum rate of 200 mg/min or 1 g/5 min (used when nicotinic effects are present, as evidenced by fasciculation of large muscles). Observe patient for hypertension. (May be needed with high exposure to carbamates.)
- If the patient is seizing, administer one of the following benzodiazepines:
  - Diazepam (Valium®) 5 mg IV. If unable to start an IV, administer diazepam 5 mg intranasally or 10 mg per rectum. May repeat PRN up to 20 mg maximum dose (d)(e).

  or

  - Lorazepam (Ativan®) 2 mg IV. If unable to start an IV, administer lorazepam 2 mg IM. May repeat once PRN (maximum dose = 4 mg) (d).

  or

  - Midazolam (Versed®) 2 mg IV. If unable to start an IV, administer midazolam 2 mg intranasally. May repeat once PRN (maximum dose = 4 mg) (d).

Chemical Treatment Guide 4A: *GREEN* ■

If treating 5 or more patients or treating self-exposure (with pinpoint pupils):

- Administer **Mark I Kit(s)** (two auto-injectors containing atropine 2 mg in one and pralidoxime 600 mg in the other; see Medical Procedure 4.54) as follows:
  - For early symptoms (severe rhinorrhea or mild to moderate dyspnea): administer one Mark I auto-injector kit. If no improvement in patient's status in 10 minutes, administer another Mark I auto-injector kit (c)(f).
  - For severe respiratory distress, coma, or seizures: administer three Mark I auto-injectors and one CANA auto-injector (diazepam 10 mg IM) (c)(f).

For all patients meeting the preceding criteria:

- Alert the emergency department to prepare for a contaminated patient.
- Do *not* induce vomiting or give furosemide (Lasix®) or morphine.
- If the patient is experiencing eye pain and/or blepharospasm, administer scopolamine 1 drop in each eye.

ALS Level 2

None.

Note

(a) If risk of exposure from fumes is high, call for a hazardous materials team. PPE (usually Level A) with SCBA must be worn in the hazardous area. PPE with a minimum of Level C protection must be worn for treatment outside the hazardous area.

(b) If advised by the Poison Information Center, every other dose of atropine can be increased to 0.06 mg/kg IV.

(c) The endpoint for treatment is manifested by patient improvement with clear lung sounds.

(d) Intranasal administration of benzodiazepines requires the use of a mucosal atomization device.

(e) Use a tuberculin or 3–5 mL syringe *without the needle* to administer diazepam (Valium®). Position the patient in a decubitus knee position or supine, with the legs held apart, and insert the lubricated syringe approximately 5 cm (approximately 2 inches) into the rectum. Inject the diazepam, remove the syringe, and tape the patient's buttocks closed.

(f) When possible, establish an IV and administer atropine, diazepam, lorazepam, and midazolam IV and pralidoxime IV drip.

Chemical Treatment Guide 5A: *RED*

- **Cyanide: hydrogen cyanide, hydrocyanic acid (AC), cyanogen chloride (CK)**
- **Hydrogen sulfide, sulfides, and mercaptans**
- **Azides**

Signs and Symptoms

Cardiovascular: initially, pulse decreases and BP rises. In later stages, tachycardia, dysrhythmias, and cardiovascular collapse can occur. There may also be palpitations and/or chest tightness.

Respiratory: can cause immediate respiratory arrest. Initially there is usually an increase in the rate and depth of respirations, which later become slow and gasping. Irritation of the respiratory tract, cough, dyspnea, tachypnea, and pulmonary edema may also occur.

CNS: can cause immediate coma. Initially there is usually weakness, headache, and confusion; seizures are common.

GI: nausea/vomiting, profuse salivation, possibly garlic taste in mouth.

Skin: pale, cyanotic, or reddish color, dermatitis, sweating.

Note

Good medical supportive care, including airway management, is paramount and should precede the use of the cyanide antidote kit. However, the rapid administration of the cyanide antidote kit is the only therapy that will reverse the life-threatening symptoms.

Supportive Care

- Remove the patient from the hazardous area (a).
- Avoid exposure to vapors emitting from soaked clothes.
- Medical Supportive Care Protocol 2.1.3. Administer high-flow O_2.
- If the patient was exposed externally, remove his/her clothing quickly and decontaminate.
- Contact the Poison Information Center (1-800-222-1222).
- If the patient is conscious, administer activated charcoal 50 g PO for oral ingestion.
- Only a physician or the Poison Information Center can authorize treatment beyond supportive care for exposure to azides.

Chemical Treatment Guide 5A: *RED* ■

ALS Level I

- If the patient is unconscious, administer sodium bicarbonate 1 mEq/kg IV.
- If the patient is exhibiting life-threatening symptoms (severe respiratory compromise or arrest, shock, seizures, coma), administer the cyanide antidote kit (3 parts) in the following order (to induce methemoglobinemia). **If symptoms are not severe, or if diagnosis is not certain, omit Steps 1 and 2 and only give sodium thiosulfate (Step 3). Paramedics who are not part of a hazardous materials team and non-rescue supervisors can only give sodium thiosulfate.**

  Option 1: Rescue Supervisor and Hazardous Materials Team Paramedic

  1. Amyl nitrite (break pearls into gauze sponge and hold under the patient's nose or BVD intake valve) for 15–30 seconds of each minute until the sodium nitrite solution is ready (b).
  2. Sodium nitrite 3% (300 mg/10 mL) 10 mL (or 0.35 mL/kg) at 2.5–5 mL/min IV.

  All Paramedics

  3. Sodium thiosulfate 25% 12.5 g (50 mL) IV.

  Option 2: All Paramedics

  - Hydroxycarbolomine 5 g (2 vials) infused over 15 minutes: Reconstitute each vial (2.5 g) with 100 mL of normal saline and then infuse the first vial over 7.5 minutes and repeat for the second vial.
- If the patient has dysrhythmias, treat PRN (see Adult Protocol 2.3).
- If hypotension persists, treat PRN (see Adult Protocol 2.4.1).
- Alert the emergency department to prepare for a contaminated patient.
- Do *not* induce vomiting.
- If the patient is seizing, administer one of the following benzodiazepines:
  - Diazepam (Valium®) 5 mg IV. If unable to start an IV, administer diazepam 5 mg intranasally or 10 mg per rectum. May repeat PRN up to 20 mg maximum dose (c)(d).

  or

  - Lorazepam (Ativan®) 2 mg IV. If unable to start an IV, administer lorazepam 2 mg IM. May repeat once PRN (maximum dose = 4 mg) (c).

  or

  - Midazolam (Versed®) 2 mg IV. If unable to start an IV, administer midazolam 2 mg intranasally. May repeat once PRN (maximum dose = 4 mg) (c).

Chemical Treatment Guide 5A: *RED*

ALS Level 2

- If symptoms persist after 20 minutes, repeat the cyanide antidote kit at 50% of the initial dose.
- If the patient becomes cyanotic after administration of the cyanide antidote kit, contact the Poison Information Center **(1-800-222-1222)** for further instructions.

Note

(a) If risk of exposure from fumes is high, call for a hazardous materials team. Refer to the appropriate hazardous materials PPE protocol, as the risk of secondary contamination is very high.

(b) If the patient has IV access and received supportive care, Step 1 may be bypassed for Step 2.

(c) Intranasal administration of benzodiazepines requires the use of a mucosal atomization device.

(d) Use a tuberculin or 3–5 mL syringe *without the needle* to administer diazepam (Valium®). Position the patient in a decubitus knee position or supine, with the legs held apart, and insert the lubricated syringe approximately 5 cm (approximately 2 inches) into the rectum. Inject the diazepam, remove the syringe, and tape the patient's buttocks closed.

Chemical Treatment Guide 6A: *PINK*

- **Ethylene glycol**
- **Methanol**

Clinical Manifestations of Ethylene Glycol Poisoning

Phase I (30 minutes to 12 hours): ethanol-like inebriation, metabolic acidosis, seizures, and coma.

Phase 2 (12 to 36 hours): tachycardia, tachypnea, hypertension, pulmonary edema.

Phase 3 (36 to 48 hours): crystalluria, acute tubular necrosis with oliguria—renal failure.

Signs and Symptoms of Methanol Exposure

Cardiovascular: dysrhythmias and hypotension.

Respiratory: respiratory insufficiency or arrest, pulmonary edema, chemical pneumonitis, and bronchitis.

CNS: CNS depression and coma, seizures, headache, muscle weakness, and delirium.

GI: GI bleeding, nausea/vomiting, and diarrhea.

Eye: chemical conjunctivitis.

Skin: problems ranging from irritation to full-thickness burns.

Supportive Care

- Remove the patient from the hazardous area.
- Medical Supportive Care Protocol 2.1.3.
- Contact the Poison Information Center (1-800-222-1222).

Chemical Treatment Guide 6A: *PINK*

ALS Level 1

- If the patient is seizing, administer one of the following benzodiazepines:
  - Diazepam (Valium®) 5 mg IV. If unable to start an IV, administer diazepam 5 mg intranasally or 10 mg per rectum. May repeat PRN up to 20 mg maximum dose (a)(b).

  or

  - Lorazepam (Ativan®) 2 mg IV. If unable to start an IV, administer lorazepam 2 mg IM. May repeat once PRN (maximum dose = 4 mg) (a).

  or

  - Midazolam (Versed®) 2 mg IV. If unable to start an IV, administer midazolam 2 mg intranasally. May repeat once PRN (maximum dose = 4 mg) (a).
- If the patient's lungs are clear, administer normal saline at a rate of 100 mL/h IV.
- If the patient's respiratory rate is twice the normal rate, administer sodium bicarbonate 8.4% 1–2 mEq/kg IV.
- If the patient has dysrhythmias, treat PRN (see Adult Protocol 2.3).
- Administer thiamine 100 mg IV.

ALS Level 2

None.

NOTE

(a) Intranasal administration of benzodiazepines requires the use of a mucosal atomization device.

(b) Use a tuberculin or 3–5 mL syringe *without the needle* to administer diazepam (Valium®). Position the patient in a decubitus knee position or supine, with the legs held apart, and insert the lubricated syringe approximately 5 cm (approximately 2 inches) into the rectum. Inject the diazepam, remove the syringe, and tape the patient's buttocks closed.

Chemical Treatment Guide 7A: *ORANGE* ■

- **Hydrofluoric acid (HF)**
- **Vicane**

Signs and Symptoms

Hypovolemic shock and collapse, tachycardia with weak pulse, acute pulmonary edema, asphyxia, chemical pneumonitis, upper airway obstruction with stridor, pain and cough, decreased LOC, nausea/vomiting, diarrhea, possible GI bleeding, and possible blindness. HF also causes severe skin burns. The damage may be severe with no outward signs, except that the patient will complain of severe pain.

Supportive Care

- Remove the patient from the hazardous area (a).
- Medical Supportive Care Protocol 2.1.3. (Ipecac is contraindicated.)
- If the patient was exposed externally, remove his/her clothing and jewelry and decontaminate with copious amounts of water.
- Contact the Poison Information Center (1-800-222-1222).
- If the patient has pulmonary edema, maintain adequate ventilation and oxygenation, and provide pulmonary suction to remove fluid. Non-cardiogenic pulmonary edema should not be treated with Lasix, but with positive end-expiratory pressure (PEEP) or a CPAP mask (see Medical Procedure 4.24).

ALS Level I

- **If the patient has burns to the eye(s):**
  - Immediately flush with copious amounts of water or normal saline.
  - Prepare an eye wash solution by mixing calcium gluconate (10%) 50 mL in normal saline 500 mL (b).
  - Apply calcium gluconate eye wash using the Morgan lens (see Medical Procedure 4.45) and continue until arrival at the receiving facility (b).
- **If the patient has burns to the skin:**
  - Immediately flush with copious amounts of water.
  - Prepare a skin gel by mixing calcium gluconate (10%) 10 mL into a 2-oz tube of KY Jelly (making a 2.5% gel) (b).
  - Apply a 2.5% calcium gluconate gel on the burned area. For burns to the hand(s), place the hand in a glove filled with this gel (b).
- **For inhalation injury:**
  - Immediately support ventilations.
  - Administer calcium gluconate (10%) 1–2 g slow IV over 5 minutes.
  - For severe respiratory depression/arrest and/or cardiac toxicity (dysrhythmia, prolonged QT interval, hypotension), administer calcium gluconate (10%) 1–2 g slow IV over 5 minutes (b).
- If the patient has dysrhythmias, treat PRN (see Adult Protocol 2.3).
- If hypotension persists, treat PRN (see Adult Protocol 2.4.1).

Chemical Treatment Guide 7A: *ORANGE* ■

ALS Level 2

- If systemic symptoms persist, repeat calcium gluconate (10%) 1–2 g slow IV over 5 minutes (b).

NOTE

(a) If risk of exposure from fumes is high, call for a hazardous materials team. Refer to the appropriate hazardous materials PPE protocol, as the risk of secondary contamination is very high.

(b) Do not use calcium carbonate, as the outcome can be disastrous.

Chemical Treatment Guide 8A: *PURPLE*

- **Ketones**
- **Phosphine**

Signs and Symptoms of Ketone Exposure

Cardiovascular: cardiac dysrhythmias and tachycardia.

Respiratory: upper respiratory tract irritation, dyspnea, tachypnea, a burning sensation in the chest and pulmonary edema.

CNS: CNS depression to coma, confusion, tinnitus, disorientation, headache, drowsiness, weakness, and seizures.

GI: pain and irritation of the mucous membranes, nausea/vomiting, and diarrhea.

Eye: chemical conjunctivitis.

Skin: irritation and dermatitis, cyanosis of extremities.

Signs and Symptoms of Phosphine Exposure

Cardiovascular: cardiovascular collapse with weak and rapid pulse. Patients may present with a reflex bradycardia.

Respiratory: mild and transient cough (only symptom at the time of exposure to most agents). A delayed onset of dyspnea, tachypnea, violent coughing, and pulmonary edema follows. Some agents work immediately on the upper airway, resulting in pain and choking, spasm of the glottis, temporary reflex arrest of breathing, and possibly upper airway obstruction spasm or edema of the glottis.

CNS: fatigue, restlessness, and decreased LOC (usually delayed signs).

GI: burning of the mucous membranes, nausea/vomiting, and abdominal pain.

Eye: chemical conjunctivitis.

Skin: irritation of moist skin areas, pallor, and cyanosis.

Note

Symptoms may be immediate or may be delayed for 5 to 72 hours.

Supportive Care

- Remove the patient from the hazardous area (a).
- Avoid exposure to vapors emitting from soaked clothes.
- Medical Supportive Care Protocol 2.1.3. Administer 100% high-flow oxygen. (Ipecac is contraindicated.)
- If the patient was exposed externally, remove his/her clothing and decontaminate as appropriate (do not use water as an initial irrigating solution for *phosphine exposure* due to possible reactivity). Provide ocular irrigation with normal saline (see Medical Procedure 4.45, Morgan Lens).
- Contact the Poison Information Center (1-800-222-1222).

Chemical Treatment Guide 8A: *PURPLE*

ALS Level 1

- If the patient is seizing, administer one of the following benzodiazepines:
  - Diazepam (Valium®) 5 mg IV. If unable to start an IV, administer diazepam 5 mg intranasally or 10 mg per rectum. May repeat PRN up to 20 mg maximum dose (b)(c).

  or

  - Lorazepam (Ativan®) 2 mg IV. If unable to start an IV, administer lorazepam 2 mg IM. May repeat once PRN (maximum dose = 4 mg) (b).

  or

  - Midazolam (Versed®) 2 mg IV. If unable to start an IV, administer midazolam 2 mg intranasally. May repeat once PRN (maximum dose = 4 mg) (b).
- If the patient has dysrhythmias, treat PRN (see Adult Protocol 2.3).
- If hypotension persists, treat PRN (see Adult Protocol 2.4.1).

ALS Level 2

None.

Note

(a) If risk of exposure from fumes is high, call for a hazardous materials team. PPE (usually Level A) with SCBA must be worn in the hazardous area. PPE with a minimum of Level C protection must be worn for treatment outside the hazardous areas.

(b) Intranasal administration of benzodiazepines requires the use of a mucosal atomization device.

(c) Use a tuberculin or 3–5 mL syringe *without the needle* to administer diazepam (Valium®). Position the patient in a decubitus knee position or supine, with the legs held apart, and insert the lubricated syringe approximately 5 cm (approximately 2 inches) into the rectum. Inject the diazepam, remove the syringe, and tape the patient's buttocks closed.

Chemical Treatment Guide 9A: *WHITE* □

- **Phenol (carbolic acid)**

Signs and Symptoms

Nausea/vomiting, diarrhea, excessive sweating, headache, dizziness, ringing in the ears, seizures, loss of consciousness, coma, respiratory depression, inflammation of the respiratory tract, shock, and death. Exposure to skin can result in severe burns, which will cause the skin to have a white, red, or brown appearance. Failure to decontaminate the skin may allow the phenol to be absorbed systemically, resulting in death.

Supportive Care

- Remove the patient from the hazardous area (a).
- Avoid exposure to vapors emitting from soaked clothes.
- Medical Supportive Care Protocol 2.1.3. (Ipecac is contraindicated.)
- If the patient was exposed externally, remove his/her clothing and decontaminate with copious amounts of water.
  - After thoroughly rinsing skin, apply vegetable oil to exposed areas. (Isopropyl alcohol may be used for *very* small skin burns only.)
  - Provide ocular irrigation with normal saline (see Medical Procedure 4.45, Morgan Lens).
- Contact the Poison Information Center (1-800-222-1222).

ALS Level I

- Assess the need for intubation (Medical Procedure 4.17 and 4.20).
- If the patient is seizing, administer one of the following benzodiazepines:
  - Diazepam (Valium®) 5 mg IV. If unable to start an IV, administer diazepam 5 mg intranasally or 10 mg per rectum. May repeat PRN up to 20 mg maximum dose (b)(c).

  or

  - Lorazepam (Ativan®) 2 mg IV. If unable to start an IV, administer lorazepam 2 mg IM. May repeat once PRN (maximum dose = 4 mg) (b).

  or

  - Midazolam (Versed®) 2 mg IV. If unable to start an IV, administer midazolam 2 mg intranasally. May repeat once PRN (maximum dose = 4 mg) (b).
- If hypotension persists, treat PRN (see Adult Protocol 2.4.1).

Chemical Treatment Guide 9A: *WHITE* □

ALS Level 2

None.

Note

(a) If risk of exposure from fumes is high, call for a hazardous materials team. Refer to the appropriate hazardous materials PPE protocol, as the risk of secondary contamination is very high.

(b) Intranasal administration of benzodiazepines requires the use of a mucosal atomization device.

(c) Use a tuberculin or 3–5 mL syringe *without the needle* to administer diazepam (Valium®). Position the patient in a decubitus knee position or supine, with the legs held apart, and insert the lubricated syringe approximately 5 cm (approximately 2 inches) into the rectum. Inject the diazepam, remove the syringe, and tape the patient's buttocks closed.

Pediatric Chemical Treatment Guide IP: *YELLOW* ☐

- **Acids and acid mists**
- **Alkaline compounds**
- **Ammonia (liquid and gas)**
- **Chlorine gas and phosgene (CG)**
- **Methylene biphenyl isocyanate, ethyl isocyanate, and methylene dilsocyanate (MDI)**
- **Mustard (sulfur mustard): Lewisite, blister agents (H, HD, HS)**

Signs and Symptoms

Low concentrations of airborne acids and alkalis can produce rapid onset of eye, nose, and throat irritation. Higher concentrations (low concentrations of ammonia) can produce cough, stridor, wheezing, and chemical pneumonia (non-cardiogenic pulmonary edema). Ingestion of acids and alkalis can result in severe injury to the upper airway, esophagus, and stomach. In addition, there may be circulatory collapse, as well as partial- or full-thickness burns.

End-stage symptoms may resemble organophosphate poisoning. However, patients will have **normal or dilated pupils** (patients *will not* have pinpoint pupils). These patients *should not* be given atropine or 2-PAM.

Supportive Care

- Remove the patient from the hazardous area (a).
- If the patient was exposed externally, remove his/her clothing and jewelry and decontaminate with copious amounts of water. Provide ocular irrigation with normal saline (do not attempt to neutralize with another solution; see Medical Procedure 4.45, Morgan Lens).
- If the patient has external burns, see Pediatric Protocol 3.9.7, Burn Injuries.
- Medical Supportive Care Protocol 3.1.3. (Ipecac, charcoal, and NG tube are contraindicated. Avoid oral airways.)
- Contact the Poison Information Center (1-800-222-1222).
- If the patient has pulmonary edema, maintain adequate ventilation and oxygenation, and provide pulmonary suction to remove fluid. Non-cardiogenic pulmonary edema should not be treated with Lasix, but with positive end-expiratory pressure (PEEP) or a CPAP mask (see Medical Procedure 4.24).

Pediatric Chemical Treatment Guide 1P: *YELLOW*

ALS Level 1

- If the patient has bronchospasm:
  - Albuterol (Ventolin®): 1 nebulizer treatment
    If < 1 year old or < 10 kg: mix 1.25 mg in 1.5 mL of normal saline (0.083%).
    If > 1 year or > 10 kg: mix 2.5 mg in 3 mL of normal saline (0.083%).
    See Medical Procedure 4.27. May repeat twice PRN (a).
- If bronchodilators are administered, may add ipratropium bromide (Atrovent®) 0.5 mg (0.5 mL) to either albuterol or levalbuterol nebulizer treatment on first nebulizer treatment only.
- If the patient has inhaled chlorine or hydrochloric acid (HCl) and has significant respiratory distress, administer sodium bicarbonate via nebulizer (8.4% 3 mL mixed with normal saline 3 mL or 4.2% in 6 mL of NS).
- If seizure continues for 5 minutes, administer one of the following benzodiazepines:
  - Diazepam (Valium®) 0.5 mg/kg (maximum dose = 10 mg) rectally. If IV access is available prior to seizure, administer diazepam (Valium®) 0.2 mg/kg IV (c)(d).

  or

  - Lorazepam (Ativan®) 0.1 mg/kg (maximum total dose = 4 mg) IM. If IV access is available prior to seizure, administer lorazepam (Ativan®) 0.1 mg/kg (maximum total dose = 4 mg) IV (c).

  or

  - Midazolam (Versed®) 0.1 mg/kg (maximum dose = 2 mg) IV (c).
- If hypotension persists, administer 20 mL/kg normal saline IV PRN (maximum total dose = 60 mL/kg).

ALS Level 2

None.

Note

(a) If risk of exposure from fumes is high, call for a hazardous materials team. Refer to the appropriate hazardous materials PPE protocol, as the risk of secondary contamination is very high.
(b) Do not give albuterol if the patient's heart rate ≥ 200.
(c) Intranasal administration of benzodiazepines requires the use of a mucosal atomization device.
(d) Use a tuberculin or 3–5 mL syringe *without the needle* to administer diazepam (Valium®). Position the patient in a decubitus knee position or supine, with the legs held apart, and insert the lubricated syringe approximately 5 cm (approximately 2 inches) into the rectum. Inject the diazepam, remove the syringe, and tape the patient's buttocks closed.

Pediatric Chemical Treatment Guide 2P: *BLUE*

- **Aromatic hydrocarbons (benzene, toluene, xylene)**
- **Arsenic compounds (heavy metal poisoning)**
- **Carbon monoxide poisoning**
- **Chlorinated hydrocarbons (methylene chloride)**
- **Ketones**

Signs and Symptoms

Mild exposure signs and symptoms: Cough, hoarseness, headache, poor concentration, irritability, agitation, anxiety, drowsiness, dizziness, weakness, tremors, transient euphoria, vision and hearing disturbances, nausea/vomiting, salivation, diarrhea, stomach pain, and chemical burns with chlorinated hydrocarbons. (For arsenic signs and symptoms, see below.)

Moderate to severe exposure signs and symptoms: Cardiovascular collapse, tachydysrhythmias (especially ventricular fibrillation), chest pain, pulmonary edema, dyspnea, tachypnea, respiratory failure, paralysis, altered mental status, seizures, excessive salivation, pale skin, cyanosis, rarely cherry-red skin with carbon monoxide, and delayed carcinogenic effects. (For arsenic signs and symptoms, see below.)

Signs and symptoms of arsenic exposure: Severe gastrointestinal fluid loss, burning abdominal pain, watery or bloody diarrhea, muscle spasm, seizures, cardiovascular collapse, tachycardia, hypotension, ventricular dysrhythmias, shock, and coma. There may be respiratory or cardiac arrest, and acute renal failure may occur with bronze urine within a few minutes.

End-stage symptoms may resemble organophosphate poisoning. However, patients will have **normal or dilated pupils** (patients *will not* have pinpoint pupils). These patients *should not* be given atropine or 2-PAM.

Products may be **flammable.**

Supportive Care

- Remove the patient from the hazardous area (a).
- Medical Supportive Care Protocol 3.1.3. (Ipecac and an NG tube are contraindicated. Avoid oral airways.)
- If the patient was exposed externally, remove his/her clothing and jewelry and decontaminate as appropriate. Provide ocular irrigation with normal saline (see Medical Procedure 4.45, Morgan Lens).
- Administer high-flow oxygen (100%) (b).
- Contact the Poison Information Center (1-800-222-1222).
- If the patient has pulmonary edema, maintain adequate ventilation and oxygenation, and provide pulmonary suction to remove fluid. Non-cardiogenic pulmonary edema should not be treated with Lasix, but with positive end-expiratory pressure (PEEP) or a CPAP mask (see Medical Procedure 4.24).

Pediatric Chemical Treatment Guide 2P: *BLUE* ■

ALS Level 1

- If the patient has dysrhythmias, treat PRN (see Pediatric Protocol 3.3) (c).
- If seizure continues for 5 minutes, administer one of the following benzodiazepines:
  - Diazepam (Valium®) 0.5 mg/kg (maximum dose = 10 mg) rectally. If IV access is available prior to seizure, administer diazepam (Valium®) 0.2 mg/kg IV (d)(e).

  or

  - Lorazepam (Ativan®) 0.1 mg/kg (maximum total dose = 4 mg) IM. If IV access is available prior to seizure, administer lorazepam (Ativan®) 0.1 mg/kg (maximum total dose = 4 mg) IV (d).

  or

  - Midazolam (Versed®) 0.1 mg/kg (maximum dose = 2 mg) IV (d).
- If hypotension persists, administer 20 mL/kg normal saline IV PRN (maximum total dose = 60 mL/kg).

ALS Level 2

None.

Note

(a) If risk of exposure from fumes is high, call for a hazardous materials team. Refer to the appropriate hazardous materials PPE protocol, as the risk of secondary contamination is very high.

(b) Document the duration of exposure to CO and when oxygen therapy was started (this information is needed to assist in making HBO decisions).

(c) Administration of epinephrine to patients in a pre-code status may not be desirable for this group of patients. A physician or the Poison Information Center should guide the administration of epinephrine in these cases.

(d) Intranasal administration of benzodiazepines requires the use of a mucosal atomization device.

(e) Use a tuberculin or 3–5 mL syringe *without the needle* to administer diazepam (Valium®). Position the patient in a decubitus knee position or supine, with the legs held apart, and insert the lubricated syringe approximately 5 cm (approximately 2 inches) into the rectum. Inject the diazepam, remove the syringe, and tape the patient's buttocks closed.

Pediatric Chemical Treatment Guide 3P: *GRAY*

- **Dinitrobenzene (DNB)**
- **Nitrogen products and other products causing methemoglobinemia**

Signs and Symptoms

Methemoglobinemia characterized by chocolate-brown-colored blood, CNS depression, headache, dizziness, ataxia, vertigo, tinnitus, dyspnea, tachypnea, violent coughing, choking, possible upper airway obstruction spasm or edema of the glottis, abdominal pain, hypotension, heart blocks, ventricular dysrhythmias, seizures (rare), pallor, cyanosis, and cardiovascular collapse.

Note

Symptoms may be immediate or may be delayed for 5 to 72 hours.

Supportive Care

- Remove the patient from the hazardous area (a).
- Medical Supportive Care Protocol 3.1.3.
- If the patient was exposed externally, remove his/her clothing and decontaminate as appropriate.
- Administer high-flow oxygen (100%).
- Contact the Poison Information Center (1-800-222-1222).
- If nitrogen product ingestion occurred, administer activated charcoal 1 g/kg (maximum dose = 50 g) PO.

ALS Level 1

- If the patient is dyspneic, is cyanotic, has normal SpO_2, and has chocolate-brown-colored blood, administer methylene blue (1%) 1–2 mg/kg slow IV over 5 minutes, followed by a normal saline 30 mL flush to decrease pain at the IV site.
- If the patient has dysrhythmias, treat PRN (see Pediatric Protocol 3.3).
- If seizure continues for 5 minutes, administer one of the following benzodiazepines:
  - Diazepam (Valium®) 0.5 mg/kg (maximum dose = 10 mg) rectally. If IV access is available prior to seizure, administer diazepam (Valium®) 0.2 mg/kg IV (b)(c).

  or

  - Lorazepam (Ativan®) 0.1 mg/kg (maximum total dose = 4 mg) IM. If IV access is available prior to seizure, administer lorazepam (Ativan®) 0.1 mg/kg (maximum total dose = 4 mg) IV (b).

  or

  - Midazolam (Versed®) 0.1 mg/kg (maximum dose = 2 mg) IV (b).
- If hypotension persists, administer 20 mL/kg normal saline IV PRN (maximum total dose = 60 mL/kg).
- Do *not* induce vomiting.

Pediatric Chemical Treatment Guide 3P: *GRAY*

ALS Level 2

- If cyanosis persists, administer methylene blue (1%) 1–2 mg/kg slow IV over 5 minutes, followed by a 30 mL flush of normal saline to decrease pain at the IV site.

NOTE

(a) If risk of exposure from fumes is high, call for a hazardous materials team. Refer to the appropriate hazardous materials PPE protocol, as the risk of secondary contamination is very high.

(b) Intranasal administration of benzodiazepines requires the use of a mucosal atomization device.

(c) Use a tuberculin or 3–5 mL syringe *without the needle* to administer diazepam (Valium®). Position the patient in a decubitus knee position or supine, with the legs held apart, and insert the lubricated syringe approximately 5 cm (approximately 2 inches) into the rectum. Inject the diazepam, remove the syringe, and tape the patient's buttocks closed.

Pediatric Chemical Treatment Guide 4P: *GREEN* ■

- **Carbamate: insecticide poisoning**
- **Organophosphate: insecticide poisoning and nerve agents (GA, GB, GD, GF, VX)**

Signs and Symptoms

The muscarinic effects are described as the classic **SLUDGE** syndrome (excessive **S**alivation, **L**acrimation, **U**rination, **D**iarrhea, **G**astrointestinal distress, and **E**mesis). Additional muscarinic effects include bronchorrhea, bronchospasm, and bradycardia. The patient will have constricted pupils (miosis, which may last as long as 2 months despite appropriate treatment) with inhalation or skin exposure. Ingestion may or may not cause miosis. However, stimulation of nicotinic receptors will produce tachycardia, muscle paralysis (apnea), muscle twitching/fasiculations, and seizures.

Supportive Care

- Remove the patient from the hazardous area (a).
- Avoid exposure to the patient's sweat, vomit, stool, and vapors emitting from soaked clothes.
- Medical Supportive Care Protocol 3.1.3. Administer high-flow O_2.
- If the patient was exposed externally, remove his/her clothing and decontaminate as appropriate (place the patient's clothes in sealed bag).
- Contact the Poison Information Center (1-800-222-1222).

ALS Level I

If treating 1–4 patients:

- If the patient is bradycardic (patients are usually tachycardic) or has excessive pulmonary secretions, administer atropine 0.05 mg/kg IV (maximum dose = 3 mg). Repeat every 5 minutes until secretions are inhibited (b)(c).
- In case of organophosphate poisoning, consider pralidoxime (Protopam®, 2-PAM®) 1–2 g mixed in 100 mL NS IV drip over 30 minutes. In severe cases, 2-PAM® may be given IV at a maximum rate of 200 mg/min or 1 g/5 min (used when nicotinic effects are present, as evidenced by fasciculation of large muscles). Observe the patient for hypertension (may be needed with high exposure to carbamates) (c).
- If seizure continues for 5 minutes, administer one of the following benzodiazepines:
  - Diazepam (Valium®) 0.5 mg/kg (maximum dose = 10 mg) rectally. If IV access is available prior to seizure, administer diazepam (Valium®) 0.2 mg/kg IV (d)(e).

  or

  - Lorazepam (Ativan®) 0.1 mg/kg (maximum total dose = 4 mg) IM. If IV access is available prior to seizure, administer lorazepam (Ativan®) 0.1 mg/kg (maximum total dose = 4 mg) IV (d).

  or

  - Midazolam (Versed®) 0.1 mg/kg (maximum dose = 2 mg) IV (d).

Pediatric Chemical Treatment Guide 4P: *GREEN*

If treating 5 or more patients <u>older than 5 years of age</u> or self-exposure (<u>with pinpoint pupils</u>):

- Administer Mark I Kit(s) (two auto-injectors containing atropine 2 mg in one and pralidoxime 600 mg in the other; see Medical Procedure 4.54) as follows:
  - For early symptoms (severe rhinorrhea or mild to moderate dyspnea): administer one Mark I auto-injector kit. If no improvement in patient's status in 10 minutes, administer another Mark I auto-injector kit (c)(f).
  - For severe respiratory distress, coma, or seizures: administer three Mark I auto-injectors and one CANA auto-injector (diazepam 10 mg IM) (c)(f).

For all patients meeting the preceding criteria:

- Alert the emergency department to prepare for a contaminated patient.
- Do *not* induce vomiting or give furosemide (Lasix®) or morphine.
- If the patient is experiencing eye pain and/or blepharospasm, administer scopolamine 1 drop in each eye.

ALS Level 2

None.

Note

(a) If risk of exposure from fumes is high, call for a hazardous materials team. PPE (usually Level A) with SCBA must be worn in the hazardous area. PPE with a minimum of Level C protection must be worn for treatment outside the hazardous areas.

(b) If advised by the Poison Information Center, every other dose of atropine can be increased to 0.06 mg/kg IV.

(c) The endpoint for treatment is manifested by patient improvement with clear lung sounds.

(d) Intranasal administration of benzodiazepines requires the use of a mucosal atomization device.

(e) Use a tuberculin or 3–5 mL syringe *without the needle* to administer diazepam (Valium®). Position the patient in a decubitus knee position or supine, with the legs held apart, and insert the lubricated syringe approximately 5 cm (approximately 2 inches) into the rectum. Inject the diazepam, remove the syringe, and tape the patient's buttocks closed.

(f) When possible, establish IV access and administer atropine, diazepam, lorazepam, and midazolam IV and pralidoxime IV drip.

Pediatric Chemical Treatment Guide 5P: *RED*

- **Cyanide: hydrogen cyanide, hydrocyanic acid (AC), cyanogen chloride (CK)**
- **Hydrogen sulfide, sulfides, and mercaptans**
- **Azides**

Signs and Symptoms

Cardiovascular: initially, pulse decreases and BP rises. In later stages, tachycardia, dysrhythmias, and cardiovascular collapse can occur. There may also be palpitations and/or chest tightness.

Respiratory: can cause immediate respiratory arrest. Initially there is usually an increase in the rate and depth of respirations, which later become slow and gasping. Irritation of the respiratory tract, cough, dyspnea, tachypnea, and pulmonary edema are also possible.

CNS: can cause immediate coma. Initially there is usually weakness, headache, and confusion; seizures are common.

GI: nausea/vomiting, profuse salivation, possibly a garlic taste in mouth.

Skin: pale, cyanotic, or reddish color, dermatitis, sweating.

Note

Good medical supportive care, including airway management, is paramount and should precede the use of the cyanide antidote kit. However, the rapid administration of the cyanide antidote kit will be the only therapy that will reverse the life-threatening symptoms.

Supportive Care

- Remove the patient from the hazardous area (a).
- Avoid exposure to vapors emitting from soaked clothes.
- Medical Supportive Care Protocol 3.1.3. Administer high-flow O_2.
- If the patient was exposed externally, remove his/her clothing quickly and decontaminate.
- Contact the Poison Information Center (1-800-222-1222).
- If the patient is conscious, administer activated charcoal 1 g/kg (maximum dose = 50 g) PO for oral ingestion.
- Only a physician or the Poison Information Center can authorize treatment beyond supportive care for exposure to azides.

Pediatric Chemical Treatment Guide 5P: *RED*

ALS Level I

- If the patient is unconscious, administer sodium bicarbonate 1 mEq/kg IV.
- If the patient is exhibiting life-threatening symptoms (severe respiratory compromise or arrest, shock, seizures, coma), administer the cyanide antidote kit (3 parts) in the following order (to induce methemoglobinemia). **If symptoms are not severe, or if diagnosis is not certain, omit Steps 1 and 2 and only give sodium thiosulfate (Step 3). Paramedics who are not part of a hazardous materials team and non-rescue supervisors can only give sodium thiosulfate.**

  Rescue Supervisor and Hazardous Materials Team Paramedic

  1. Amyl nitrite (break pearls into gauze sponge and hold under the patient's nose or BVD intake valve) for 15–30 seconds of each minute until the sodium nitrite solution is ready (b).
  2. Sodium nitrite 3% (300 mg/10 mL) 0.33 mL/kg at 2.5 slow IV over 5 minutes.

  All Paramedics

  3. Sodium thiosulfate 25% 1.65 mL/kg IV **(contraindicated for hydrogen sulfide exposure).**
- If the patient has dysrhythmias, treat PRN (see Pediatric Protocol 3.3).
- If hypotension persists, administer 20 mL/kg normal saline IV PRN (maximum total dose = 60 mL/kg).
- Alert the emergency department to prepare for a contaminated patient.
- Do *not* induce vomiting.
- If seizure continues for 5 minutes, administer one of the following benzodiazepines:
  - Diazepam (Valium®) 0.5 mg/kg (maximum dose = 10 mg) rectally. If IV access is available prior to seizure, administer diazepam (Valium®) 0.2 mg/kg IV (c)(d).

  or

  - Lorazepam (Ativan®) 0.1 mg/kg (maximum total dose = 4 mg) IM. If IV access is available prior to seizure, administer lorazepam (Ativan®) 0.1 mg/kg (maximum total dose = 4 mg) IV (d).

  or

  - Midazolam (Versed®) 0.1 mg/kg (maximum dose = 2 mg) IV (d).

Pediatric Chemical Treatment Guide 5P: *RED*

ALS Level 2

- If symptoms persist after 20 minutes, repeat the cyanide antidote kit at 50% of the initial dose.
- If the patient becomes cyanotic after the cyanide antidote kit, contact the Poison Information Center (1-800-222-1222) for further instructions.

Note

(a) If risk of exposure from fumes is high, call for a hazardous materials team. Refer to the appropriate hazardous materials PPE protocol, as the risk of secondary contamination is very high.

(b) If the patient has IV access and received supportive care, Step 1 may be bypassed for Step 2.

(c) Intranasal administration of benzodiazepines requires the use of a mucosal atomization device.

(d) Use a tuberculin or 3–5 mL syringe *without the needle* to administer diazepam (Valium®). Position the patient in a decubitus knee position or supine, with the legs held apart, and insert the lubricated syringe approximately 5 cm (approximately 2 inches) into the rectum. Inject the diazepam, remove the syringe, and tape the patient's buttocks closed.

Pediatric Chemical Treatment Guide 6P: *PINK*

- **Ethylene glycol**
- **Methanol**

Clinical Manifestations of Ethylene Glycol Poisoning

Phase I (30 minutes to 12 hours): ethanol-like inebriation, metabolic acidosis, seizures, and coma.

Phase 2 (12 to 36 hours): tachycardia, tachypnea, hypertension, pulmonary edema.

Phase 3 (36 to 48 hours): crystalluria, acute tubular necrosis with oliguria—renal failure.

Signs and Symptoms of Methanol Exposure

Cardiovascular: dysrhythmias and hypotension.

Respiratory: respiratory insufficiency or arrest, pulmonary edema, chemical pneumonitis, and bronchitis.

CNS: CNS depression and coma, seizures, headache, muscle weakness, and delirium.

GI: GI bleeding, nausea/vomiting, and diarrhea.

Eye: chemical conjunctivitis.

Skin: problems ranging from irritation to full-thickness burns.

Supportive Care

- Remove the patient from the hazardous area.
- Medical Supportive Care Protocol 3.1.3.
- Contact the Poison Information Center (1-800-222-1222).

Pediatric Chemical Treatment Guide 6P: *PINK*

ALS Level 1

- If seizure continues for 5 minutes, administer one of the following benzodiazepines:
  - Diazepam (Valium®) 0.5 mg/kg (maximum dose = 10 mg) rectally. If IV access is available prior to seizure, administer diazepam (Valium®) 0.2 mg/kg IV (a)(b).

  or

  - Lorazepam (Ativan®) 0.1 mg/kg (maximum total dose = 4 mg) IM. If IV access is available prior to seizure, administer lorazepam (Ativan®) 0.1 mg/kg (maximum total dose = 4 mg) IV (a).

  or

  - Midazolam (Versed®) 0.1 mg/kg (maximum dose = 2 mg) IV (a).
- If the patient's lungs are clear, administer normal saline at a rate of 100 mL/h IV.
- If the patient's respiratory rate is twice the normal rate, administer sodium bicarbonate 8.4% 1–2 mEq/kg IV.
- If the patient has dysrhythmias, treat PRN (see Pediatric Protocol 3.3).
- Administer thiamine 100 mg IV.

ALS Level 2

None.

Note

(a) Intranasal administration of benzodiazepines requires the use of a mucosal atomization device.

(b) Use a tuberculin or 3–5 mL syringe *without the needle* to administer diazepam (Valium®). Position the patient in a decubitus knee position or supine, with the legs held apart, and insert the lubricated syringe approximately 5 cm (approximately 2 inches) into the rectum. Inject the diazepam, remove the syringe, and tape the patient's buttocks closed.

Pediatric Chemical Treatment Guide 7P: *ORANGE*

- **Hydrofluoric acid (HF)**
- **Vicane**

Signs and Symptoms

Hypovolemic shock and collapse, tachycardia with weak pulse, acute pulmonary edema, asphyxia, chemical pneumonitis, upper airway obstruction with stridor, pain and cough, decreased LOC, nausea/vomiting, diarrhea, possible GI bleeding, and possible blindness. HF also causes severe skin burns. The damage may be severe with no outward signs, except that the patient will complain of severe pain.

Supportive Care

- Remove the patient from the hazardous area (a).
- Medical Supportive Care Protocol 3.1.3. (Ipecac is contraindicated.)
- If the patient was exposed externally, remove his/her clothing and jewelry and decontaminate with copious amounts of water.
- Contact the Poison Information Center (1-800-222-1222).
- If the patient has pulmonary edema, maintain adequate ventilation and oxygenation, and provide pulmonary suction to remove fluid. Non-cardiogenic pulmonary edema should not be treated with Lasix, but with positive end-expiratory pressure (PEEP) or a CPAP mask (see Medical Procedure 4.24).

ALS Level I

- **If the patient has burns to the eye(s):**
  - Immediately flush with copious amounts of water or normal saline.
  - Prepare an eye wash solution by mixing calcium gluconate (10%) 50 mL in normal saline 500 mL (b).
  - Apply calcium gluconate eye wash using a Morgan lens (see Medical Procedure 4.45) and continue until arrival at the receiving facility (b).
- **If the patient has burns to the skin:**
  - Immediately flush with copious amounts of water.
  - Prepare a skin gel by mixing calcium gluconate (10%) 10 mL into a 2-oz tube of KY Jelly (making a 2.5% gel) (b).
  - Apply a 2.5% calcium gluconate gel on the burned area. For burns to the hand(s), place the hand in a glove filled with this gel (b).

Pediatric Chemical Treatment Guide 7P: *ORANGE*

- **For inhalation injury:**
  - Immediately support ventilations.
  - Administer calcium gluconate (10%) 1 mL mixed with 3 mL NS via nebulizer (b).
  - For severe respiratory depression/arrest and/or cardiac toxicity (dysrhythmia, prolonged QT interval, hypotension), administer calcium gluconate (10%) 100 mg/kg (maximum dose = 1 g) via slow IV over 5 minutes (b).
- If the patient has dysrhythmias, treat PRN (see Pediatric Protocol 3.3).
- If hypotension persists, administer 20 mL/kg normal saline IV PRN (maximum total dose = 60 mL/kg).

ALS Level 2

- If systemic symptoms persist, repeat calcium gluconate (10%) 100 mg/kg (maximum dose = 1 g) via slow IV over 5 minutes (b).

Note

(a) If risk of exposure from fumes is high, call for a hazardous materials team. Refer to the appropriate hazardous materials PPE protocol, as the risk of secondary contamination is very high.

(b) Do not use calcium carbonate, as the outcome can be disastrous.

Pediatric Chemical Treatment Guide 8P: *PURPLE*

- **Ketones**
- **Phosphine**

Signs and Symptoms of Ketone Exposure

Cardiovascular: cardiac dysrhythmias and tachycardia.

Respiratory: upper respiratory tract irritation, dyspnea, tachypnea, a burning sensation in the chest and pulmonary edema.

CNS: CNS depression to coma, confusion, tinnitus, disorientation, headache, drowsiness, weakness, and seizures.

GI: pain and irritation of the mucous membranes, nausea/vomiting, and diarrhea.

Eye: chemical conjunctivitis.

Skin: irritation and dermatitis, cyanosis of extremities.

Signs and Symptoms of Phosphine Exposure

Cardiovascular: cardiovascular collapse with weak and rapid pulse. Some patients may have a reflex bradycardia.

Respiratory: mild and transient cough (only symptom at the time of exposure to most agents). A delayed onset of dyspnea, tachypnea, violent coughing, and pulmonary edema follows. Some agents work immediately on the upper airway, resulting in pain and choking, spasm of the glottis, temporary reflex arrest of breathing, and possibly upper airway obstruction spasm or edema of the glottis.

CNS: fatigue, restlessness, and decreased LOC (usually delayed signs).

GI: burning of the mucous membranes, nausea/vomiting, and abdominal pain.

Eye: chemical conjunctivitis.

Skin: irritation of moist skin areas, pallor, and cyanosis.

Note

Symptoms may be immediate or may be delayed for 5 to 72 hours.

Supportive Care

- Remove the patient from the hazardous area (a).
- Avoid exposure to vapors emitting from soaked clothes.
- Medical Supportive Care Protocol 3.1.3. Administer 100% high-flow oxygen. (Ipecac is contraindicated.)
- If the patient was exposed externally, remove his/her clothing and decontaminate as appropriate (do not use water as an initial irrigating solution for *phosphine exposure* due to possible reactivity). Provide ocular irrigation with normal saline (see Medical Procedure 4.45, Morgan Lens).
- Contact the Poison Information Center (1-800-222-1222).

Pediatric Chemical Treatment Guide 8P: *PURPLE*

- For phosphine ingestions, administer activated charcoal 1 g/kg (maximum dose = 50 g) PO.
- If the patient has pulmonary edema, maintain adequate ventilation and oxygenation, and provide pulmonary suction to remove fluid. Non-cardiogenic pulmonary edema should not be treated with Lasix, but with positive end-expiratory pressure (PEEP) or a CPAP mask (see Medical Procedure 4.24).

ALS Level 1

- If seizure continues for 5 minutes, administer one of the following benzodiazepines:
  - Diazepam (Valium®) 0.5 mg/kg (maximum dose = 10 mg) rectally. If IV access is available prior to seizure, administer diazepam (Valium®) 0.2 mg/kg IV (b)(c).

  or

  - Lorazepam (Ativan®) 0.1 mg/kg (maximum total dose = 4 mg) IM. If IV access is available prior to seizure, administer lorazepam (Ativan®) 0.1 mg/kg (maximum total dose = 4 mg) IV (b).

  or

  - Midazolam (Versed®) 0.1 mg/kg (maximum dose = 2 mg) IV (b).
- If the patient has dysrhythmias, treat PRN (see Pediatric Protocol 3.3).
- If hypotension persists, treat PRN.

ALS Level 2

None.

Note

(a) If risk of exposure from fumes is high, call for a hazardous materials team. PPE (usually Level A) with SCBA must be worn in the hazardous area. PPE with a minimum of Level C protection must be worn for treatment outside the hazardous areas.

(b) Intranasal administration of benzodiazepines requires the use of a mucosal atomization device.

(c) Use a tuberculin or 3–5 mL syringe *without the needle* to administer diazepam (Valium®). Position the patient in a decubitus knee position or supine, with the legs held apart, and insert the lubricated syringe approximately 5 cm (approximately 2 inches) into the rectum. Inject the diazepam, remove the syringe, and tape the patient's buttocks closed.

Pediatric Chemical Treatment Guide 9P: *WHITE* □

- **Phenol (carbolic acid)**

Signs and Symptoms:

Nausea/vomiting, diarrhea, excessive sweating, headache, dizziness, ringing in the ears, seizures, loss of consciousness, coma, respiratory depression, inflammation of the respiratory tract, shock, and death. Exposure to skin can result in severe burns, which will cause the skin to have a white, red, or brown appearance. Failure to decontaminate the skin may allow the phenol to be absorbed systemically, resulting in death.

Supportive Care

- Remove the patient from the hazardous area (a).
- Avoid exposure to vapors emitting from soaked clothes.
- Medical Supportive Care Protocol 3.1.3. (Ipecac is contraindicated.)
- If the patient was exposed externally, remove his/her clothing and decontaminate with copious amounts of water.
  - After thoroughly rinsing the skin, apply vegetable oil to exposed areas. (Isopropyl alcohol may be used for *very* small skin burns only.)
  - Provide ocular irrigation with normal saline (see Medical Procedure 4.45, Morgan Lens).
- Contact the Poison Information Center (1-800-222-1222).

ALS Level 1

- Assess the need for intubation (Medical Procedures 4.17 and 4.20).
- If seizure continues for 5 minutes, administer one of the following benzodiazepines:
  - Diazepam (Valium®) 0.5 mg/kg (maximum dose = 10 mg) rectally. If IV access is available prior to seizure, administer diazepam (Valium®) 0.2 mg/kg IV (b)(c).

  or
  - Lorazepam (Ativan®) 0.1 mg/kg (maximum total dose = 4 mg) IM. If IV access is available prior to seizure, administer lorazepam (Ativan®) 0.1 mg/kg (maximum total dose = 4 mg) IV (b).

  or
  - Midazolam (Versed®) 0.1 mg/kg (maximum dose = 2 mg) IV (b).
- If hypotension persists, administer 20 mL/kg normal saline IV PRN (maximum total dose = 60 mL/kg).

Pediatric Chemical Treatment Guide 9P: *WHITE* □

ALS Level 2

None.

Note

(a) If risk of exposure from fumes is high, call for a hazardous materials team. Refer to the appropriate hazardous materials PPE protocol, as the risk of secondary contamination is very high.

(b) Intranasal administration of benzodiazepines requires the use of a mucosal atomization device.

(c) Use a tuberculin or 3–5 mL syringe *without the needle* to administer diazepam (Valium®). Position the patient in a decubitus knee position or supine, with the legs held apart, and insert the lubricated syringe approximately 5 cm (approximately 2 inches) into the rectum. Inject the diazepam, remove the syringe, and tape the patient's buttocks closed.

8.2 Adult Hazardous Material Exposure (Biological Agents)

This protocol is to be used for those patients suspected of exposure to biological agents via any route of exposure (e.g., inhalation, absorption). It gives specific considerations for each type of exposure as well as general treatment guidelines. **Scene safety should be of primary concern, with special attention being paid to the need for personal protective equipment.** Additional assistance may be necessary (e.g., hazardous materials team, police).

Because many biological agents are spread through an airborne route, **scene safety must include use of protective masks by all personnel,** and must include containment of the unknown substance to prevent its airborne spread. Any victim who has a cough, respiratory symptoms, or a flu-like syndrome should be considered as potentially infectious to others by the respiratory route, until proven otherwise. Both patients and healthcare workers should wear protective masks. If a patient needs low-flow oxygen therapy, it may be given by nasal cannula under a protective mask. If a patient needs high-flow oxygen therapy, it may be given by non-rebreather mask, which should not be covered by a protective mask; instead, the healthcare workers must wear protective masks.

Symptoms that would develop after a biological weapon (BW) attack would be delayed and nonspecific, making the initial diagnosis difficult. A BW attack should be considered if any of the following factors are present:

- Large epidemic with unprecedented number of ill or dying
- HIV-positive individuals who demonstrate first susceptibility ("canary in a coal mine")
- High volumes of patients complaining primarily of respiratory symptoms that are severe and are associated with an unprecedented mortality rate
- A cause of infection that is unusual or impossible for the particular region (such as the Ebola virus, which is rarely seen outside Africa)
- Multiple, yet simultaneous outbreaks
- An epidemic caused by a multidrug-resistant pathogen, previously unknown
- Sick or dead animals of multiple types
- Identification of the delivery vehicle for the agent
- Prior intelligence reports or claims by aggressors of a BW attack

Signs and Symptoms

After a characteristic incubation period following aerosol exposure, most BW agents present as an initial influenza syndrome characterized by the following signs and symptoms:

- Fever
- Chills
- Malaise
- Headache
- Myalgia

8.2 Adult Hazardous Material Exposure (Biological Agents)

Some BW agents rapidly develop into a pulmonary syndrome characterized by the following signs and symptoms:

- Dyspnea
- Cyanosis
- Chest pain
- Radiological abnormalities
- Liver involvement, indicated by rising liver enzymes, with or without jaundice
- Encephalitis (may occur with some viral agents), typified by photophobia, confusion, and nuchal rigidity
- Maculopapular, vesicular pustular, or ulcerative skin lesions, with or without bleeding abnormalities
- Unexplained death or flaccid paralysis (may indicate a biological toxin)

A history should be obtained from the patient and bystanders, to include the following information:

- Duration of symptoms
- Pertinent medical history
- Patient's recent history of travel
- Infectious contacts
- Employment
- Activities over the preceding 3–5 days

If a biological agent exposure is suspected, call for a hazardous materials team. In this instance, refer to the appropriate hazardous materials PPE protocol, to protect against secondary contamination. All patients who have been exposed to hazardous materials must be properly decontaminated prior to initiation of extensive medical treatment and transportation to the hospital.

Contact the Poison Information Center (1-800-222-1222) for consultation regarding specific therapy, and then contact the receiving emergency department for confirmation of ALS Level 2 orders.

It is imperative that the emergency department be made aware early that a contaminated patient is being transported so that proper preparations can be made to receive the patient.

8.2.1 Anthrax

Bacillus anthraces is a gram-positive, rod-shaped organism that becomes infectious when it converts into a spore and enters the host. The spore germinates inside a macrophage, which is then transported to regional lymph nodes. There, local production of toxins causes edema and necrosis of the tissue, leading to bacteremia, toxemia, and death. Symptoms vary with the method of exposure:

- **Cutaneous Anthrax:** Skin lesions appear in 1–5 days, consisting of 1- to 2-cm vesicles with regional edema and lymphadenitis. Most patients with small lesions will be afebrile. Lesions develop into a painless necrotic ulcer with a black eschar base.
- **Gastrointestinal Anthrax:** Signs and symptoms include fever, nausea/vomiting, abdominal pain, bloody diarrhea, sometimes rapidly developing ascites, and possibly acute abdomen. Oropharyngeal cases show primary involvement of the tonsils.
- **Inhalation Anthrax:** A 6-day incubation period is followed by fever, myalgias, cough, and fatigue. Initial improvement is followed by abrupt onset of respiratory distress, shock, and death in 24–36 hours. Physical findings are nonspecific, pneumonia is rare, and 50% of cases have associated hemorrhagic meningitis.

Supportive Care

- Remove the patient from the hazardous area (a).
- If the patient was exposed externally, remove his/her clothing and decontaminate as appropriate.
- Medical Supportive Care Protocol 2.1.3.
- Contact the Poison Information Center (1-800-222-1222).

ALS Level 1

None.

ALS Level 2

If there is a high suspicion of significant exposure to anthrax, then Medical Control or the Poison Information Center may order preventive treatment with oral ciprofloxacin (Cipro®) 500 mg PO bid or doxycycline 100 mg PO bid.

NOTE

(a) If risk of exposure is high, call for a hazardous materials team. Refer to the appropriate hazardous materials PPE protocol, as the risk of secondary contamination is very high.

8.2.2 Botulism

The botulinum toxins are a group of seven related neurotoxins produced by the bacillus *Clostridium botulinum*. When inhaled, these toxins produce a clinical picture very similar to that associated with foodborne intoxication, although the time to onset of paralytic symptoms may actually be longer than for foodborne cases, and may vary by type and dose of toxin. The clinical syndrome produced by one or more of these toxins is known as "botulism." Botulism toxin is also a licensed medicine that is used for the treatment of dystonias and can be found in some hospital pharmacies.

Signs and Symptoms

The onset of symptoms of inhalation botulism may vary from 24–36 hours to several days following exposure. Symptoms include the following:

- Bulbar palsies produce loss of function in nerves originating in the brain stem, causing the following symptoms:
  - Blurred vision
  - Mydriasis
  - Diplopia
  - Ptosis
  - Photophobia
  - Dysphagia
  - Dysphonia
- Following bulbar palsies, skeletal muscles become weak, leading to a symmetrical descending paralysis (head-to-toe).
- These symptoms may progress acutely to respiratory failure and death within 24 hours.
- Patients usually remain awake and alert.

Supportive Care

- Medical Supportive Care Protocol 2.1.3 or Pediatric Protocol 3.1.3.
- Contact the Poison Information Center (1-800-222-1222).

ALS Level 1

None.

ALS Level 2

None.

8.2.3 Cholera

Vibrio cholerae is a short, curved, motile, gram-negative, non-sporulating rod. Cholera is the prototype toxigenic diarrhea, which is secretory in nature. Transmission of the pathogen occurs through direct and indirect fecal contamination of water or foods, and by heavily soiled hands or utensils. *V. cholerae* can survive for as long as 24 hours in sewage, and as long as 6 weeks in certain types of relatively impure water containing organic material. Because cholera does not easily spread from human to human, for this pathogen to be an effective biological weapon, major drinking water supplies would have to be heavily contaminated.

Cholera is an acute infectious disease, characterized by sudden onset with nausea, vomiting, profuse diarrhea with "rice water" appearance, rapid loss of body fluids, toxemia, and frequent collapse. If untreated, mortality may by 50%.

Signs and Symptoms

The following signs and symptoms occur within 12 to 72 hours of exposure:

- Intestinal cramping
- Painless diarrhea
- Vomiting
- Malaise
- Headache
- Low-grade fever

Supportive Care

- Remove the patient from the hazardous area.
- Medical Supportive Care Protocol 2.1.3. Consider fluid replacement.
- Contact the Poison Information Center (1-800-222-1222).

ALS Level 1

None.

ALS Level 2

In-hospital treatment may include the use of tetracycline 500 mg qid for 3 days or doxycycline 300 mg once or 100 mg bid for 3 days. If the organism is tetracycline resistant, use ciprofloxacin 500 mg bid for 3 days or erythromycin 500 mg qid for 3 days.

8.2.4 Plague

The plague is spread to humans from either the bite of an infected flea or inhalation of the organism. Infection occurs in three forms:

- **Bubonic:** involves lymph nodes closest to the bite of infected flea.
- **Pneumonic:** an infection of the lungs.
- **Septicemia:** a generalized infection in the blood, caused by the bacteria escaping through the lymph nodes or lungs.

Signs and Symptoms

Two to three days after inhaling the plague organism, the patient will develop the following signs and symptoms:

- High fever
- Myalgia
- Chills
- Headache
- Cough with bloody sputum
- Signs of overwhelming infection (including pneumonia)

Chest X-ray may show patchy infiltrates or consolidation, with a rapidly progressing pneumonia causing dyspnea, stridor, and cyanosis. The patient will experience eventual respiratory failure and circulatory collapse; laboratory evidence will show disseminated intravascular coagulation (DIC).

Supportive Care

- Remove the patient from the hazardous area (a).
- Respiratory isolation is mandatory for the first 48 hours of treatment.
- Medical Supportive Care Protocol 2.1.3.
- Contact the Poison Information Center (1-800-222-1222).

ALS Level 1

None.

ALS Level 2

- Antibiotic treatment must be started within 24 hours of the onset of symptoms. In-hospital treatment may include the use of streptomycin 15 mg/kg IM bid for 10 days or doxycycline 200 mg IV initially, followed by 100 mg bid for 10 days. For plague meningitis, administer chloramphenicol 12.5–18.75 mg/kg qid.
- If there is a high suspicion of significant exposure to plague, then Medical Control or the Poison Information Center may order preventive treatment with oral ciprofloxacin (Cipro®) 500 mg PO bid or doxycycline 100 mg PO bid.

Note

(a) If risk of exposure is high, call for a hazardous materials team. Refer to the appropriate hazardous materials PPE protocol, as the risk of secondary contamination is very high.

8.2.5 Q Fever

Q fever is caused by a rickettsia organism, *Coxiella burnetii*, that is highly infectious and resistant to heat and drying. Its natural reservoir is sheep, cattle, and goats. Humans acquire the disease by inhalation of aerosols contaminated with the organism. Following a 10- to 20-day incubation, Q fever generally occurs as a self-limiting febrile illness lasting 2 days to 2 weeks, and is characterized by headaches, fatigue, and myalgias. Pneumonia occurs in 50% of all patients, with half of these patients (25% total) presenting with a cough (usually non-productive) or rales.

Signs and Symptoms

- High-grade fever
- Rigors
- Severe headache
- Photophobia
- Myalgias
- Nausea/vomiting
- Diarrhea

Supportive Care

- Remove the patient from the hazardous area.
- Medical Supportive Care Protocol 2.1.3. Decontaminate as appropriate.
- Contact the Poison Information Center (1-800-222-1222).

ALS Level 1

None.

ALS Level 2

Most cases will resolve even without antibiotic therapy. To shorten the duration of the illness, in-hospital treatment may include the use of tetracycline 500 mg qid or doxycycline 100 mg bid for 5 to 7 days.

8.2.6 Ricin

Ricin is a potent cytotoxin that is derived from the beans of the castor plant and is a by-product in castor oil production. When inhaled as a small-particle aerosol, this toxin may produce pathologic changes within 8 hours and severe respiratory symptoms followed by acute hypoxic respiratory failure in 36–72 hours. When ingested, ricin causes severe gastrointestinal symptoms, followed by vascular collapse and death. This toxin may also cause disseminated intravascular coagulation, microcirculatory failure, and multiple-organ failure if given intravenously.

Signs and Symptoms

After inhalation:

- Fever
- Chest tightness
- Cough
- Shortness of breath
- Nausea
- Joint pain within 4 to 8 hours of exposure
- Necrosis of the lower airway epithelium and severe pulmonary edema
- Death within 36–72 hours

After ingestion:

- Nausea
- Vomiting
- Severe diarrhea
- Gastrointestinal hemorrhage with necrosis of the liver, spleen, and kidneys
- Shock leading to death within 3 days

After injection:

- Marked death of muscles and lymph nodes near the site of injection
- Multiple-organ failure, leading to death

8.2.6 Ricin

Supportive Care

- Remove the patient from the hazardous area (a).
- Medical Supportive Care Protocol 2.1.3. Decontaminate as appropriate.
- Contact the Poison Information Center (1-800-222-1222).

ALS Level 1

None.

ALS Level 2

If ingested, aggressive gastric lavage and activated charcoal should be administered in the hospital.

Note

(a) Risk of exposure via the airborne route is high. Refer to the appropriate hazardous materials PPE protocol, as the risk of secondary contamination is very high.

8.2.7 Smallpox

Smallpox is caused by the *Variola* virus. Although the fully developed cutaneous eruption of smallpox is unique, earlier stages of the rash could be mistaken for varicella. Secondary spread of infection constitutes a nosocomial hazard from the time of onset of a smallpox patient's exanthem until scabs have separated. Quarantine with respiratory isolation should be applied to secondary contacts for 17 days post-exposure.

Signs and Symptoms

- Fever
- Rigors
- Headache
- Malaise
- Nausea/vomiting
- Back ache
- Approximately 15% of patients develop delirium.
- Approximately 10% of light-skinned patients exhibit an erythematous rash.
- Two to three days later, an enanthem appears concomitantly with a discrete rash about the face, hands, and forearms.
- Following eruptions on the lower extremities, the rash spreads to the trunk over the next week.
- Lesions quickly progress from macules to papules, and eventually to pustular vesicles.
- With smallpox, lesions are more abundant on the extremities and face, as opposed to varicella (chickenpox), in which lesions on various segments of the body remain generally synchronous in their stage of development and primarily start on the trunk and spread to the extremities.

Supportive Care

- ◆ Remove the patient from the hazardous area (a).
- ◆ Medical Supportive Care Protocol 2.1.3. Decontaminate as appropriate.
- ◆ Contact the Poison Information Center (1-800-222-1222).

ALS Level 1

None.

ALS Level 2

Immune globulin for variola and the vaccines (vaccinia and VIG) may be obtained through the CDC.

Note

(a) Risk of exposure via the airborne route is high. Refer to the appropriate hazardous materials PPE protocol, as the risk of secondary contamination is very high.

8.2.8 Staphylococcal Enterotoxin B

Staphylococcal enterotoxin B (SEB) is a fever-producing exotoxin produced by the bacteria *Staphylococcus aureus*. This toxin commonly causes food poisoning in improperly handled foods that have an overgrowth of the staph organism and then are ingested. SEB symptoms will vary with the route of exposure (inhaled versus ingested).

Signs and Symptoms

From 3–12 hours after **aerosol exposure,** there will be a sudden onset of the following signs and symptoms:

- Fever (103–106°F), lasting 2 to 5 days
- Chills
- Headache
- Myalgia
- Nonproductive cough, which may persist for up to 4 weeks
- In some patients, shortness of breath and retrosternal chest pain

If **ingested,** symptoms include the following:

- Nausea
- Vomiting
- Diarrhea

High exposure can lead to septic shock and death.

Supportive Care

- Remove the patient from the hazardous area.
- Medical Supportive Care Protocol 2.1.3. Decontaminate as appropriate.
- Contact the Poison Information Center (1-800-222-1222).

ALS Level 1

None.

ALS Level 2

None.

8.2.9 Trichothecene Mycotoxins (T2)

The trichothecene mycotoxins are nonvolatile compounds produced by filamentous fungi (molds). They are relatively insoluble in water, but are highly soluble in ethanol, methanol, and propylene glycol. Exposure usually occurs through inhalation, ingestion, and/or absorption. Aerosol attack in the form of "yellow rain" will present as droplets of yellow fluid contaminating clothes and the environment.

Signs and Symptoms

Exposure to skin:

- Skin pain
- Pruritus
- Redness
- Vesicles
- Necrosis
- Sloughing of epidermis

Exposure to airway:

- Nose and throat pain
- Nasal discharge
- Itching and sneezing
- Cough
- Dyspnea
- Wheezing
- Chest pain
- Hemoptysis

Severe poisoning by any route:

- Prostration
- Weakness
- Ataxia
- Collapse
- Shock
- Death

Supportive Care

- Remove the patient from the hazardous area.
- Medical Supportive Care Protocol 2.1.3. Decontaminate as appropriate.
- Contact the Poison Information Center (1-800-222-1222).

ALS Level 1

None.

ALS Level 2

If ingested, aggressive gastric lavage and activated charcoal should be administered in the hospital.

8.2.10 Tularemia

Francisella tularensis is a nonmotile, gram-negative coccobacillus that typically causes disease in animals. Humans can become infected by either handling diseased animal fluids or by being bitten by infected deerflies, mosquitoes, or ticks. The organism can also remain viable for weeks in a number of media and is easily spread by aerosol. After infection, bacteremia results, with a secondary spread to the lungs and other organs.

Signs and Symptoms

The following signs and symptoms will appear within 2–10 days of inhalational exposure:

- Fever
- Chills
- Headache
- Generalized muscle pain
- Nonproductive cough
- Pneumonia

If the organism was ingested or inoculated, symptoms will also include regional lymphadenopathy, with or without cutaneous ulcers.

Clinical diagnosis is both difficult and problematic. Physical findings are usually nonspecific, although chest X-ray may reveal pneumonic process, mediastinal lymphadenopathy, or pleural effusion. Routine culture is possible but hazardous to lab personnel. Diagnosis can be established retrospectively by serology.

Supportive Care

- Remove the patient from the hazardous area (a).
- Medical Supportive Care Protocol 2.1.3. Decontaminate as appropriate.
- Contact the Poison Information Center (1-800-222-1222).

ALS Level 1

None.

ALS Level 2

- Antibiotic therapy for 10 days includes streptomycin 1 g q 12 hours IM or 15 mg/kg IM bid. If not available, administer gentamicin 3 mg/kg/day.
- Prophylaxis with tetracycline or doxycycline is effective if warning of BW attack is provided or if there is a high suspicion of significant exposure, as ordered by Medical Control or the Poison Information Center.

Note

(a) If risk of exposure is high, call for a hazardous materials team. Refer to the appropriate hazardous materials PPE protocol, as the risk of secondary contamination is very high.

8.2.11 Venezuelan Equine Encephalitis (VEE)

VEE virus is a mosquito-borne alphavirus that is endemic in certain parts of the world (Central and South America, Mexico, and Florida), where it infects horses, mules, and donkeys. If this agent was intentionally released as an aerosol, disease might occur simultaneously in both horses and humans, but this pattern would not be commonly recognized.

Signs and Symptoms

After exposure, a sudden onset of symptoms begins in 1–5 days:

- Generalized malaise
- Spiking fever (up to 104°F)
- Rigors
- Severe headache
- Photophobia
- Myalgias in the legs and lumbosacral area
- Nausea and vomiting
- Cough
- Sore throat
- Diarrhea

These symptoms last up to 3 days, and then are followed by a period of weakness and lethargy. Most patients recover in 1–2 weeks. Some patients, especially children, may develop signs of CNS infection, with meningismus, convulsions, coma, and paralysis. There is a 20% mortality rate in children who develop encephalitis.

Supportive Care

- Remove the patient from the hazardous area (a).
- Medical Supportive Care Protocol 2.1.3 or Pediatric Protocol 3.1.3.
- Contact the Poison Information Center (1-800-222-1222).

ALS Level 1

None.

ALS Level 2

None.

Note

(a) Risk of exposure via the airborne route is low. However, patients should be isolated from mosquitoes for 72 hours to prevent spread by vectors.

8.2.12 Viral Hemorrhagic Fevers

The VHF are a diverse group of illnesses caused by a variety of RNA viruses; they demonstrate a wide range of morbidity and mortality. These viruses include:

- Ebola
- Marburg
- Dengue
- Yellow fever
- Crimean-Congo fever
- Hantaan viruses
- Lassa fever

Each of these viruses has a unique history and is capable of being spread in most cases by an aerosol or formite (except dengue virus). VHF agents, especially Marburg and Ebola, have allegedly been considered for weaponization. The clinical syndrome that these viruses cause in humans is called VHF.

Signs and Symptoms

- Fever
- Easy bleeding
- Petechiae
- Hypotension and shock
- Flushing of the face and chest
- Edema
- Malaise
- Myalgias
- Headache
- Vomiting
- Diarrhea

8.2.12 Viral Hemorrhagic Fevers

Supportive Care

- Remove the patient from the hazardous area (a)(b).
- Medical Supportive Care Protocol 2.1.3 or Pediatric Protocol 3.1.3.
- Contact the Poison Information Center (1-800-222-1222).

ALS Level 1

None.

ALS Level 2

None.

Note

(a) Risk of exposure via the airborne route is high. Refer to the appropriate hazardous materials PPE protocol, as the risk of secondary contamination is very high.

(b) Risk of exposure from a symptomatic patient via blood or body secretions is high. Full PPE with masks, goggles, sleeves, and gowns is appropriate. If the patient is not severely ill, IV access should be delayed until hospital arrival. If IV access is needed for immediate patient resuscitation, extra care is appropriate to protect the healthcare worker, and IV attempts should not be made on combative patients or in a moving vehicle.

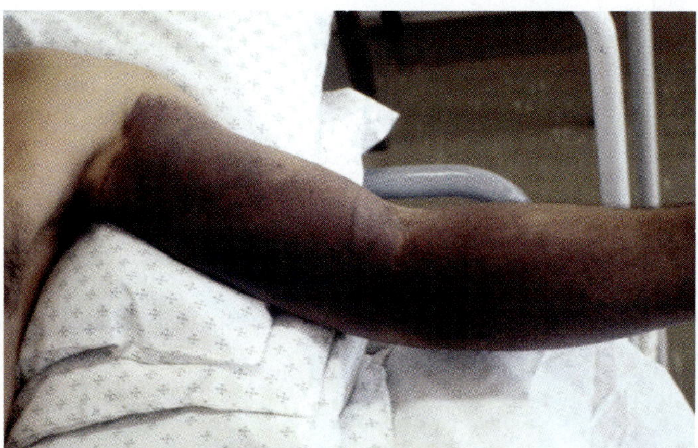

Viral hemorrhagic fevers cause the blood vessels and tissues to seep blood.

8.3 Adult Hazardous Material Exposure (Radiological Agents)

This protocol is to be used for those patients suspected of exposure to radiological agents via any route of exposure (e.g., ingestion, absorption). It gives specific considerations for each type of exposure as well as general treatment guidelines. Scene safety should be of primary concern, with special attention being paid to the need for personal protective equipment. If a radiological agent exposure is suspected, call for a hazardous materials team. In this instance, refer to the appropriate hazardous materials PPE protocol to protect against secondary contamination. All patients who have been exposed to hazardous materials must be properly decontaminated prior to initiation of extensive medical treatment and transportation to the hospital.

Contact the Poison Information Center (1-800-222-1222) for consultation regarding specific therapy, and then contact the receiving emergency department for confirmation of ALS Level 2 orders.

It is imperative that the emergency department be made aware early that a contaminated patient is being transported so that the proper preparations can be made to receive the patient.

Types of Radiation Injury

- **External irradiation** occurs when all or part of the body is exposed to penetrating radiation from an external source. Following external exposure, an individual is not radioactive and can be treated like any other patient.
- **Contamination** means that radioactive materials in the form of gases, liquids, or solids are released into the environment and contaminate people externally, internally, or both. An external surface of the body, such as the skin, can become contaminated quite easily. If radioactive materials get inside the body through the lungs, gut, or wounds, the contaminant can become deposited internally.
- **Incorporation** refers to the uptake of radioactive materials by body cells, tissues, and target organs such as bone, liver, thyroid, or kidney. Incorporation cannot occur unless contamination has occurred.

These three types of accidents can happen in combination and can be complicated by physical injury or illness.

8.3 Adult Hazardous Material Exposure (Radiological Agents)

Irradiation of the whole body or some specific body part does not constitute a medical emergency, even if the amount of radiation received is high. The effects of irradiation usually are not evident for days or weeks; thus, while medical treatment is needed, it is not needed on an emergency basis. In contrast, **contamination accidents must be considered medical emergencies,** because they might lead to internal contamination and subsequent incorporation. Incorporation can result in adverse health effects several years later if the amount of incorporated radioactive material is high.

Treatment priorities are established as follows:

- Treat life-threatening problems first.
- Limit the radiation dose to both victims and healthcare personnel (time, distance, shielding).
- Control the spread of radioactive contaminants.

Serious medical problems should have priority over concerns about radiation, such as radiation monitoring, contamination control, and decontamination. However, attention should be given to PPE for medical personnel.

8.3.1 Radiation Exposure/Contamination

Radiation exposure/contamination may be a health risk to both the patient and the rescuer, depending on the type of radiation, time of exposure, distance from the radioactive source, and level of shielding from the radioactive source. Not all exposures will require medical treatment, however. In exposures where traumatic injuries are not present, the following steps should be taken.

Supportive Care

- Remove the patient from the hazardous area (a)(b).
- Decontaminate as appropriate (b).
- Medical Supportive Care Protocol 2.1.3 or Pediatric Protocol 3.1.3 PRN.
- Contact the Poison Information Center (1-800-222-1222).

ALS Level 1

None.

ALS Level 2

Additional treatment should be administered in the hospital.

NOTE

(a) Use of radiological monitoring devices is essential, as risk of exposure may be high. Call for a hazardous materials team.

(b) In mild to moderate exposures without traumatic injuries, self-decontamination may be recommended for the patient at his/her home. Self-decontamination should include removing one's clothing, placing the clothes into a plastic bag, and showering with soap and water.

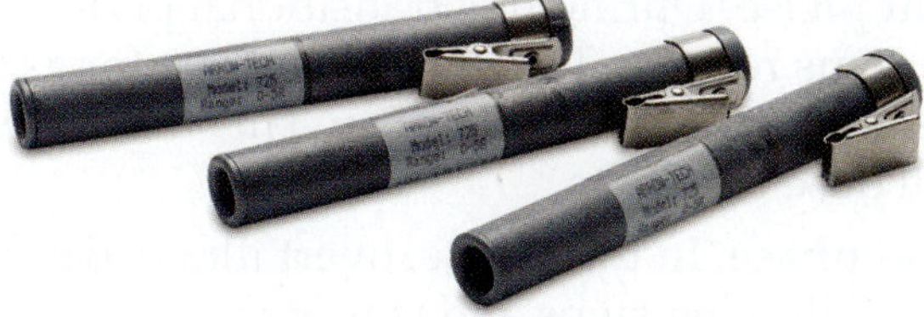

Personal radiological monitoring device.

8.3.2 Acute Radiation Syndrome

Acute radiation syndrome (ARS) is an acute illness that follows a roughly predictable course over a period of time ranging from a few hours to several weeks after exposure to ionizing radiation. It occurs if enough radiation reaches enough sensitive tissue. The following factors are important in determining whether ARS will develop:

- High dose
- High dose rate
- Whole-body exposure
- Penetrating irradiation

Other factors to be considered include age (young and old), sex, genetics, and medical history. Regardless of the source of radiation, if the dose is high enough, it will produce the same effect.

Signs and Symptoms

Signs and symptoms that develop in the ARS occur in four distinct phases:

- **Prodromal phase**. Depending on the total amount of radiation absorbed, patients may experience a variety of symptoms, including:
  - Loss of appetite
  - Nausea
  - Vomiting
  - Fatigue
  - Diarrhea

  After high radiation doses, the following additional symptoms may develop:
  - Prostration
  - Fever
  - Respiratory difficulties
  - Increases in excitability

  This is the stage at which most victims seek medical care.
- **Latent phase**. During this transitional period, many of the initial symptoms resolve. This phase may last for as long as 3 weeks, depending on the original dose. This time interval decreases as the initial dose increases.
- **Illness phase**. In this phase, overt illness develops, often characterized by the following signs and symptoms:
  - Infection
  - Bleeding
  - Electrolyte imbalance
  - Diarrhea
  - Changes in mental status
  - Shock
- **Recovery or death phase**. This phase follows the period of overt illness, which may take weeks or months to resolve.

8.3.2 Acute Radiation Syndrome

Supportive Care

- Remove the patient from the hazardous area.
- Medical Supportive Care Protocol 2.1.3 or Pediatric Protocol 3.1.3. Decontaminate as appropriate.
- Contact the Poison Information Center (1-800-222-1222).

ALS Level 1

None.

ALS Level 2

Additional treatment should be administered in the hospital.

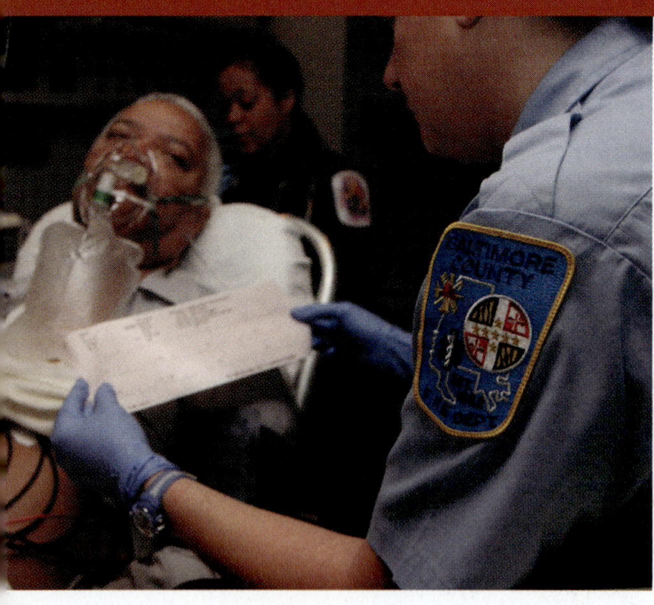

Forms

All forms referenced in *Florida Regional Common EMS Protocols* can be found online at http://www. Florida. EMSzone.com. These forms can be printed and used both in the classroom and in the field.

Visit http://www. Florida.EMSzone.com to find the following forms:

- F.1 Florida Protocol Forms
  - F.1.1 Dive Accident: Rapid Field Neurologic Exam Record
  - F.1.2 Dive Accident: Signs and Symptoms Checklist
  - F.1.3 Dive History/Profile
  - F.1.4 Emergency Worker Rehabilitation Sheet
  - F.1.5 Employer's Exposure Information Form
  - F.1.6 Infectious Disease Exposure Report Form
  - F.1.7 Stroke Alert Checklist
  - F.1.8 Trauma Telemetry Report
- F.2 Mass Casualty Incident Forms
  - F.2.1 Command Field Operating Guide
  - F.2.2 Medical Field Operating Guide
  - F.2.3 Medical Supply Field Operating Guide
  - F.2.4 Triage Field Operating Guide
  - F.2.5 Treatment Field Operating Guide
  - F.2.6 Treatment Log
  - F.2.7 Transport Field Operating Guide
  - F.2.8 Hospital Transport Log
  - F.2.9 Medical Communication Field Operating Guide
  - F.2.10 Hospital Capability Worksheet
  - F.2.11 Staging Field Operating Guide
  - F.2.12 Unit Staging Log
  - F.2.13 MCI-WMD/Terrorist Event Field Operating Guide

Photographic Credits

Chapter 1

Opener Courtesy of Michael Hohl

Chapter 2

Opener Courtesy of Michael Hohl; **page 75** Courtesy of Leonard V. Crowley, M.D., Biology Department, Century College; **page 130** © Comstock Images/Getty Images; **page 133** © Elisa Locci/ShutterStock, Inc.; **page 146** Courtesy of Carol B. Guerrero; **page 156** Courtesy of Neil Malcom Winkelmann

Chapter 3

Opener Courtesy of Michael Hohl; **page 186, page 198** Courtesy of Health Resources and Services Administration, Maternal and Child Health Bureau, Emergency Medical Services for Children Program; **page 233** Courtesy of Dey, L.P.; **page 238** Courtesy of Ronald Dieckmann, M.D.; **page 240** © Lonni Aylett/Dreamstime.com; **page 247** © Innershadows/Dreamstime.com; **page 257** © PhotoCreate/ShutterStock, Inc.

Chapter 4

Opener Courtesy of Michael Hohl; **page 292** Courtesy of Philips Respironics, Murrysville, PA; **page 293** Courtesy of Marianne Gausche-Hill, MD, FACEP, FAAP; **page 301** Courtesy of ZOLL Medical Corporation; **page 304** Courtesy of Advanced Circulatory Systems, Inc.; **page 308** Cyanokit® is a registered trademark of Merck Santé (France), an affiliate of Merck KGaA, Darmstadt, Germany. The product is not yet approved by the FDA in the U.S.; **page 313** Courtesy of Armstrong Medical Ind.; **page 321** Courtesy of Nicholas Palmieri; **page 324** The Morgan Lens courtesy of MorTan, Inc.; **page 327** Courtesy of

David Clark Company Incorporated; **page 340** Courtesy of Dey, L.P.; **page 349** MAD® photograph courtesy of Wolfe Tory Medical, Inc.

Chapter 5

Opener Courtesy of Michael Hohl

Chapter 6

Opener © AbleStock

Chapter 7

Opener Courtesy of Michael Hohl

Chapter 8

Opener © Brian Hendricks/ShutterStock, Inc.; **page 470** Courtesy of U.S. Department of Transportation; **page 489** Courtesy of Dr. Saeed Keshavarz/RCCI (Research Center of Chemical Injuries)/IRAN; **page 548** Courtesy of Professor Robert Swanepoel/National Institute for Communicable Disease, South Africa; **page 551** Courtesy of Fluke Biomedical

Unless otherwise indicated, all photographs and illustrations are under copyright of Jones and Bartlett Publishers, LLC, courtesy of Maryland Institute for Emergency Medical Services Systems, or have been provided by the American Academy of Orthopaedic Surgeons.